Latest Scientific Findings in Ruminant Nutrition - Research for Practical Implementation

Edited by László Babinszky

Published in London, United Kingdom

Latest Scientific Findings in Ruminant Nutrition - Research for Practical Implementation
http://dx.doi.org/10.5772/10.5772/intechopen.1001764
Edited by László Babinszky

Contributors
Aemiro Kehaliew, Asfaw Bisrat, Ayele Abebe, Azmat Alam Khan, Bala Krishna Rao Dabbir, Bethlehem Mekonnen, Busisiwe Gunya, Diego Maredi Matabane, Diriba Geleti, Fekede Feyissa, Geberemariyam Terefe, Gebeyehu Goshu, Getu Kitaw, Gezahegn Kebede, Hoda Javaheri Barfourooshi, Jones Wilfred Ng'ambi, Kasa Biratu, Katalin Somfalvi-Tóth, László Babinszky, Mani Saravanan, Mesfin Dejene, Monnye Mabelebele, Mulugeta Walelegne, Razia Kausar, Róbert Tóthi, Safdar Imran, Showkeen Muzamil, Snober Irshad, Somu Yogeshpriya, Sreenivasa Reddy Rajavolu, Subramanian Sivaraman, Syed Mudasir Ahmad, Szilvia Orosz, Tesfaye Getachew, Tesfaye Zewdie, Tlou Grace Manyelo, Tsegaab Bekele, Veronika Halas, Zulfqarul Haq

First published in London, United Kingdom, 2024 by IntechOpen
IntechOpen is the global imprint of INTECHOPEN LIMITED, registered in England and Wales, registration number: 11086078, 167-169 Great Portland Street, London, W1W 5PF, United Kingdom

British Library Cataloguing-in-Publication Data
A catalogue record for this book is available from the British Library

Additional hard and PDF copies can be obtained from orders@intechopen.com

Latest Scientific Findings in Ruminant Nutrition - Research for Practical Implementation
Edited by László Babinszky
p. cm.

This title is part of the Veterinary Medicine and Science Book Series, Volume 21
Topic: Animal Nutrition
Series Editor: Rita Payan Carreira
Topic Editor: Manuel Gonzalez Ronquillo

Print ISBN 978-0-85466-977-6
Online ISBN 978-0-85466-976-9
eBook (PDF) ISBN 978-0-85466-978-3
ISSN 2632-0517

For EU product safety concerns:
IN TECH d.o.o., Prolaz Marije Krucifikse Kozulić 3, 51000 Rijeka, Croatia,
info@intechopen.com or visit our website at intechopen.com.

IntechOpen Book Series

Veterinary Medicine and Science

Volume 21

Aims and Scope of the Series

Paralleling similar advances in the medical field, astounding advances occurred in Veterinary Medicine and Science in recent decades. These advances have helped foster better support for animal health, more humane animal production, and a better understanding of the physiology of endangered species to improve the assisted reproductive technologies or the pathogenesis of certain diseases, where animals can be used as models for human diseases (like cancer, degenerative diseases or fertility), and even as a guarantee of public health. Bridging Human, Animal, and Environmental health, the holistic and integrative "One Health" concept intimately associates the developments within those fields, projecting its advancements into practice. This book series aims to tackle various animal-related medicine and sciences fields, providing thematic volumes consisting of high-quality significant research directed to researchers and postgraduates. It aims to give us a glimpse into the new accomplishments in the Veterinary Medicine and Science field. By addressing hot topics in veterinary sciences, we aim to gather authoritative texts within each issue of this series, providing in-depth overviews and analysis for graduates, academics, and practitioners and foreseeing a deeper understanding of the subject. Forthcoming texts, written and edited by experienced researchers from both industry and academia, will also discuss scientific challenges faced today in Veterinary Medicine and Science. In brief, we hope that books in this series will provide accessible references for those interested or working in this field and encourage learning in a range of different topics.

Meet the Series Editor

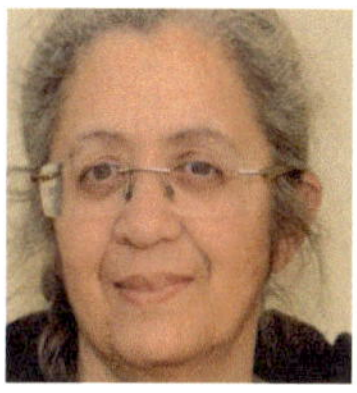

Rita Payan Carreira earned her Veterinary Degree from the Faculty of Veterinary Medicine in Lisbon, Portugal, in 1985. She obtained her Ph.D. in Veterinary Sciences from the University of Trás-os-Montes e Alto Douro, Portugal. After almost 32 years of teaching at the University of Trás-os-Montes and Alto Douro, she recently moved to the University of Évora, Department of Veterinary Medicine, where she teaches in the field of Animal Reproduction and Clinics. Her primary research areas include the molecular markers of the endometrial cycle and the embryo–maternal interaction, including oxidative stress and the reproductive physiology and disorders of sexual development, besides the molecular determinants of male and female fertility. She often supervises students preparing their master's or doctoral theses. She is also a frequent referee for various journals.

Meet the Volume Editor

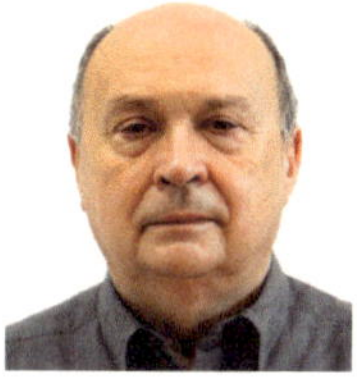

Dr. László Babinszky is Professor of Animal Nutrition and Professor Emeritus at both the University of Debrecen and the Hungarian University of Agriculture and Life Sciences, Kaposvár Campus, Hungary. He obtained his Ph.D. from Wageningen University, the Netherlands. Throughout his career, Dr. Babinszky has contributed significantly to academia and research across multiple institutions in Hungary, the Netherlands, Austria, and Germany. He has authored more than 300 publications, including peer-reviewed papers and book chapters. He has also edited five print books and four e-books. His expertise is recognized internationally, as evidenced by his long-standing membership in various prestigious committees, such as the American Society of Animal Science (ASAS, USA), where he has served for 27 years. Additionally, he serves on the editorial boards of numerous international journals, including *Acta Agriculturae Scandinavica Section A: Animal Science*. Dr. Babinszky is also a sought-after lecturer, having been invited to speak at universities across Europe, the United States, Canada, Australia, New Zealand, and China.

Contents

Preface

Ruminants (Ruminantia) are a suborder of mammals (Mammalia) that belong to the order of even-toed ungulates (Artiodactyla). The word "ruminant" comes from the Latin ruminare, which means "to chew over again."

Ruminants were domesticated 8,000–10,000 years ago and still play a significant role in human life today. Ruminants and the products derived from them are an important food source worldwide. Large ruminants (such as cattle and buffalo) and small ruminants (such as sheep and goats) are vital not only because they provide animal-derived protein important for human nutrition but also because they primarily consume high-fiber feed that is unsuitable for human consumption.

It is essential to emphasize that the products of these animals (meat and milk) are not only important for their high biological value protein content but also because they contain numerous micronutrients (e.g., vitamin B_{12}, essential fatty acids) that are biologically more accessible to humans than those found in plant-based foods.

Furthermore, these animals also serve as tools for ecosystem management, and in some countries, their ownership provides social status and livelihood. They also supply important industrial and pharmaceutical raw materials.

In general, ruminant animals contribute positively to human wellbeing by converting inedible plant materials, such as grasslands and fibrous feedstuffs, into valuable sources of food energy and nutrients. Dairy cattle, in particular, are considered the most efficient ruminants in converting feed protein and energy into animal-derived food products like milk and dairy goods.

As the global population continues to grow, the demand for beef and milk is expected to rise accordingly. In 2023, global milk production reached 9,657 million tons, marking a 15% increase compared to the previous year. Various projections predict further growth in this area in the coming decades. To meet this increasing demand for meat and milk, it is necessary to improve the sustainability of ruminant livestock farming.

Several strategies can be applied to enhance the sustainability of ruminant breeding systems, such as selecting appropriate ruminant breeds, improving the efficiency of housing systems and manure management technologies, ensuring the proper health status of livestock farms, and mitigating the negative effects of climate change. In addition, it is crucial to develop efficient feeding systems because their application allows for the sustainable and profitable production of high-quality animal-derived foodstuffs that are safe for human consumption.

This book presents the latest scientific findings in ruminant (cattle, sheep, and goats) nutrition. It focuses on feeding solutions that can sustainably improve the quality of animal-derived products to enhance consumer health. It also demonstrates how feeding methods can reduce harmful emissions of nitrogen, phosphorus, and methane. Furthermore, the book addresses the pressing issue of climate change, particularly the effects of heat stress on ruminants, and offers innovative solutions for mitigating these impacts through improved feeding and forage production methods.

Additionally, the book highlights the critical importance of animal health in ensuring the production of safe and high-quality food raw materials. It also touches upon the intersection of nutrition and the leather industry, exploring how the nutritional status of sheep influences the quality of their leather.

This book is designed for researchers, academics, university students, and practitioners who are engaged in ruminant nutrition and sustainable agriculture.

I would like to thank the chapter authors for their excellent contributions. I am also grateful to the staff at IntechOpen for their technical assistance in publishing the book, especially Publishing Process Manager Dorian Salatić and Commissioning Editor Lucija Tomicic-Dromgool.

Dr. László Babinszky
Professor,
Faculty of Agricultural and Food Sciences and Environmental Management,
Department of Animal Nutrition and Physiology,
University of Debrecen,
Debrecen, Hungary,

Hungarian University of Agriculture and Life Sciences,
Kaposvár Campus,
Institute of Physiology and Nutrition,
Department of Farm Animal Nutrition,
Kaposvár, Hungary

Chapter 1

New Trends in the Treatment of Hypokalemia in Cows

Bala Krishna Rao Dabbir and Sreenivasa Reddy Rajavolu

Abstract

Of all the mineral cations, potassium (K) is an essential nutrient for animals, and it is the third most common mineral in the body. Potassium has a role in maintaining normal cardiac and renal function, neuronal transmission, muscular contraction, and acid-base balance. The main thrust of this chapter is to review the physiology, pathology, pharmacology, occurrence, etiology, clinical signs of hypokalemia and its diagnostic and therapeutic approach in cows. The ambulatory measures to minimize the agony and preventive strategies to reduce the incidence of hypokalemia were discussed. Beside the potassium salt therapy, the inclusion of Taurine in the therapeutic regime was rational and to be appreciated.

Keywords: hypokalemia, pathophysiology, causes, diagnosis, treatment, taurine, prevention

1. Introduction

The main cation in intracellular fluid is potassium. It is essential for controlling osmotic pressure, maintaining acid-base balance, transmitting nerve impulses, contracting muscles, especially the heart muscle, and performing several cell membrane tasks as a component of the sodium-potassium pump. Additionally, necessary for glycogenesis, potassium facilitates the conversion of adenosine triphosphate to pyruvic acid by transferring phosphate. Potassium is also essential for many fundamental cellular enzymatic processes, including protein synthesis, amino acid absorption, and glucose metabolism [1, 2].

Alterations in the equilibrium between intracellular and extracellular potassium can result in hyperkalemia or hypokalemia despite the unaltered total body potassium content. Internal potassium balance is most typically impacted by disturbances in the acid-base balance [3–5]. The transport of hydrogen ions into the cells counteracts the elevated concentration of hydrogen ions in the extracellular fluid that results from metabolic acidosis. To maintain electro-neutrality, potassium ions must exit the intracellular compartment, which raises the concentration of potassium in plasma. Similar to this, potassium may be redistributed from the extracellular to the intracellular compartment in metabolic alkalosis, leading to hypokalemia [3, 5]. Maintaining the resting membrane potential depends on the ratio of extracellular to intracellular potassium [1]. Recently, isoflupredone acetate was administered intramuscularly to lactating dairy cows in conjunction with ketosis to cause a state of severe muscle weakness, recumbency, and hypokalemia [6]. Theileriosis, recumbency, traumatic reticulo-peritonitis, excessive use of isoflupredone acetate in the treatment of ketosis, excessive bicarbonate administration in the treatment of ruminal lactic acidosis, ileus, botulism, and abomasal displacement were the main causes of hypokalemia [7]. The parenteral administration of dextrose or insulin may result in hypokalemia [8].

Animal cells contain potassium as the primary cation (positive ion), whereas sodium is the primary cation outside of animal cells. The membrane potential, which is the differential in electric potential between the inside and exterior of cells, is caused by the concentration differences of these charged particles. Ion pumps in the cell membrane regulate the potassium and sodium levels in the membrane. An action potential, or "spike" of electrical discharge, can be produced by the cell thanks to the potential in the cell membrane that potassium and sodium ions cause. For bodily processes including neurotransmission, muscle contraction, and heart function, cells must be able to generate electrical discharge. In addition, potassium is a necessary mineral for controlling blood pressure, acidity levels, and water balance [9].

It is well knowledge that potassium homeostasis and acid-base balance are related. Generally speaking, hypokalaemia (lower blood pH) is linked to lower plasma potassium concentration, whereas acidaemia (lower blood pH) is linked to higher plasma potassium concentration (hyperkalaemia) [10].

The objective of this chapter is to describe the pathophysiology, diagnosis and therapy through intravenous and/or oral route (powder and bolus) of potassium formulations. A further aim is to demonstrate the role of taurine in potassium homeostasis and measures to prevent hypokalemia in the cows.

1.1 Absorption and excretion

In the rat, Rajendran and Geoffrey [11] noted that despite the colon's great potential for K+ secretion and absorption, its function in preserving K+ homeostasis is frequently disregarded. For a long time, it was believed that the main processes for K+ absorption in the colons of humans and animals were solvent drag and/or passive diffusion. Nonetheless, it is now evident that electro neutral K+ absorption in the animal colon is mediated by apical H+, K+-ATPase, in conjunction with basolateral K+-Cl− co-transport and/or K+ and Cl− channels functioning in tandem. The rat colon's K+ absorption is indicative of both ouabain-sensitive and -insensitive apical H+, K+-ATPase activities. H+, K+-ATPases that are ouabain-sensitive and -insensitive found in crypt cells and surface cells, respectively. Colonic H+, K+-ATPase is made up of the subunits α (HKCα) and β (HKCβ), which when co-expressed in HEK293 cells that show ouabain-insensitive H+, K+-ATPase activity; in Xenopus oocytes. On the other hand, HKCα co-expressed with the gastric β-subunit shows ouabain sensitive H+, K+-ATPase activity. Apical H+, K+-ATPase activity, HKCα specific mRNA and protein expression, and K+ absorption are all improved by aldosterone. Conversely, apical K+ channels that work in tandem with the baso-lateral Na+-K+-2Cl− co-transporter induce active K+ secretion [11].

1.2 Causes of hypokalemia

1.2.1 Lactation stress

In the lactating cow, 75% of potassium elimination is via the urine, 13% in feces and 12% in the milk **Table 1** [12]. In the hypokalemic cow, this may be concentrated

Serial number	Disorders	Causes	References
1	Physiological or metabolic	Lactational stress, summer stress	[6, 12–16]
2	Pathological	Left displaced abomasum, right displaced abomasum, abomasal volvulus, abomasal impaction, clinical mastitis, dystocia, retained placenta, and hepatic lipidosis, prolonge anorexia, diarrohea	[7, 17–20]
3	Induced	Frequent administration of cortisones with minerlocoticoid activity, calcium, mifex, calcium, borogluconate, dextrose, insulin, bicarbonates	[7, 8]

Table 1.
Showing causes of hypokalemia.

in the first 45 days of lactation [13] or 60 days [6]. In general, the younger cow seems to be more at risk than older cows [14].

Large milk producers have lower mean serum potassium concentrations than small milk producers [15]. These high milk producers are also more likely to experience hypokalemia during the early stages of lactation due to increased potassium loss in milk and a noticeable negative energy balance [16].

1.2.2 Summer stress

Nutritionists discovered a link between heat stress and potassium loss, with cows that stayed in the shade losing five times less potassium than the group of cows that had no shade. Heat-stressed cows also ate less during the daytime, thus also reducing their potassium intake [21].

1.2.3 Frequent administration calcium magnesium phosphite

The authors observed that the infusion of Calcium 1.86% w/v (as Calcium Gluconate I.P.) in (Miphocal or Mifex brands), Anhydrous Dextrose I.P. 20% w/v and Magnesium Hypophosphite 5.0% w/v were indiscriminately administered by para veterinarians to cure downers to more than 25 cows, resulted in 22.5–3 mM of potassium and 2 mM of calcium per liter respectively.

Tamer and Chandra Deep [17] report the development of hypocalcemia and hyperkalemia attributable to magnesium infusion in a pre-eclamptic human patient (**Table 1**).

1.2.4 Pathology

A nursing dairy cow with left or right displaced abomasum, abomasal volvulus, abomasal impaction, clinical mastitis, dystocia, retained placenta, and hepatic lipidosis is likely to have hypokalemia, which is defined as serum or plasma potassium concentration < 3.9 mEq/L [17–19]. In cows, hypokalemia is frequently seen as a result of prolonged anorexia and other main gastrointestinal and urinary system disorders [20, 22].

1.2.5 Clinical signs of hypokalemia

Following their initial period of rigidity and disinclination to move, the majority of animals exhibit the following clinical symptoms:

1. Depression characterized by a lack of resistance to manipulation and generalized weakness.

2. Diminished muscle tone in different parts of the body from tail to tongue.

3. Bradycardia.

4. An unusual neck alignment (an S-shaped neck) (**Figure 1**).

5. Recumbency.

6. Generalized intestinal and stomach stasis, resulting in minimal defecation and ruminal atony.

2. Diagnosis of hypokalemia

Confirming a hypokalemia diagnosis requires serum biochemical investigation. A prompt and precise diagnosis is necessary to save the recumbent cowl, determine the prognosis, and choose the dosage and method of potassium chloride administration. Serum potassium levels below 2.5 mM/L indicate severe hypokalemia, which will cause most cows to be less alert, recumbent. Moderate hypokalemia is indicated by a serum potassium content of 2.5–3.5 mM/L. Some of these cows also are recumbent,

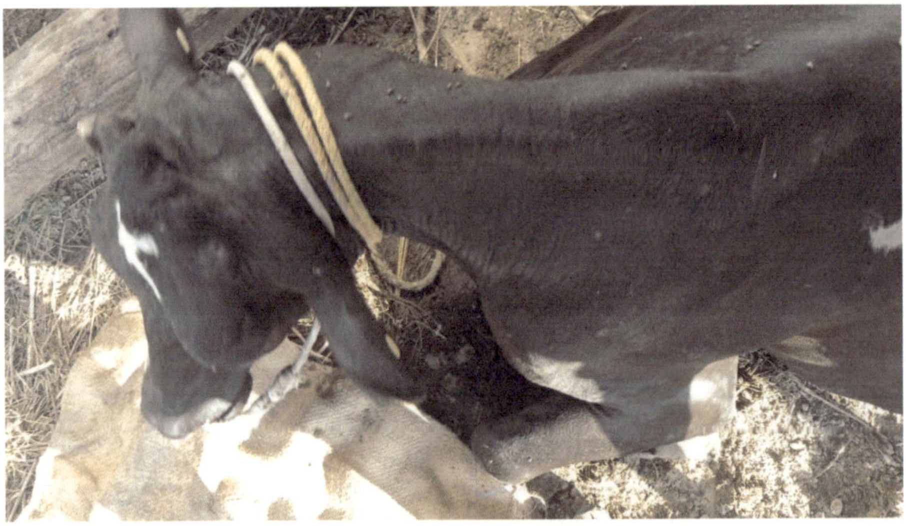

Figure 1.
Showing hypokalemic cow (photo courtesy—Dr. Manjunath, Mangalore).

and reduced gut motility. Serum potassium concentrations can be measured, but measurements of sodium, chloride, calcium, and phosphorus concentrations as well as serum CK and AST activity may be y useful in deciding the drug therapy. Aciduria can occur when the potassium concentration in the urine drops [13].

2.1 Strides in the estimation of serum and blood potassium

2.1.1 Potentiometric direct measurement

Since the development of commercially available electrodes for sodium and potassium ions and electrodes selective for univalent cations over a decade ago, the determination of sodium and potassium in biological fluids has been the subject of substantial research (**Table 2**). This electrode, a glass electrode that is sodium ion selective, and a reference electrode are all included in a small-volume cell. Since a potassium ion specific electrode is the gold standard for clinical potassium measurements and can be miniaturized for small blood volumes, can be used to measure potassium in the blood sample. Anantibiotic, valinomycin, selectively binds potassium and it, is pumped into a membrane inside the ion specific electrode. When valinomycin comes in contact with a potassium-containing solution, potassium binds to it, creating a potential difference relative to a reference and building up a charge. Thus, by measuring this voltage, one would be able to ascertain the potassium concentration in a sample solution. Potassium is relatively low in concentration, thus amplification of the signal will be necessary to successfully detect it at clinically relevant concentration [23].

2.1.2 Rapid quantitative turbid-metric spot test analysis of potassium in the blood serum

The market offers a quantitative turbid metric spot test method for determining potassium concentration in the blood serum. Potassium is precipitated using sodium tetraphenylborate, a traditional analytical reagent, in basic media. Using a

Serial number	Design	Principle	References
1	Potentiometric direct measurement	Valinomycin, selectively binds potassium and it, is pumped into a membrane inside the ion specific electrode. When valinomycin comes in contact with a potassium-containing solution, potassium binds to it, creating a potential difference relative to a reference and building up a charge	[23]
2	Turbid-metric	Potassium is precipitated using sodium tetraphenylborate. The turbidity is measured with spectrophotometer	[24]
3	Smartphone-enabled quantification of potassium in the blood plasma	Turbid metric principle	[25]
4	Equipment-free detection of K+	Microfluidic paper-based analytical devices	[26]

Table 2.
Showing various diagnostic techniques'.

micro-turbid metric cell created for this purpose, the turbidity is measured directly in this solution without any additional dilution. The buffer and the solution of the analytical reagent were combined with the blood serum. At 700 nm, the turbidity is measured with a spectrophotometer in the working concentration range, the calibration curve is a straight line with a correlation coefficient of 0.9998. The analytical outcomes achieved using this technique is in contrast those obtained using an electrode that selectively use ionized potassium ions [24].

2.1.3 Smartphone-enabled quantification of potassium in the blood plasma

A novel technique for measuring the K+ concentration, [K+], in the blood plasma using an optical attachment that was specially made for a smartphone. Turbidity is the basis for the development of the approach. Measurement of blood plasma solutions using sodium tetraphenylborate, a recognized reagent that cause potassium to precipitate. A unique image-processing technique is used to analyze the photo taken with a smartphone camera. This allows the data to be converted from RGB to HSV color space and the mean value of the light-intensity component (V) to be calculated. Photographs of blood plasma with varying K+ concentrations analyzed show a relationship between V and [K+]. The outcome with those obtained using an ion-selective electrode device and atomic absorption spectroscopy, the method's correctness is verified. When employing the treated blood plasma calibration, the method's accuracy was within ±0.18 mM and precision was within ±0.27 mM in the [K+] range of 1.5–7.5 mM. Good correlation was observed between the data collected by the smartphone approach and the ion-selective electrode device in spike test conducted on a fresh blood plasma. The method's inexpensive cost and smartphone integration make it advantageous for measuring [K+] on demand and in remote locations with restricted hospital access [25].

2.1.4 Equipment-free K+ detection on microfluidic paper-based analytical devices using ionic dye in ion-selective capillary sensor

A microfluidic paper-based analytical device (μPAD) is linked to an ion-selective capillary sensor to enable remote potassium ion (K+) analysis. The concept is based on two sequential steps: first, the analyte ion is selectively substituted with an ionic dye, and this dye is subsequently detected in a distance-based paper readout. To perform the first step, the capillary sensor holds the polyvinyl chloride membrane film layer in place after it has been plasticized with dioctylsebacate. This layer has potassium ionophorevalinomycin on its inner wall, a lipophilic cation-exchanger, and the ionic indicator Thioflavin T (ThT) dye. When the sample is introduced into the film membrane, K+ in the aqueous sample solution is quantitatively removed, and ThT is substituted. This solution was placed onto the inlet region of a μPAD to flow the ThT down a channel formed by wax printing, resulting in the electrostatic binding of ThT to the cellulose carboxylic groups, converting the ion exchange signal into a distance-based analysis. The starting K+ concentration This solution was applied to the μPAD's intake region, allowing ThT to flow through a channel created by wax printing. ThT then electrostatically bound to the carboxylic groups in cellulose, transforming the ion exchange signal into a distance-based analysis. The initial K+ concentration determines the quantity of ThT in the aqueous solution after ion-exchange; hence, the sample K+ concentration is reflected in the distance of the ThT-colored area. An identifiable response in the K+ concentration range of 1–6 mM was generated by the ion exchange process when it was operated in what is referred to as a "exhaustive sensing mode," which is not achievable with the traditional optode sensing mode. Because there are no hydrogen ions present, the equilibrium competition of the capillary sensor is entirely pH-independent, in contrast to conventional optodes that have a pH-sensitive signal. Studies using mixed and separate solutions have shown that K^+ has extremely high selectivity over Na^+ and Ca^{2+} [26].

3. Various treatment options

3.1 Nonspecific treatment

Any concurrent or pre-existing ailment needs to be properly managed. A downer cow should receive good nursing care, be comfortable, and not be bothered. Maintaining the cow's constant access to water and nutrition is especially crucial. Regular milking and turning from one side to the other is necessary for dairy cows. Any equipment that aids in the animal's emergence is beneficial, but timing is crucial. Because weak animals are more likely to be injured due to a lack of muscle tone, premature attempts may exacerbate or even induce a musculoskeletal problem. After the serum potassium content returns to the normal level, using a flotation tank (Aqua cow Rise System) is quite beneficial [27].

3.2 Nursing the downer cow

Only when the cow has a good chance of recovering and there is a capable person nearby who is willing to dedicate the necessary time and energy to offer proper nursing care may a downed cow be nursed. The downer cow's chances of recovering completely are increased with proper nursing, but this can be labour- and time-intensive. If you are unable to provide the cow proper nursing care, you should think about euthanizing it right away [28].

3.3 Guideline for tending to a downtrodden cow

1. Give the cow comfortable, clean, dry bedding so that when it tries to stand, it has a non-slip surface [28].

2. Ensure a steady supply of wholesome food and clean water,

3. Every 3–4 hours, move the cow from side to side.

4. Make sure the cow is periodically moved and that her weight is not always on one side if she is unable to switch sides on her own. She should also flex and lengthen her hind limbs each time.

5. Remove the milk by hand from the udder.

6. Consistently encourage the cow to stand; only use a lifting hoist equipment to help her do so.

7. Never let a cow dangle inside a hoisting mechanism [28].

3.4 Specific treatment

The severity of the hypokalemia should determine the oral or intravenous potassium therapy. It is crucial to keep in mind that a potassium deficiency be 200–400 mEq is represented by every 1 mEq/L reductions in serum potassium. Nevertheless, this computation may overestimate or underestimate the potassium shortage. Individuals with mild to moderate hypokalemia (potassium concentration of 2.5–3.5 mEq/L), may just require oral potassium replacement. If potassium levels are less than 2.5 mEq/L, intravenous potassium should be given, very slowly and call for the attendance of a veterinarian.

3.5 Injectable formulations

Potassium injections should never be given intravenously; instead, they should be diluted with 500 ml of regular saline injections, with a pace of between 0.1 and 0.2 mEq/kg/h being the ideal range. A maximum injection rate of 0.5 mEq/kg/h is recommended for intravenous supplementation; at replacement fluid flow rates, this translates to 20–40 mEq/L of fluid.

Dosage: The dose should be frequently adjusted for the animal, and continuous monitoring of plasma concentration should be performed. When the severity of hypokalemia is known, an administration regime is recommended:

1. Mild hypokalemia: serum concentration 3.0–3.5 $K+$ mEq/l | quantity of potassium chloride per kg/weight administered for 24 hours: 2–3 mEq.

2. Moderate hypokalemia: serum levels 2.5–3.0 $K+$ mEq/l | quantity of potassium chloride/kg/weight administered for 24 hours: 3–5 mEq.

3. Severe hypokalemia: serum concentration $\leq$ 2.5 $K+$ mEq/l | quantity of potassium chloride per kg/weight administered for 24 hours: 5–10 mEq.

If the serum potassium concentration is not known, 20–40 mEq/l potassium chloride should be added to the solution for intravenous perfusion.

One millimole is equivalent to one milli equivalent (mEq) or 39.1 milligram of potassium. Potassium chloride sterile aqueous solution is widely accessible in the market for this use, often at a concentration of 2 mEq K/mL. As an alternative, adding 1 g of KCI powder to fluids meant for intravenous delivery yields about 13 mEq of $K+$ [26].

3.6 Potassium chloride injection

Potassium chloride injection is available in the market globally as vials and ampoule potassium chloride concentrate is used for electrolyte and fluid replenishment. It must be diluted before use. Potassium chloride can rehydrate the cow and restore electrolyte balance. 10 ml and 20 ml single-dose vials are a administration & dosage: intravenous. Before being administered, it must be diluted with water or another acceptable fluid to the proper strength. Potassium chloride, 2 mEq (149 mg), is present in each milliliter of sterile aqueous solution available in the market.

3.7 Potassium acetate injections Hospira, Inc.

Potassium acetate in water, sterile, nonpyrogenic, concentrated solution for injection is known as acetate injection, USP (2 mEq/mL). As an electrolyte replenisher, the fluid is given intravenously following dilution. It cannot be given without diluting it. Bicarbonate (HCO3—) can also be generated from acetate (CH3COO—), a source of hydrogen ion acceptors, through the liver's metabolic conversion process. It has been demonstrated that this can happen quickly, even in cases of severe liver disease. Potassium acetate (196 mg/mL) yields 2 mEq of potassium (K+) and acetate (CH3COO—) respectively. To alter the pH, acetic acid may be added to the solution. With a range of 5.5–8.0, the pH is 6.2. The specific gravity is 1.089 and the osmolar concentration is 4 mOsmol/mL (calculated). A maximum infusion rate of 1 mEq/kg/h is recommended [29, 30].

3.8 Oral formulation

According to Sweeney [31] oral potassium supplementation is better than intravenous since it is less expensive, easier to administer, and allows for higher doses to be given with fewer risk of side effects (**Table 3**). Given that potassium is needed in cattle with whole-body K depletion and chloride is needed in cattle with alkalaemia and pH-induced compartmental shift of K to the intracellular space, oral potassium chloride administration appears to offer the best salt formulation for treating cows with hypokalemia [14].

<table>
<tr><th></th><th>Drug/s</th><th>Presentation</th><th>Dose</th><th>Remarks</th><th>References</th></tr>
<tr><td>1</td><td>Potassium 60 g</td><td>Powder</td><td>Two doses</td><td>Effective in mild to moderate hypokalemia</td><td>[19]</td></tr>
<tr><td>2</td><td>Potassium chloride 60 sodium chloride 30</td><td>Solution</td><td>Sodium chloride 60 g Potassium chloride 30</td><td>Both salts are dissolved in 15 liters of water and given as drench in mild hypokalemia</td><td>[31]</td></tr>
<tr><td>3</td><td>Potassium chloride 52 g</td><td>Bolus</td><td>One</td><td rowspan="3">Plasma potassium concentrations for all preparations increased within 30 minutes and the increase lasted for 12 hours.. The feed intake increased in 50% of cows within 2 hours after potassium application, which may contribute to the increase of plasma potassium concentration</td><td rowspan="3">[32]</td></tr>
<tr><td>4</td><td>Potassium propionate52</td><td>500 g gel</td><td>One</td></tr>
<tr><td>5</td><td>Potassium chloride powder52</td><td>Solution</td><td>One</td></tr>
<tr><td>6</td><td>Potassium acetate</td><td>10% solution</td><td>BID for daily for 1 days</td><td>Treatment continued till recovery</td><td>[29]</td></tr>
<tr><td>7</td><td>Potassium chloride: 51 wt.%
$CaCl_2$ $2H_2O$: 25 wt-%
Water: 15 wt.%</td><td>Bolus</td><td>One or two</td><td>In the moderate hypokalemic cow, a bolus administration resulted in reconstitution of mean and medium plasma potassium concentration to normal (reference range 3.5–5.0 mmol/l) within an hour following administration. In severe hypokalemia, one more bolus was given with no adverse effect</td><td>[33]</td></tr>
</table>

	Drug/s	Presentation	Dose	Remarks	References
8	Dipotassium phosphate 100 g of phosphate 1 and 83 g of potassium	Bolus	two boluses once daily for a maximum of 3–5 days	Recovery within 3 days	[34]
	Potassium chloride 24 g Sodium carbonate Potassium carbonate Taurine 6 Propylene glycol 200 ml	Powder and liquid	Both were together administered and repeated after 10 hours if necessary	Recovery within 3–12 hours' stabilizes the potassium, provides energy palatable	[35]

Table 3.
Various oral treatment methods of hypokalemia.

3.9 Powder formulations

Since potassium chloride tastes bad when taken orally, giving cows access to it usually does not lead to enough voluntary consumption. Second, some of the advantages of supplementing may be offset by increased potassium excretion in the urine, which is linked to increased urine flow during intravenous replacement fluid administration. If a free-choice oral electrolyte solution consisting of 60 g sodium chloride and 30 g potassium chloride diluted in 15 L of water is made available to patients with minor cases of hypokalemia, it will be easily ingested and help correct the modest deficiency [31] Wittek et al. [32] conducted a comparative study on three oral potassium formulations and discovered that the cows treated for hypokalemia received 52 g of potassium in three different formulations: group B was given a potassium chloride bolus (released over 12 hours); group G was given potassium propionate gel (released over 2 hours); and group S was given potassium chloride solution (available immediately). They discovered that the amounts of potassium in plasma for all preparations rose in less than 30 minutes and continued to rise for 12 hours. Within two hours of the potassium administration, 50% of the cows' feed intake increased, which could have contributed to the rise in plasma potassium content.

3.10 Potassium acetate

Narayana et al. [29] successfully treated the downer cows, creeper cow and cattle with leg weakness with Potassium acetate 10 g b.i.d. orally, and 10% solution 100 ml intravenously/day until signs of recovery which was in a week to a month.

3.11 Bolus formulations

3.11.1 The bolus formulation is easy to administer with a Balling gun and is easy to pack and transport

Wilhelm-Olany [33] conducted a trial with a following composition bolus with ingredients.

Potassium chloride: 51 wt.%

$CaCl_2$ $2H_2O$: 25 wt.%
Water: 15 wt.%
Magnesium oxide: 9 wt.%.

There were 45–48 g of potassium per piece in the bolus formulation, or roughly 85–91 g of potassium chloride. Bolus is administered orally with a Balling gun. An hour after bolus injection, the mean and medium plasma potassium concentrations in the moderately hypokalemic cow were returned to normal (reference range 3.5–5.0 mmol/l). One extra bolus was administered in cases of severe hypokalemia with no negative consequences.

3.12 Kalitop (Resco Product, Belgium)

3.12.1 Each bolus contains 70 g of potassium

3.12.1.1 Dosage and administration

Two Kalitop bolus together in 1 application, and 2 boluses 12 hours later if necessary. Orally with the help of a bolus applicator or Balling gun.

3.12.1.2 Potassium Bolus (J Farm, Poland)

Potassium bolus for the dairy cow; includes 66 g of potassium in each bolus reduction of the risk of hypokalaemia.

Indications:

- A cow with prolonged inappetence (>2 days) after labour, especially with recurrent ketosis
- The cow receiving more than one injection of corticosteroid that have mineralocorticoid activity

Properties:

- rapid disintegration and assimilation
- reduction of the risk of hypokalemia
- counteraction of depression gastrointestinal tract motility and stimulation of appetite
- all ingredients are digestible

Composition:
Potassium chloride, magnesium stearate.
Instruction for proper use:
Give 1 bolus into the cow's mouth by using applicator.
After 8–12 hours repeat the administration of 1 bolus, if needed.
Shelf life: 18 months from the manufacturing date.

Packaging: Each 150 g bolus is secured in a plastic tube. There are four boluses in one paper box.

3.12.1.3 K-Phos Boost Bolus

Since the symptoms of hypophosphatemia and hypokalemia are similar and manifest in the early postpartum period, Solvet Animal Health (Calgary, Alberta, Canada) has created a dipotassium phosphate (K_2PO_4) bolus called "K Phos-Boost" to treat both conditions. Dipotassium phosphate (K_2HPO_4) makes up each 230-gram K Phos-Boost Bolus (Solvet Animal Health, Calgary, Alberta, Canada), which provides 100 g of phosphate and 83 g of potassium per bolus. In the rumen, the bolus dissolves entirely in 30 minutes. For dairy cows lacking in potassium and phosphorus, the suggested published dose is 131 g of potassium and 198 g of phosphate per day for a period of 1–5 day. When cows ingest two boluses of dipotassium phosphate, they get 200 g of phosphate and 166 g of potassium daily. This is in good agreement with the daily dosage that have been published. Therefore, two boluses once daily for a maximum of 3–5 days is the recommended dose [34].

Dosage: Administer using the K-Phos Boost branded applicator. Give 2 boluses orally, once daily for up to 3 days. Allow access of water.

In severe hypokalemic cows with a serum potassium concentration of less than2.5 mmol/L one dose of intravenous injection followed after 12 hours by either oral powder or Bolus potassium formulation saved the cows from certain death [36].

The oral delivery of potassium chloride in solution through the use of a bottle or a drenching gun or a stomach tube may irritate the mucous membranes of the oral cavity and the esophagus as a result of its caustic action [37].

3.12.1.4 Nutri-Pot

It turned out that drenching the Nutri-Pot (A) and Nutri-Pot (B) mixture was a simple and secure process. In addition to acting as a lubricant and demulcent, propylene glycol supplied instant energy and facilitated the rapid absorption of potassium. Increased feed absorption and consequent milk production were linked to improvements in the clinical state [35].

Generally, hypokalemia in cows with anorexia and debility when oral formulations, replenish the serum potassium but do not provide sufficient energy for speedy recovery.

Higher or frequent oral dose is not recommended, because they can lead to osmotic diarrhea, excessive salivation, muscular tremors of the legs, and excitability. Hypokalemia is usually associated with acidosis. It was hypothesized that formulation that overcomes acidosis, provides energy, improves and stabilizes cell membranes and regulates osmosis will pave a way for a speedy recovery.

Nutri-pot that was presented in two parts [36] 50 g of powder part containing 12 g of elemental potassium and 4 gram bicarbonate sodium and potassium 6 gram of taurine and liquid part containing 200 ml propylene glycol), was conducted. In 84 clinical cases 40 without taurine and another 44 with taurine, at the veterinary hospital, during 2022–2023. In Rayachoti of Andhra Pradesh. The second dose was repeated if necessary. Taurine-enriched formulation group recovered and returned to normal milk within 3 days than the formulation without taurine took 5–7 days to return to normal milk [36].

Nutri-pot is the proprietary product of Instar Health care, Kadapa. The formulation provided sufficient energy, increased palatability, enhanced absorption, countered acidosis, lessened gastric irritation, stabilized membranes and balanced the influx and outflux of potassium in the cells of the heart muscle, and skeletal muscles of limbs and neck. The role of taurine in membrane function and stabilization has greatly increased the importance of dietary taurine. Taurine apparently, normalize the content of potassium and calcium ions in vivo and in vitro. The action of taurine appears 50 be membrane-based [38] as it has detoxifying, antioxidant, and membrane-stabilizing properties apparently due to its molecular structure [39, 40].

3.12.1.5 Role of taurine in the formulation

It is assumed that taurine-containing formulations may stabilize the translocation of potassium from intracellular to extracellular and vice versa, since hypokalemia is caused by abnormalities of potassium concentration in plasma and can result from changes in external potassium balance (intake vs. excretion) or internal potassium balance (intracellular to extracellular) [38]. The antioxidant and metabolic enzyme activity were regulated by dietary K+ and taurine, which also reduced stress and balanced energy needs. The best growth performance, ionic homeostasis, and stress reduction were shown by GIFT tilapia fed a diet containing 0.5% taurine and 0.2% K+. This suggests that taurine plays a critical role in enhancing the wellbeing of fish raised in low-salinity, potassium-deficient water [41]. Taurine nutritional supplements enhance potassium ionic equilibrium [42, 43].

Evidence for the role of taurine in membrane function and stabilization exemplifies the potential importance of dietary taurine. It is said that most actions of taurine appear to be membrane-based because it has detoxifying, antioxidant, and membrane-stabilizing properties apparently due to its molecular structure. Taurine was shown to normalize the content of potassium and calcium ions in vivo and in vitro [38]. In excitable tissues, taurine (2-aminoethane sulfonic acid) is widely distributed. Its many physiological and pharmacological effects are little understood in terms of its underlying mechanisms. However, taurine's physicochemical characteristics imply that it interacts with membrane phospholipids to change the characteristics of membrane-associated proteins as well as membrane functions like ion binding and conductance [37–39].

4. Prevention of hypokalemia

Early lactation cow can suffer from negative potassium balance due to greater potassium excretion, greater secretion of potassium in milk, and increased perspiration losses during heat stress. With the inclusion of a higher amount of potassium in the early lactation diet, some studies showed an increase in milk production, 3.5% fat corrected milk, and the milk fat, which was not associated with an increase in dry matter intake. Potassium supplementation in the form of potassium carbonate has also increased milk fat percentages, partly explained by reduced ruminal synthesis of bio-hydrogenation intermediates known to inhibit milk fat synthesis. The lowering of bio-hydrogenation intermediates that inhibit milk fat synthesis is likely mediated through the alkalizing effects of some potassium supplements to increase ruminal fluid pH(I) Harrison et al. [44] recommend formulating for 1.6% K, and to increase to1.8 to 2% for heat stress. Harrison [44] advised formulating for 1.6% K and raising to 1.8–2%. In order to help achieve a DCAD of >35 mEq/100 g of dry matter, sodium levels can be raised. The maximum amount of sodium in the dry matter ratio is 0.8%.

4.1 Potassium carbonate administration

In order to enhance the buffering capacity of rations, boost the supply of K during heat stress, and balance electrolytes in the ration for optimal lactational performance, potassium carbonate has been added to feed as a feed supplement. Potassium carbonate, however, can heat feed and induce caking. A novel product has been developed by Milk Specialties Global (Eden Prairie, MN), which used 204 g of bye pass fat to coat 68 g of potassium carbonate as a premix. According to Kayla et al.'s study [45], feeding the novel product to a milking Holstein dairy cow on a regular basis did not cause any palatability issues.

The effects of adding electrolyte and ascorbic acid to feed under heat stress in buffalo were investigated by Sunil Kumar et al. [46]. They added ascorbic acid polyphosphate at 10 g/animal/d, potassium carbonate at 12.5 g/animal/d, and sodium bicarbonate at 15 g/animal/d as supplements and noted a reduction in heat stress.

4.2 Various Additives to minimize hypokalemia

4.2.1 Additional supplementation of potassium salts to animals at risk

Potassium must be given orally to the inoperant cow as part of the fluid and electrolyte treatment regimen. Supplementing animals deemed to be at risk is the focus of prevention. Oral potassium supplementation is recommended for dairy animals that are persistently anorectic and receiving treatment with isoflupredone acetate, intravenous dextrose, and insulin. While there is no definitive recommended dosage for a normal patient deemed at risk, 100 g twice a day appears to be a safe starting point [8].

4.2.2 Additional supplementation of propylene glycol

The easiest way to keep cows from developing hypokalemia is to make sure they are getting enough dry matter to eat. Propylene glycol supplementation in the early nursing cow diet enhanced energy status, reduced body weight loss, and had negligible effects on feed intake and milk production; nevertheless, it may have decreased the amount of protein and fat in the milk [35].

4.2.3 Additives to enhance the dry matter intake

Utilizing additives to balance rumen functioning: Few additions have a consistent effect on conditioning rumen functionality. This is due to the fact that every addition is dependent upon the circumstances established by the cow's overall ration consumption as well as her physical and general health. Every additive must therefore be assessed using a methodology unique to each farm. Generally speaking, the most widely utilized additions are yeast, sodium bicarbonate, and yeast derivatives. Other, less common ones are clays, algae, probiotics, enzymes, and various salts. When receiving two or more cortisone injections with mineralo-corticoid action, one should always give an oral powder or bolus.

4.2.4 Iodised oil to combat the thermal stress

In case of hypokalemia occur during thermal stress, inject 5 ml containing 150 mg of iodisedoil, at brisket region for 3 consecutive days will overcome the thermal stress for 60 days without detrimental effect on thyroid [47].

4.3 Thermo CAD heat stress pack

ThermoCAD Heat Stress Pack, an Altech, Hubbard product in hot weather, 4–8 oz. per head per day as a top-dress, as part of a TMR, or as the grain portion of a dairy or beef diet. In addition, water and forage are required. Cattle in dairy and beef feedlots that are nursing should utilize the ThermoCAD Heat Stress Pack when the weather is warm and conducive to heat stress. Tasco (Ascophyllumnodosum) is a unique blend with minerals, vitamins, electrolytes, and feed additives called ThermoCad, which is intended to assist sustain dry matter intake and replace essential nutrients that are necessary for effective heat stress abatement.

5. Conclusion

"From the latest scientific findings presented in this chapter, the following most important conclusions can be drawn:

1. The cows with serum or plasma potassium concentrations less than 3.9 mEq/L are considered hypokalemia.

2. Hypokalemia can arise from induced, physiological, or pathological conditions.

3. Extended periods of anorexia, lying down, twitches in the muscles, melancholy, fluctuations in body temperature, and an odd neck posture (an S-shaped neck) are some of the prominent symptoms.

4. The turbid metric approach is a quick, simple, and cost-effective way to estimate serum potassium at the field level.

5. A maximum delivery rate of 0.5 mEq/kg/h is recommended for severe hypokalemia when serum concentration ≤ 2, 5 K+ mEq/parenteral injections; at replacement fluid flow rates, this often equates to 20–40 mEq/L of fluid.

6. Beside the potassium salt therapy, we emphasize the inclusion of Taurine in the therapeutic regime.

6. Future research and recommendation

As a cytoprotective molecule, taurine is involved in many different processes, including energy production, neuromodulation, calcium homeostasis, and osmoregulation. These processes supports the taurine's anti-oxidant properties and the molecular mechanisms underlying its action in a variety of pathological conditions linked to oxidative stress. In fact, taurine shows promise as a treatment for conditions connected to the central nervous system, circulatory system, skeletal muscle, and metabolism. The multilayered characterization of taurine therapeutic targets with the use of next-generation sequencing will provide comprehensive insights into taurine's prospective clinical applications [47–49].

It is worthwhile to research the inclusion of taurine in the oral and injectable potassium chloride formulations to lower the dosage and speed up the healing process of hypokalemia in the dairy cow.

Acknowledgements

Our profound gratitude to Dr. Santimalla Siva Reddy, Assistant Director, Veterinary Hospital, Rayachoti, India, for assessing Nutri-Pot in hypokalemic cows and sharing his research, and to Dr. Paranjyothikanni, Ph.D. Director, Bangalore Allergic Centre, Bangalore, for his invaluable suggestions in preparing this manuscript. For editing the script, I would like to thank Dr. K. Narayana, a retired professor of veterinary pharmacology at the veterinary college in Bangalore.

Declaration of interest

The writers affirm that there is not any conflict of interest that would be seen as compromising this review's objectivity.

Author details

Bala Krishna Rao Dabbir[1*] and Sreenivasa Reddy Rajavolu[2]

1 Sreepathi Veterinary Services, Kadapa, India

2 Instar Health care, Kadapa, India

*Address all correspondence to: bdabbir@gmail.com

References

[1] Goff JP. Macro-mineral physiology and application to the feeding of the dairy cow for prevention of milk fever and other peri-parturient mineral disorders. Animal Feed Science and Technology. 2006;**126**: 237-257

[2] Schaefer TJ, Wolford RW. Disorders of potassium. Emergency Medicine Clinics of North America. 2005;**23**(3): 723-747, viii-ix

[3] Brobst D. Review of the pathophysiology of alterations in potassium homeostasis. Journal of the American Veterinary Medical Association. 1986;**188**:1019-1025

[4] Guyton AC, Hall JE. Renal regulation of potassium, calcium, phosphate, and magnesium. In: Textbook of Medical Physiology, editor. 9th ed. WB Saunders: Philadelphia; 1996. pp. 375-380

[5] Lunn DP, McGuirk SM. Renal regulation of electrolyte and acid-base balance in ruminants. Veterinary Clinics of North America: Food Animal Practice. 1980;**6**:1-28

[6] Sielman ES, Sweeney RW, Whitlock RH, Reams RY. Hypokalemia syndrome in dairy cows: 10 cases (1992-1996). JAVMA-Journal of the American Veterinary Medical Association. 1997;**210**(2):240-243

[7] Bairwa JK, Venkatesakumar E, Sivaraman S, Madheswaran. Demographic study of hypokalemic syndrome in dairy cows in and around Namakkal, Tamil Nadu. The Pharma Innovation Journal. 2023;**SP-12**(7): 1951-1954

[8] Nicolas S, Gilles F. Hypokalemia syndrome in cattle, acid-base and potassium homeostasis. Seminars in Nephrology. 2013;**33**:257-264

[9] DrugBank Accession Number DB1449

[10] Lee Hamm L, Hering-Smith K, Nakhoul N. Acid-base and potassium homeostasis. Seminars in Nephrology. 2013;**33**:257-264

[11] Rajendran VM, Geoffrey IS. Colonic potassium absorption and secretion in health and disease. Comprehensive Physiology. 2022;**8**(4):1513-1536

[12] Ward GM. Potassium metabolism of domestic ruminants: A review. Journal of Dairy Science. 1966;**49**: 268-276

[13] Peek SF, Divers TJ, Guard C, Rath AP, Rebhun WC. Hypokalemia, muscle weakness, and recumbency in dairy cattle. Veterinary Therapeutics. 2000;**1**(4):235-244

[14] Constable PD. Hypokalemia in Adult Cattle - Metabolic Disorders - MSD Veterinary Manual. Rahway, NJ, USA: Merck & Co., Inc.; 2022

[15] Rowlands GJ, Manston R, Pocock RM. Relationships between stage of lactation and pregnancy and blood composition in a herd of dairy cows and the influences of seasosnal changes in management on these relationships. The Journal of Dairy Research. 1975;**42**: 349-362

[16] Constable P, Walter Grünberg W, Rudolf SR, Henry R. Clinico-pathologic variables associated with hypokalemia in lactating dairy cows with abomasal displacement or volvulus. Journal of the American Veterinary Medical Association. 2013;**242**:826-835

[17] Tamer H, Chandan Deep T. Hypocalcemia and hyperkalemia during magnesium infusion therapy in a pre-eclamptic patient. Clinical Case Reports. 2015;**3**(10):827-883

[18] Peek SF, Divers. Hypokalemia. In: Rebhun's Diseases of Dairy Cattle. 2nd ed. Oxford, United Kingdom: Elsevier – Health Sciences Division; 2008. pp. 601-602

[19] Constable PD. Fluids: Electrolytes. In: Brumbaugh GW, editor. Clinical Pharmacology: Veterinary Clinics of North America, Food Animal Practice. 19th ed. Philadelphia: W. B. Saunders Company; 2003. pp. 1-40

[20] Wittek T, Constable PD, Morin DE. Abomasal impaction in Holstein-Friesian cows: 80 cases. Journal of the American Veterinary Medical Association. 2005; **227**:287-289

[21] Mallonee PG, Beede D, Collier RJ, Wilcox CM. Production: Physiological responses of dairy cows to varying dietary potassium during heat stress. Journal of Dairy Science. 1985;**68**(6): 1479

[22] Kalaitzakis E, Panousis N, Roubies N, Kaldrymidon E, Karatzias H. Macromineral status of dairy cows with concurrent left abomasal displacement and fatty liver. New Zealand Veterinary Journal. 2010;**58**:307-311

[23] Miyada DS, Inami K, Matsuyama G. Clinical Chemistry. 1971;**17**(1):27-30

[24] Tubino M, Rafael LD, Nelci F. Rapid quantitative turbidi metric spot test analysis of potassium in blood serum. Journal of the Brazilian Chemical Society. 2004;**15**(5):635-639

[25] Hidayat AS, Horino H, Rzeznicka II. Smartphone-enabled quantification of potassium in blood plasma. Sensors. 2021;**21**(4751):4-11

[26] Soda Y, Citterio D, Bakker E. Equipment-free detection of K^+ on microfluidic paper-based analytical devices based on exhaustive replacement with ionic dye in ion-selective capillary sensors. ACS Sensors. 2019;**4**(3): 670-677. DOI: 10.1021/acssensors.8b01

[27] Constable PD. Hypokalemia in adult cattle. In: Aiello SE, editor. Merck Veterinary Manual. 11th ed. New Jersey: Merck & Co., Inc; 2016. pp. 1004-1005

[28] Brochure. How to Manage a Down Cow. Australia: Dairy Australia Limited; 2016. pp. 1–6

[29] Narayana K, Setty DRL, Sastry KNV, Thandaveshwar MG. Downer cow syndrome. Indian Veterinary Journal. 1977;**54**:148-153

[30] Veltri KT, Mason C. Medication-induced hypokalemia. P T. 2015;**40**(3): 185-119

[31] Sweeney RW. Treatment of potassium balance disorders. Veterinary Clinics of North America: Food Animal Practice. 1999;**15**(3): 609-617

[32] Wittek T, Müller AE, Wolf F, Schneider S. Comparative study on 3 oral potassium formulations for treatment of hypokalemia in dairy cows. Journal of Veterinary Internal Medicine. 2019;**33**: 1814-1821

[33] Wilhelm-Olany AR. Effects of oral supplementation of potassium chloride in hypokalemic dairy cows by use of a bolus formulation on metabolism, abomasal position and vaginal discharge characteristics [PhD thesis]. Berlin: FreienUniversität; 2019

[34] Verhoef W, Zuidhof S, Ross JA, Beaugrand K, Olson M. Evaluation of a novel dipotassium phosphate bolus for treatment of metabolic disorders in dairy cattle. Frontiers in Veterinary Science. 2023;**10**:1274183. DOI: 10.3389/fvets.2023.1274

[35] Liu Q, Wang C, Yang WZ, Zhang WW, Yang XM, He DC, et al. Effects of feeding propylene glycol on dry matter intake, lactation performance, energy balance and blood metabolites in early lactation dairy cows. Animal. 2009;**3**(10):1420-1142

[36] Santimalla VSR, Rajavolu SR, Dabbir BKR. Oral treatment of hypokalemia with potassium chloride and propylene glycol in cows. International Journal of Pharmaceutical Chemistry Analysis. 2023;**10**(3):202-204

[37] Mann S, Feist M, Weber BK, Zoller DK, Metzner M. Balling gun-induced trauma in cattle: Clinical presentation, diagnosis and prevention. The Veterinary Record. 2013;**172**(26):685

[38] Huxtable RJ, Sebrineg LA. Towards a Unifying Theory for the Actions of Taurine. Vol. 1. Amsterdam: Elsevier Science Publishers; 1986. pp. 481-485

[39] Shustova TI, Mashkova NY, Cherkashina EM, Dokshina GA. Effect of taurine on potassium, calcium and sodium levels in the blood and tissues of rats. Voprosy Meditsinskoi Khimii. 1986;**32**(4):113-116

[40] Uysal M. Erythrocyte lipid per oxidation and (Na-K)-ATPase activity in cholesterolfed rabbits. International Journal for Vitamin and Nutrition Research. 1986;**56**:307-310

[41] Qi B, Yamagami T, Naruse Y, Sokejima S, Kagamimori S. Effects of taurine on depletion of erythrocyte membrane Na-K ATPase activity due to ozone exposure or cholesterol enrichment. Journal of Nutritional Science and Vitaminolog. 1995;**41**:627-634

[42] Anindita B, Santosh Kumar P, Sairam K. Supplementation of taurine improves ionic homeostasis and mitochondrial function in the rats exhibiting post-traumatic stress disorder-like symptoms. European Journal of Pharmacology. 2021;**908**(5):174361

[43] Velselvi R, Dasgupta S, Varghese T, Sahu NP, Tripathi G, Panmei H, et al. Taurine and/or inorganic potassium as dietary osmolyte counter the stress and enhance the growth of GIFT reared in ion imbalanced low saline water. Food Chemistry: Molecular Sciences. 2022;**4**(30):1-12

[44] Harrison JH, White R, Kincai R, Jenkins TE, Block E. Potassium in the early lactation dairy cow and its impact on milk and milk fat production. WCDS Advances in Dairy Technology. 2011;**23**:313-319

[45] Kayla M, Hultquist PAS, David P, Casper PAS. Palatability evaluation of free fatty acid encapsulated potassium carbonate as a feed ingredient for lactating dairy cows fed a total mixed ration. The Professional Animal Scientist. 2016;**32**(3):328-332

[46] Sunil Kumar BV, Singh G, Meur SK. Effects of addition of electrolyte and ascorbic acid in feed during heat stress in buffaloes. Asian-Australasian Journal of Animal Sciences. 2010;**23**(7):880-888

[47] Randhawa SS, Chhabra S, Randhawa CS, Zahid U, Dhaliwal PS. A note on treatment of hyperthermia in

crossbred cattle. Asian Pacific Journal of Tropical Biomedicine. 2014;**4**(Suppl 1): S272-S274

[48] Huxtable RJ. Physiological actions of taurine. Physiological Reviews. 1992; **72**(1):101-163

[49] Baliou S, Adamaki M, Ioannou P, Pappa A, Panayiotidis M, Spandidos D, et al. Protective role of taurine against oxidative stress (review). Molecular Medicine Reports. 2021;**24**(605):21-20

Chapter 2

Impact of Unsaturated Fat Supplementation on Mammary Gland Growth and Development in Dairy Animals

Hoda Javaheri Barfourooshi

Abstract

The dairy industry plays a pivotal role in promoting food security across human societies globally by providing high-quality protein sources, primarily raw milk, sourced from animal husbandry. A key factor contributing to the economy of the dairy industry is the enhancement of both the quality and quantity of milk produced in dairy farms. One of the strategies used to increase milk production is the use of fats in livestock feeding. Despite the long history of adding fats to animal diets, information on the effects of varying types and amounts of fat consumption at different stages of animal breeding remains scarce. Unsaturated fats, particularly polyunsaturated fatty acids, are commonly used in dairy farms. In addition to their nutritional value in providing energy for animals, they have been shown to have positive effects on growth and overall health. This has led to their categorization as functional foods. These compounds increase milk production by promoting the growth and development of mammary tissue through changing gene expression. This section aims to present a brief summary of the impact of consuming unsaturated fats on the growth and development of the mammary gland.

Keywords: polyunsaturated fatty acid, mammary gland, functional foods, Holstein cow, Saanen goat

1. Introduction

The significance of milk as a nutrient is widely recognized in both academic and business settings. Ancient records found on stone tablets in the Great Sahara, located in North Africa, demonstrate that the importance of milk and dairy products has been understood since 4000 BC. Even today, the role of these substances in meeting the nutritional needs of human societies in terms of energy, high-quality protein, minerals, and key vitamins is well-defined [1].

The capacity for milk production is primarily determined by the number of milk-producing cells. Any manipulation of these cells can directly impact the amount of milk production [2]. Accordingly, the factors that influence the number of epithelial cells have the most significant effect on milk production. Mammary gland growth control is a complex process influenced by many hormones and external factors, such as photoperiods and diet [3].

Fat supplements have long been crucial for providing energy to dairy animals. However, the use of unsaturated oils instead of saturated fats not only avoids the adverse effects of the latter but also offers a range of benefits [4]. In recent years, unsaturated fatty acids have emerged as the primary regulators in biological tissues. Given their role as the key components of cell membranes, the composition of fatty acids greatly influences the function of cell membranes. Moreover, the presence of fatty acids in diverse biological systems and processes, such as the immune system, blood coagulation and vascular resistance, enzyme activities, cell proliferation and differentiation, and the expression of receptors, has been widely acknowledged. Omega-3 family fatty acids, owing to their unique biological properties like long chain length and the presence of double bonds on carbon number three, are considered potent regulators in these pathways [5].

Polyunsaturated fatty acids play a critical role in many physiological actions, particularly in stimulating cell growth. As such, feeding foods containing omega-3 and omega-6 fatty acids at the end of the first pregnancy is highly recommended. This period is crucial for mammary gland growth as it promotes an increase in parenchymal tissue relative to the surrounding stroma, thereby positively and stimulatingly affecting the growth, proliferation, and organization of mammary gland tissue. Notably, enhancing the growth and development of mammary gland tissue can lead to improved production performance in the animal. It is expected that the supplementation of dairy animal feed with polyunsaturated fatty acids during the physiologically critical periods for mammary gland growth will increase both the quantity and quality of milk produced. To achieve the optimal results, this feeding practice must be implemented during the appropriate developmental stage of the animal. Such an approach has the potential to be an effective strategy for enhancing milk production and quality in the dairy industry.

2. Mammary gland growth

The mammary gland is an epithelial skin appendage comprising different tissues and cell types that undergo significant morphological and functional changes throughout the reproductive cycle in association with growth, functional differentiation, and regression [6]. The growth and development of mammary tissue can be categorized into distinct stages, including: (1) mammogenesis, which encompasses the growth and differentiation of ductal and alveolar mammary tissue; (2) colostrogenesis, the transfer of immunoglobulins to mammary secretions before parturition; (3) lactogenesis, the initiation of the secretion of a suitable volume of prepartum milk; (4) lactation, which involves the continuous production and secretion of milk; and (5) regression, which entails the cessation of lactation and the return of the mammary gland to a less differentiated state [7].

The lactating mammary gland comprises parenchymal and stromal connective tissues. The former consists of epithelial structures, such as ducts and alveoli that are closely associated with the stromal connective tissue. The stroma is characterized by cellular and noncellular components, with the cellular constituents encompassing fibroblasts, endothelial cells of blood vessels, and leukocytes that accumulate in the tissue. The noncellular parts comprise collagen and other connective tissue proteins.

Significant white fat tissue is formed in the mammary gland during the early stages of fetal development and remains until pregnancy in the animal, representing an extra-parenchymal tissue that forms part of the developing stroma of the gland [8].

2.1 Growth and development of the mammary gland during pregnancy

The mammary gland's function is the primary determinant of milk production per animal. The differences in milk production between dairy and beef cattle are predominantly attributed not only to the increase in parenchymal mammary mass of dairy animals but also to the heightened activity of most secretory cells alone [3]. The structural development of the mammary gland can be classified into five (or six) stages: (1) development during the embryonic period, (2) development during the prepuberty period, (3) development during the postpuberty period, (4) development during pregnancy, (5) development during lactation [8], and (6) development during regression [9].

Mammary growth resumes during pregnancy after entering the isometric growth stage following puberty. Milk-secreting cells develop solely during pregnancy, and the amount of milk produced is directly dependent on the number of secretory cells and their functional differentiation. As such, factors that maintain or increase the number of existing alveoli during the lactation period, along with those that affect the functional differentiation of these cells, significantly affect milk production. Thus, this period is pivotal in determining the number of secretory cells and future milk production in the mammary gland. During the second half of pregnancy, the size of the alveoli continues to increase, and new alveoli are added until a vast area of the mammary gland is covered. Alveolar cells gradually undergo the necessary biochemical and structural changes to begin abundant milk secretion, lactogenesis, at the time of parturition. Although it was previously believed that terminally differentiated cells do not multiply, recent observations have shown that cells continue to proliferate during the initial phases of lactogenesis. At this time, epithelial cells exhibit a net appearance in the apical region of the cell, resulting from the abundance and accumulation of secretory vesicles. In fully differentiated cells, the basal-lateral part of the cytoplasm appears darker in staining and is devoted to absorbing precursors and synthesizing proteins and lipids. The cytoplasm of the apical region, which is full of Golgi apparatus, structures, processes and packages proteins and lactose for secretion from the cell [2, 8].

2.1.1 Metabolic changes during pregnancy

In the last 3 to 4 weeks of pregnancy, a rapid growth of the fetus occurs, along with mammary gland development and favorable metabolic adjustments for the mobilization of fat and other nutrients. However, during this period, nutrient intake is reduced, and the metabolism of glucose and fatty acids undergoes significant changes. Metabolic adaptations occur in other tissues of the mother's body to ensure the supply of glucose required by the uterus and lactating mammary gland, even under conditions of maternal nutritional changes. Hormonal changes that occur before parturition are also well-defined. The adaptive changes start in the prenatal period and continue after parturition and lactation. These changes involve increased lipolysis, decreased lipogenesis, increased gluconeogenesis, increased glycogenolysis, increased consumption of fats, and decreased consumption of glucose as energy sources. They also involve increased mobilization of protein reserves, increased absorption of minerals and mobilization of mineral reserves, increased feed consumption, and increased absorption capacity for nutrients [10]. Extensive metabolic and hormonal adjustments occur during the transition period from late pregnancy to early lactation. During this period, the plasma concentration of insulin decreases, and the responsiveness of muscle and skeletal tissue to insulin decreases. These adaptations may be crucial factors in the initiation of catabolic activities of the transition period [11].

2.1.2 Metabolic changes during the transition period

The transition period in dairy breeds, which includes about 3 weeks before to 3 weeks after calving, is widely considered a sensitive and critical stage [12]. During this period, significant changes occur in the nutritional, behavioral, physiological, and anatomical patterns of livestock, particularly in the mammary, reproductive, immune, metabolic, and digestive systems. Appropriate management during this period is essential to ensure that the animal moves from the nonproductive to the productive stage with full health. The future performance and health of dairy cattle depends on successfully navigating this period [13].

2.2 Mammary gland growth and development during lactation

Mammary milk production is a two-step process called lactogenesis. The first stage commences during the final trimester of pregnancy, characterized by the limited structural and functional differentiation of the alveolar epithelium. The second stage follows immediately before parturition and is characterized by the completion of structural and biochemical differentiation, coinciding with the onset of milk production and secretion [3]. During lactation, mammary epithelial cells become highly specialized in the production of milk proteins, including casein and whey proteins [14]. The number and activity of these cells determine the shape of the lactation curve and, consequently, the volume of milk produced [15]. Notably, an increase in mammary cell growth can have severe and permanent effects on milk production in response to frequent milking in early-stage dairy cows [16]. The growth of the mammary gland is minimal when lactation is fully established. The relative contribution of hypertrophy and hyperplasia to this phenomenon remains unclear. Approximately 40% of the parenchymal tissue comprises closely packed alveoli, while the remainder comprises alveoli that are greatly expanded in the stromal matrix [2, 8]. The number of cells reflects the sum of the relative rates of cell proliferation and death. The mammary gland grows when the rate of cell proliferation exceeds the rate of cell death, and when the rate of cell death exceeds the rate of cell proliferation, it diminishes [15].

2.2.1 Metabolic changes during lactation

In the first 3 to 4 weeks after calving, there is a slight increase in dry matter intake, accompanied by a rapid drop in nutrients to support milk production. During this period, there is continued rapid growth of mammary tissue and hypertrophy of key digestive and metabolic organs. Metabolically, the cow mobilizes its nutrient reserves, primarily from fat tissue, labile proteins, and bones. A crucial adjustment during this period is the stabilization of the homeostatic control mechanisms of essential nutrients such as glucose and calcium to support lactation. This process is known as homeorhesis and is considered a long-term adaptation to a change in stage, such as a transition from non-lactating to lactating or non-ruminant to ruminant. It involves a coordinated set of changes in metabolism that enables the animal to cope with the challenge and adapt to the new stage. Any inefficiency in a metabolic process can undoubtedly affect the efficiency of other processes as well [10].

3. Genes involved in the growth and development of the mammary gland

Growth factors are central to the growth and development of many cells. These factors, which include EGF, IGF, FGF, and TNF-α, play a unique role in controlling growth [17]. The production of IGF-I is regulated by both growth hormone and nutritional status [18]. The concentration of IGF-I mRNA, which is essential for growth, is higher in the stromal part of the mammary gland compared to its epithelial parts, indicating that the stromal segment is responsible for the local synthesis of IGF-I. During pregnancy, as the population of IGF receptors increases, the role of IGFs in mammary gland growth becomes more pronounced. Moreover, the synergistic effects of IGFs, EGF, and TGF-α on cow udder growth have been observed in some studies. The growth factors EGF and TGF-α have a stimulating effect on mammary gland growth, and their activity increases significantly in the presence of IGF-I, indicating a mainly supportive role in intensifying growth stimulation. The regulation of mammary functions during pregnancy is also attributed to these growth factors [19].

IGFBP1 to IGFBP6 are six structurally related proteins that regulate the activity of IGFs. These IGF-binding proteins modulate the transport of IGFs to specific cells and tissues, enhancing their access to receptors, by prolonging the half-life of IGF. One of the vital functions of IGFs is to inhibit cell death in some cells, where programmed cell death is due to apoptosis, and growth factors play a crucial role in its regulation [20].

4. Nutritional solutions

Adequate consumption compounds providing net energy and metabolizable protein are crucial for the healthy functioning of cows [21]. However, during the transition period, animals face increased challenges due to the heightened demand for nutrients and the reduced capacity of their digestive system. Inadequate nutrition during the dry period can lead to postpartum problems such as metabolic diseases, susceptibility to infections, infertility, and reduced milk production [11]. Despite the high energy demand during late pregnancy and early lactation, cows cannot consume enough feed to satisfy their metabolic and production needs. To address this issue, it is advisable to incorporate energy-dense compounds, such as fat, into their diet during this period.

4.1 The importance of fats in animal nutrition

Fats are a rich source of energy for animals, owing to their high energy and storage properties [22]. Incorporating fat supplements into animal diets increases the energy density, resulting in improved lactation performance and metabolic efficiency in lactating cows. Other benefits of using fat supplements include improved reproductive efficiency and reduced incidence of metabolic abnormalities. Inadequate energy consumption during the prenatal period and early lactation is linked to increased risk of metabolic abnormalities and poor reproductive performance [23]. The essentiality of certain fats for optimal growth and development in animals and humans has been studied for almost 80 years, and the theory of their necessity is well-established. There is growing evidence that long-chain fatty acids with polyunsaturated bonds can modulate the expression of genes that regulate cell growth and differentiation [24]. When incorporating unsaturated fats into the diet of ruminants, it is important to be aware of the permissible limit of consumption of these fats in their unprotected form, which is up to 5%. If there is a need to consume more than this amount, it is recommended to use protected fats in order to avoid disturbing the rumen function and endangering the health of the animal.

4.1.1 The role of fatty acids in the growth and development of mammary tissue

Although the lipogenic activities of adipose tissue in non-lactating ruminants in response to long-chain fatty acids have been studied, few studies have examined the effects of these compounds on mammary gland and adipose tissue in lactating animals. The effect of fatty acids on the different tissue is summarized in **Table 1**.

Consumption of oilseeds in the middle of lactation by dairy cows has a suppressive effect on *de novo* production of lipids in the mammary gland, while no such effect is observed in goats [25].

Mammary epithelial cells grow and organize only when they come into contact with the fat pad. This interaction is influenced by specific fatty acids produced by the fat pad that can trigger changes in epithelial development. Unsaturated fatty acids, especially, stimulate the growth of mammary epithelial cells and can enhance the external effects of other growth factors such as IGF-I and EGF [8, 36]. A diet lacking essential fatty acids can stunt ductal growth and alveolar regression, while a diet rich in unsaturated fats can increase parenchymal growth and tumorigenesis. The growth of epithelial cells can be stimulated by unsaturated fatty acids and their derivatives. Furthermore, unsaturated fatty acids and their derivatives can enhance the proliferative effects of EGF. Fatty acids derived from adipocytes can regulate epithelial growth and potentially morphogenesis through direct and indirect mechanisms involving lipids and their derivatives [37].

Studies have shown that polyunsaturated fatty acids can increase prepubertal mammary growth in sheep. Additionally, studies using bovine and human mammary epithelial cells have suggested that mammary growth may be influenced by retinoids and conjugated linoleic acid (CLA) [2]. The fatty acid composition in adipose tissue reflects the long-term consumption of fatty acids through food. Altering the stored fatty acids in mammary gland fat is crucial for storing and releasing the fatty acids required for the differentiation, proliferation, and normal morphogenesis of mammary epithelial cells [26].

Omega-3 fatty acids have been shown to have a wide range of effects on cellular activity. These fatty acids are a source of energy production while also determining the physicochemical properties of cell membranes. Further, they act as substrates for the production of signaling molecules or acting mediators and moderate the regulation of gene expression. Therefore, omega-3 fatty acids have significant impacts on physiological activity and pathological processes through different mechanisms [38].

In most mammalian species, the histological appearance of the parenchymal tissue is similar, with wide areas of alveolar cavity and compressed stromal tissue between alveoli visible from late pregnancy until lactation. The relative area occupied by the epithelium and the alveolar cavity space is similar, with approximately 40% for each, and the remaining 20% is covered by stromal tissue. Alveolar cells undergo

Author	Subjects	Supplement type	Time of consumption	Effect
Bernard et al. [25]	Cow/Goat	Oilseeds	Middle of lactation	Suppress *de novo* lipid production/No effect.
Bagga et al. [26]	Women	Fish oil	Daily for 3 months	Increasing ω-3/ω-6 ratio approximately fourfold.
McFadden et al. [27]	Prepubertal ewe lamb	Formaldehyde-protected sunflower seed supplement	From 7 to 22 week of age	Increasing mammary parenchymal weight, parenchymal dry fat-free tissue, and DNA content.
Javaheri Barfourooshi et al. [28]	Cow	Fish oil	Dry period and early lactation	Increasing the mammary gland relative percentage of epithelial area.
Javaheri Barfourooshi et al. [29]	Primiparous Saanen goat	Roasted soybean and extruded flaxseed	Two months before kidding to 4 months after parturition	Improving the volume, environment, and size of mammary halves.
Mach et al. [30]	Cow	Rapeseed, soybean, linseed, or a mixture of three oils (unprotected)	Middle of lactation	Downregulation of gene sets related to cell development and remodeling, apoptosis, nutrient metabolic process, and immune system response.
Javaheri Barfourooshi et al. [31]	Cow	Fish oil	Dry period and early lactation	Decreasing of relative expression of IGF-I and TNF-α genes, increasing of relative expression of Bcl-2 gene, increasing the ratio of Bcl-2/Bax gene expression.
Seti et al. [32]	Human colorectal cancer cell line	Alpha-Linolenic acid (ALA) and Linoleic acid (LA)	24 hours (treatment time of cells)	A potential mitogenic effect on cells, reduction in apoptotic activity.
Manna et al. [33]	Rat (carcinogenic model)	Fish oil	7 weeks of age to 32 weeks of age	Increase in Bax immunolabeling and reduction of Bcl-2 immunopositivity and TUNEL-positive apoptotic cells.
Lennie et al. [34]	Human (Patients with heart failure)	Polyunsaturated fat/Omega-3	4 days	Reduction of sTNF-R1 and sTNF-R2.
Huang et al. [35]	Barrows	Linseed	Growing-finishing period	Increasing the expression of PPARγ in longissimus muscle and spleen, reduction in TNF-α gene expression level in longissimus muscle, spleen, and adipose tissue and serum concentration of TNF-α.

Table 1.
Effect of polyunsaturated fatty acids on the different tissue in human or animals.

progressive biochemical and structural differentiations necessary for the initiation of abundant milk secretion (lactogenesis) at parturition [8, 39].

Studies conducted on laboratory animals have shown that polyunsaturated fatty acids stimulate the growth of mammary parenchymal tissue by promoting the proliferation of epithelial cells, while saturated fats inhibit growth. In ruminants, unsaturated fatty acids have a stimulating effect on the growth of mammary epithelial tissue in the prepubertal age, despite an increase in dietary energy. It has also been demonstrated that lambs receiving diets containing unsaturated fatty acids exhibit increased mammary growth before puberty and a larger amount of empty fat pad, which allows for further development of parenchymal parts [27]. In a recent study, Javaheri Barfourooshi et al. [28] showed that incorporating fish oil into the diet of Holstein cows during the dry period and the first 2 months of lactation led to an increase in the percentage of epithelial cells and a decrease in the stromal tissue of the mammary gland compared to cows consuming palm oil (**Figure 1**).

It is important to note that histological assessments alone are insufficient to accurately measure the effects of treatments that may affect the total number of cells in the entire mammary gland. Akers and Capuco [3] demonstrated differences in the relative proportions of well-differentiated alveolar epithelial cells, which were related to higher milk production in Holstein cows compared to similar Hereford cows. Differences in the relative proportions of luminal versus stromal space have been shown to correspond with differences in milk production; that is, more luminal space per stromal tissue is associated with increased milk production.

Furthermore, the increase in the number of epithelial cells per alveolus in cows consuming fish oil suggests that the number of epithelial cells per alveolus was higher than in those receiving palm oil. Additionally, the number of alveoli with a diameter ranging between 50 and 90 micrometers in cows consuming fish oil increased

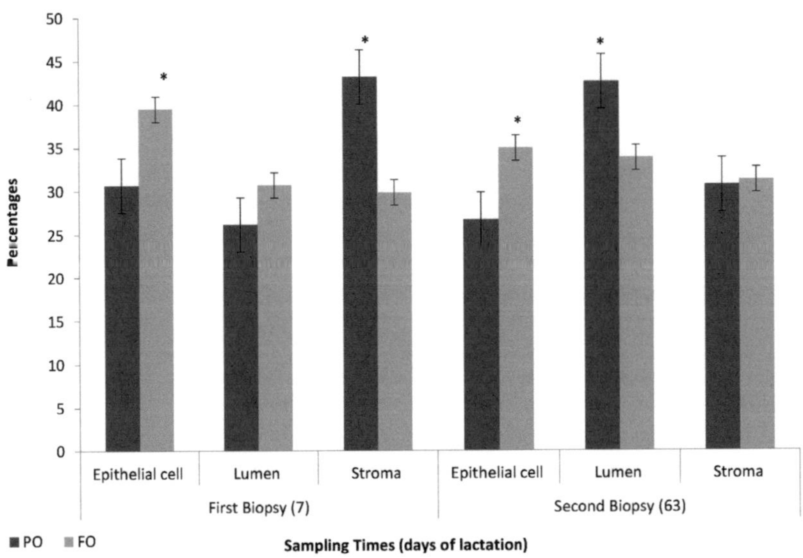

Figure 1.
*Percentage of different parts of alveoli (LSMEANS±SEM) at the first and second biopsy (7 and 63 DIM, respectively) for two diets, palm oil (PO) and fish oil (FO). * Referred to significance at $p < 0.05$ level.*

significantly compared to those consuming palm oil, leading to uniformity in the size of the alveoli. This can increase the surface-to-volume ratio in the alveoli, which may be one of the possible reasons for higher milk production in this group [28].

Comparable results were obtained in Saanen goats that consumed extruded flax-seeds and roasted soybeans in their late pregnancy and early lactation diets, relative to goats that consumed palm oil or a diet without any fat source (Javaheri Barfourooshi, unpublished data). These changes were also visible in the context of mammary gland morphology, as the volume, circumference, and other dimensions of the mammary gland of goats that consumed extruded flaxseed and roasted soybeans were compared to those that received palm oil and those that did not receive any fat supplements in their diet [29]. These histological findings have indicated that the consumption of diets containing unsaturated fatty acids promotes the growth and development of the epithelial parts of the mammary gland. At the time of parturition, the mammary gland tissue had a fully mature structure with active epithelial cells, compared to the groups that consumed saturated fat or a fat-free diet (**Figure 2**).

It has been demonstrated that consuming a diet deficient in essential fatty acids leads to ductal growth damage and alveolar regression, while a diet rich in unsaturated acids increases the growth of epithelial cells. Research has shown that unsaturated fatty acids increase mammary gland growth during prepuberty in sheep [2].

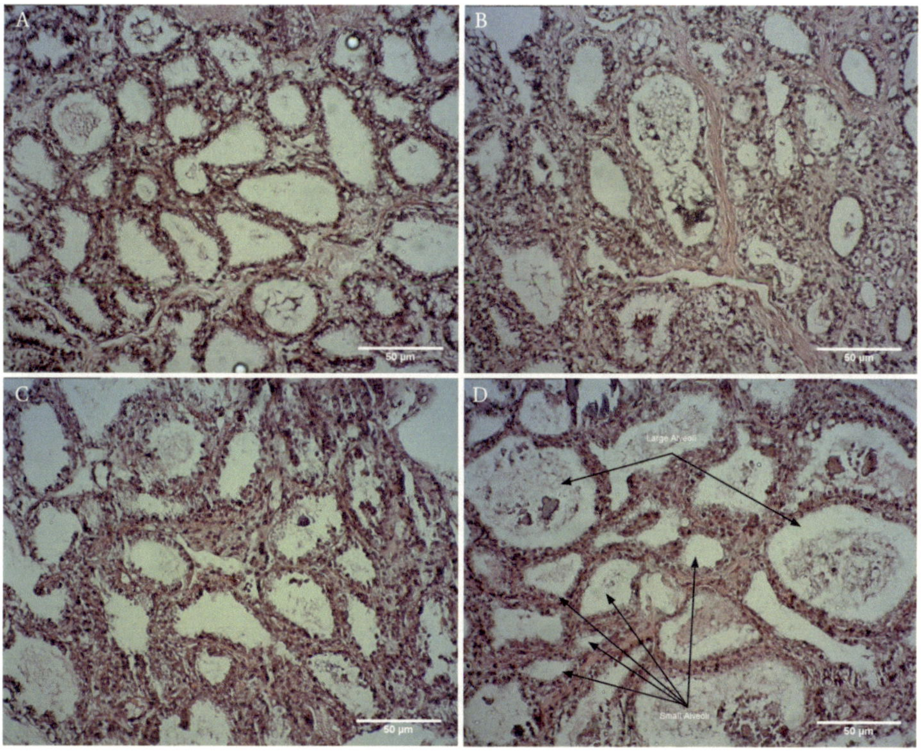

Figure 2.
Mammary tissue sections for palm oil (PO) and fish oil (FO) groups at two different biopsy times. (A) FO mammary tissue section in the first biopsy, (B) PO mammary tissue section in the first biopsy, (C) FO mammary tissue section in the second biopsy, and (D) PO mammary tissue section in the second biopsy. The arrows show large and small alveoli.

In the context of dairy cow farming, it has been observed that incorporating unsaturated fatty acids into their diet induces significant alterations in the transcription of various genes in the mammary gland. Such findings are of notable interest as they provide insight into the complex mechanisms underlying milk production in dairy cows. Similar to the changes made in milk production and composition, the effects of unsaturated fatty acid supplementation on gene expression may also change with the stage of lactation and different amounts of protein and energy in the cow's diet [30].

Nutritional status is known to regulate blood insulin-like growth factor-I (IGF-I) and insulin-like growth factor-binding proteins (IGFBPs) levels. During food deprivation, the somatotropin-IGF-I axis does not pair, leading to an increase in somatotropin levels and a decrease in IGF-I levels. The uncoupling of the ST-IGF-I axis causes somatotropin to increase the availability of nutrients by affecting the lipolysis of adipose tissue for non-mammary tissues while minimizing the consumption of nutrients by the mammary gland [19].

Several studies have reported the stimulatory effects of IGF-I on DNA synthesis or on increasing the number of cells *in vitro* in the mammary gland of ruminants. The growth-stimulating effect of IGF-I depends on the period of time when the tissue is affected by it, rather than the amount of IGF-I. In the mammary tissue of nonpregnant sheep or in early pregnancy, this effect is minimal, but in late pregnancy, its effect (tissue responsiveness to IGF-I) reaches its maximum value. While it is now known that growth factors affect the control of the cell cycle machinery both positively (IGF-I) and negatively (TGF-β), the mechanisms by which hormones capable of initiating mammary development control growth factors that may mediate their effects are still mostly unknown [40]. In some *in vitro* studies, IGF-I and IGF-II have been shown to be powerful mitogens for normal mammary epithelial cells, as well as mammary tumors in rodents, sheep, and cattle. Both IGF-I and IGF-II are expressed in the mammary fat plate of sheep, confirming the previous theory that IGFs produced in the mammary act as paracrine mitogens for the mammary epithelium. The interaction between the stromal and epithelial parts of the mammary gland has significant effects on cell growth and morphogenesis. Based on these results, it is suggested that the proliferating epithelium exerts a positive feedback on its surrounding stroma, likely through the local release of diffusible factors, to increase the expression of IGF-I and IGF-II [41].

The growth of mammary epithelial cells and the *ex vivo* effects of growth factors such as IGF-I and EGF have been the focus of multiple studies with regard to the impact of fatty acids, particularly unsaturated fatty acids. The fat pad of the mammary gland is believed to mediate the effects of synthetic hormones on the development of the mammary epithelium [42]. It is postulated that synthetic hormones alter the expression of growth factors, such as IGF-I, which then act through specific receptors on epithelial cells, resulting in either positive or negative effects on epithelial cell proliferation. The fat pad's response to multiple signals might be altered by interacting with the epithelium, for example, by producing IGFBP or other growth factors. Proliferative responses are correlated with a higher concentration of mammary IGF-I protein and a lower concentration of mammary IGFBP-3 protein. As a result, proliferative processes are linked to a net increase in the biological supply of IGF-I in the mammary gland [43].

Few studies have delved into the effect of polyunsaturated omega-3 fatty acids on the proteins of the IGF pathway. These studies have shown that such fatty acids reduce proteins related to carcinogenesis and growth and increase the proteins linked to the negative regulatory effect on the IGF pathway, such as IGFBP-3 [44].

Mach et al. [30] have reported that the consumption of diets rich in unsaturated fatty acids affects the transcription of several genes related to cell growth, cell cycle, regeneration, apoptosis, and mTOR and JAK/STAT signaling pathways [40].

Adipocytes are primarily responsible for the expression of IGF-I in the mammary gland, and its expression is at its highest in the mammary tissue of heifers at the end of pregnancy, reaching its lowest level during lactogenesis and galactopoiesis [45]. With the onset of lactation, the expression of genes involved in milk component production is upregulated, while genes related to cell proliferation are inhibited. In goats, the growth and development of mammary tissue persist to a small extent during early lactation; in contrast, mammogenesis is completed at the time of parturition in sheep [46].

Javaheri Barfourooshi et al. [31] conducted a study on Holstein cows and found that fish oil, rich in polyunsaturated fatty acids, affects the expression and early production of IGF-I and, thereby, the proliferation and development of mammary epithelial cells. Fish oil significantly increased the number of epithelial cells and decreased the stroma in the mammary tissue of cows during the first week of lactation compared to palm saturated fat. However, while higher IGF-I was observed in the cows receiving palm oil, this may not necessarily indicate higher impact on mammary tissue, as IGF-I's effects are influenced by various binding proteins (IGFBPs) [31].

Similarly, in a separate study conducted by Javaheri Barfourooshi et al. (unpublished data) on Saanen goats in their first pregnancy, it was discovered that the administration of fat supplements led to the maintenance of high expression of IGF-I throughout the entire period, with a greater effect observed during peak production. Sustaining high IGF-I expression levels may contribute to the modulation of apoptosis and stimulation of cell survival. The expression of the IGFBP-3 gene changed concurrently with the expression of the IGF-I gene, indicating that IGFBP-3 plays an intermediate role in controlling the growth, development, and activity of milk secretory cells. IGF-I and IGFBP-3 gene expression was not significantly different among goats at the time of parturition. However, during the first weeks of lactation until peak production, the activity of IGF-I in the goats consuming saturated fat, omega-3, and omega-6 stimulated cell development and preserved parenchymal tissue, resulting in better performance of the cells. In the absence of fat, a certain level of IGFBP-3 helped to maintain the existing situation to control the death of secretory cells and maintain the secretory activity of parenchymal tissue cells. The majority of IGFBPs in the mammary gland are in the form of IGFBP-3, and its concentration in blood and milk decreases during the lactation period compared to prepartum and postpartum stages [47].

Javaheri Barfourooshi et al. (unpublished data) found the impact of different fat sources on the expression of IGFBP-3 and IGFBP-5 genes during early and mid-lactation periods in Saanen goats. The study discovered that the expression of the IGFBP-3 gene decreased during early lactation and continued until mid-lactation, particularly for goats consuming omega-3 and omega-6 (**Figure 3**).

Histological studies revealed that goats consuming omega-3 and omega-6 sources had a higher ratio of parenchymal tissue to stroma and more compressed secretory cells as well as more parenchymal cells compared to those consuming saturated fat and those not receiving any type of fat supplement. The increasing trend of IGFBP-3 gene expression at the end of the lactation period for goats consuming unsaturated fat and its decreasing trend in those consuming saturated fat may be due to the maintenance of the function of IGF-I in controlling apoptosis. The expression of the IGFBP-5 gene was higher in goats consuming omega-3 compared to other goats. Over time, the changes in the expression of the IGFBP-5 gene for goats receiving omega-3

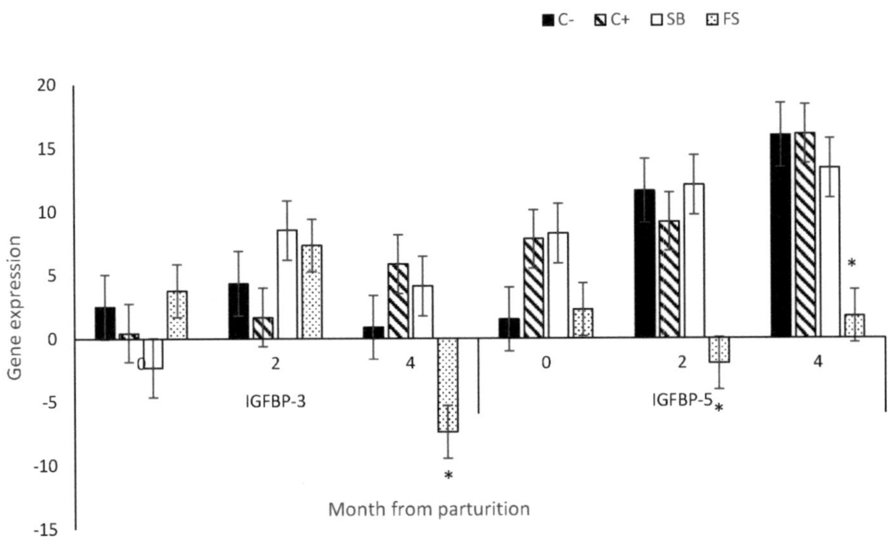

Figure 3.
*Changes in IGFBP-3 and IGFBP-5 gene expression in Saanen goats during three sampling periods (0: time of parturition, 2: 2 months after kidding, 4: 4 months after kidding). C–: negative control group; C+: positive control group (palm oil); SB: omega-6 group (roasted soybean); FS: omega-3 group (extruded flaxseed). * Significance was considered at the level of 5% ($p < 0.05$).*

and palm fat were completely opposite to the previous two genes, with its value increasing as it approached the production peak and decrease at the end of the period. In contrast, the trend of changes in this gene for goats consuming roasted soybeans and those not receiving fat supplements was the opposite of goats receiving omega-3 and palm oil.

IGFs play a critical role in inhibiting programmed cell death in some cells, with growth factors playing a vital role in regulating apoptosis [20]. Fatty acids affect both systemic physiological processes and intracellular events such as gene expression, apoptosis, signal transduction, and cell proliferation [32]. TNF-α inhibits the stimulation of IGF-I in DNA synthesis. Therefore, by removing IGFBP-3, the ability of IGF-I to increase DNA synthesis is weakened. The deletion of IGFBP-3 results in a decrease in base DNA synthesis, indicating that a certain level of IGFBP-3 is required for cell proliferation [20]. Additionally, the expression of the IGFBP-5 gene in mammary gland epithelial cells suggests that this protein is suitable for inhibiting IGF-I activity. Studies have also shown that IGFBP-5 regulates apoptosis by modulating IGFs [48].

Javaheri Barfourooshi (unpublished data) conducted a study on Saanen goats to investigate the expression of the Bcl-2 and Bax genes, which are anti- and pro-apoptotic factors, respectively. The study was conducted during peak lactation periods to examine the potential effects of dietary factors on gene expression. The results of the study indicated that the relative expression of the Bcl-2 gene increased and then decreased in goats receiving palm oil and omega-6. In contrast, the expression of the Bax gene increased significantly during peak lactation for goats receiving palm oil and omega-6, with lower expression levels in those consuming omega-3. The expression ratio of these two genes (Bax/Bcl-2) increased for goats receiving palm oil and omega-6 as the lactation peak approached, followed by a decrease in 4 months after parturition. However, this ratio was higher in goats receiving omega-6 than in those receiving palm oil. The increase in Bax gene expression during peak lactation in goats consuming omega-6 compared to other goats indicates an acceleration in the rate of the apoptosis process at this time. This leads to an earlier and more intense apoptosis process, resulting in the earlier cell death of epithelial cells and alveolar structures that produce milk. Consequently, this leads to a shorter duration of maximum milk production compared to the normal state. These findings suggest that the consumption of omega-6 in the diet may have an adverse effect on milk production in Saanen goats during peak lactation.

Previous studies have indicated that the expression of Bax protein in the mammary gland of goats is low during peak lactation and increases at the end of lactation and during the dry period. Additionally, it has been reported that docosahexaenoic acid (DHA), an omega-3 fatty acid, can stimulate the expression of Bcl-2 protein [49]. Another study revealed that feeding mice with fish oil resulted in morphological changes in the breast tissue, including changes in the size of the nucleus of the epithelial cells of the mammary gland, as well as distinct morphological changes in chromatin and nucleus [33]. Furthermore, omega-3 fatty acids have been reported to control the regression function and decrease apoptosis by upregulating the expression of Bcl-2 family genes [50].

Javaheri Barfourooshi et al. [31] conducted a study on the mammary gland of dairy cows that consumed fish oil. The study observed an increase in the expression of anti-apoptotic genes and a decrease in the expression of apoptosis-initiating genes. Therefore, they suggested that the consumption of fish oil and other omega-3 sources could delay the process of apoptosis that naturally occurs in the cells of the mammary epithelial tissue as the peak of lactation approaches. In their study, the expression of the Bcl-2 gene in the cows consuming fish oil tended to increase over time, and the expression of the Bcl-2/Bax ratio increased as the peak of production approached in the cows consuming fish oil. Conversely, the opposite trend was observed in the group receiving saturated palm oil. The expression of anti-apoptotic genes increased, while the expression of pro-apoptotic genes decreased in the cows consuming fish oil. Therefore, they concluded that by postponing the process of apoptosis that naturally occurs in the epithelial cells of the mammary gland during the peak of lactation, the alveolar structures that produce milk can be preserved, leading to higher milk production for a more extended period in cows consuming fish oil (**Table 2**) [31].

In Saanen goats, the consumption of omega-6 has been found to result in a significant increase in TNF-α level compared to other groups, potentially leading to PGE2

Gene Symbol	PO	FO	SEM	P value		
				Treatment	Time	Treatment× Time
Bax	1.62	1.59	0.08	0.75	0.38	0.89
Bcl-2	1.67	1.70	0.02	0.29	0.05	0.67
Bcl-2/Bax	1.04	1.07	0.06	0.58	0.58	0.66
Cox-2	1.45	1.44	0.05	0.87	0.27	0.26
TNF-α	1.69	1.60	0.04	0.06	0.17	0.64

[1]Expression of genes is based on the logarithm in Section 10.
PO: Palm oil group; FO: Fish oil group.

Table 2.
Mammary gland apoptotic gene expression [1] in cows during 8 weeks after parturition.

production. Moreover, at the peak of production, the level of TNF-α was higher in goats consuming omega-6 than other goats, with goats receiving palm oil ranking second (Javaheri Barfourooshi et al., unpublished data). These conclusions were drawn based on the research conducted by Lennie et al. [34], that saturated fat has also been reported to elevate the level of inflammatory markers. A study conducted by Lennie et al. [34] found that the increase in the level of omega-6 compared to omega-3 and the imbalance between them is directly related to the increase in the level of inflammatory markers. Furthermore, their experiments compared the relationship between fatty acid consumption and the level of the inflammatory marker TNF-α in a group of heart patients. The excessive consumption of saturated fatty acid and trans fatty acid (unsaturated) was directly linked to increase TNF-α levels in cardiac patients. In contrast, Javaheri Barfourooshi et al. [31] reported that the expression of TNF-α in cows consuming fish oil was considerably lower than those consuming palm oil. Various animal species have demonstrated that omega-3 fatty acids with polyunsaturated bonds can reduce TNF-α production [47]. These fatty acids may regulate the expression of TNF-α through the activation of one or more transcription factors such as PPARγ [35].

Due to the limited number of studies investigating the effect of these fatty acids on the healthy mammary tissue of pregnant and lactating animals, it is challenging to provide a definitive opinion on this matter and identify the exact mechanisms involved. More research is needed in this area to gain a better understanding of the relationship between fatty acid consumption and the inflammatory response in lactating animals.

5. Conclusion

The following most important conclusions can be drawn from the latest research results discussed in this chapter.

1. Adding unsaturated fat sources, particularly sources containing omega-3 fatty acids such as fish oil or extruded flaxseed, to the diet during critical periods of mammary gland development (such as late first pregnancy or dry period) can stimulate the proliferation and development of alveolar epithelial cells.

2. By delaying the natural process of apoptosis in the mammary tissue, it preserves the milk-producing units for a longer period of time, leading to increased milk production and persistency of lactation.

3. Omega-3 fatty acids have been found to reduce the production of pro-inflammatory cytokine TNF-α in the mammary tissue. While maintaining the health of the mammary gland, they also significantly reduce the microbial load of milk.

4. The produced milk has a higher health index for human consumption due to having significant amounts of omega-3 fatty acids, offering countless benefits to the consumer.

Further research is needed to ascertain the optimal dosage and duration of unsaturated fat supplementation for maximum benefit.

Acknowledgements

University of Tehran financially supported the study [28] under the grant number 7108017/6/18.

Animal Science Research Institute of Iran (ASRI), Agricultural Research Education and Extension Organization (AREEO), and Ministry of Agriculture of Iran financially supported the study [33, 42, unpublished data], Project code: 01-13-13-022-95014.

Author details

Hoda Javaheri Barfourooshi
Department of Animal Production Management, Animal Science Research Institute of Iran (ASRI), Agricultural Research Education and Extension Organization (AREEO), Karaj, Iran

*Address all correspondence to: hoda.javaheribarfourooshi@gmail.com; h_javaheri@asri.ir

References

[1] Bauman DE, Mather IH, Wall RJ, Lock AL. Major advances associated with the biosynthesis of milk. Journal of Dairy Science. 2006;**89**(4):1235-1243. DOI: 10.3168/jds.s0022-0302(06)72192-0

[2] Sejrsen K, Purup S, Vestergaard M, Foldager J. High body weight gain and reduced bovine mammary growth: Physiological basis and implications for milk yield potential. Domestic Animal Endocrinology. 2000;**19**(2):93-104. DOI: 10.1016/s0739-7240(00)00070-9

[3] Akers RM, Capuco AV, Keys JE. Mammary histology and alveolar cell differentiation during late gestation and early lactation in mammary tissue of beef and dairy heifers. Livestock Science. 2006;**105**(1-3):44-49. DOI: 10.1016/j.livsci.2006.04.026

[4] Palmquist DL, Jenkins TC. A 100-year review: Fat feeding of dairy cows. Journal of Dairy Science. 2017;**100**(12):10061-10077. DOI: 10.3168/jds.2017-12924

[5] Moallem U. The effects of extruded flaxseed supplementation to high-yielding dairy cows on milk production and milk fatty acid composition. Animal Feed Science and Technology. 2009;**152**(3-4):232-242. DOI: 10.1016/j.anifeedsci.2009.04.018

[6] Rossiter H, Barresi C, Ghannadan M, Gruber F, Mildner M, Fodinger D, et al. Inactivation of VEGF in mammary gland epithelium severely compromises mammary gland development and function. The FASEB Journal. 2007;**21**(14):3994-4004. DOI: 10.1096/fj.07-8720com

[7] Barrington GM, Besser TE, Gay CC, Davis WC, Reeves JJ, McFadden TB, et al. Regulation of the immunoglobulin G1 receptor: Effect of prolactin on in vivo expression of the bovine mammary immunoglobulin G1 receptor. Journal of Endocrinology. 1999;**163**(1):25-31. DOI: 10.1677/joe.0.1630025

[8] Akers RM. Mammary development, anatomy, and physiology. In: Lactation and the Mammary Gland. Wiley Online Books; 2016. pp. 45-65. DOI: 10.1002/9781119264880.ch2

[9] Malewski T, Kaminski S, Zwierzchowski L. Gene expression profiling of mouse mammary gland: Transition from pregnancy to lactation. Animal Science Papers and Reports. 2005;**23**(3):159-169

[10] Lean IJ, Van Saun R, DeGaris PJ. Energy and protein nutrition management of transition dairy cows. The veterinary clinics of North America. Food Animal Practice. 2013;**29**:337-366. DOI: 10.1016/j.cvfa.2013.03.005

[11] Holtenius K, Agenas S, Delavaud C, Chilliard Y. Effects of feeding intensity during the dry period. 2. Metabolic and hormonal responses. Journal of Dairy Science. 2003;**86**:883-891. DOI: 10.3168/jds.s0022-0302(03)73671-6

[12] Drackley JK. Biology of dairy cows during the transition period: The final frontier? Journal of Dairy Science. 1999;**82**(11):2259-2273. DOI: 10.3168/jds.s0022-0302(99)75474-3

[13] Badiei A. Practical indicators of transition period evaluation in dairy cows. In: Proceedings of the 15th Iranian Veterinary Congress, Society of Veterinarians of Iran, Iran, Tehran. 2008. Available from: https://civilica.com/doc/59027

[14] Wakao H, Schmitt-Ney M, Groner B. Mammary gland-specific nuclear factor in present in lactating rodent and bovine mammary tissue and composed of a single polypeptide of 89 kDa. The Journal of Biological Chemistry. 1992;**267**(23):16365-16370. DOI: 10.1016/s0021-9258(18)42011-x

[15] Capuco AV, Ellis SE, Hale SA, Long E, Erdman RA, Zhao X, et al. Lactation persistency: Insights from mammary cell proliferation studies. Journal of Animal Science. 2003;**81**(Suppl. 3):18-31. DOI: 10.2527/2003.81suppl_318x

[16] Wall EH, McFadden TB. The effects of milk removal or four-times-daily milking on mammary expression of genes involved in the insulin-like growth factor-I axis. Journal of Dairy Science. 2010;**93**(9):4062-4070. DOI: 10.3168/jds.2010-3162

[17] Ohlsson C, Moha S, Sjogren K, Tivesten A, Isgaard J, Isaksson O, et al. The role of liver-derived insulin-like growth factor–I. Endocrine Reviews. 2009;**30**(5):494-535. DOI: 10.1210/er.2009-0010

[18] Luo J, Qin F, Deng C, Li F, Li W, Yue X. Polymorphisms of IGF-IR gene and their association with economic traits in two indigenous Chinese dairy goat breeds. Gene. 2019;**695**:51-56. DOI: 10.1016/j.gene.2019.01.039

[19] Cohick WS. The role of the IGF system in mammary physiology of ruminants. Domestic Animal Endocrinology. 2022;**79**:106709. DOI: 10.1016/j.domaniend.2021.106709

[20] Leibowitz BJ, Cohick WS. Endogenous IGFBP-3 is required for both growth factor-stimulated cell proliferation and cytokine-induced apoptosis in mammary epithelial cells. Journal of Cellular Physiology. 2009;**220**(1):182-188. DOI: 10.1002/jcp.21748

[21] Drackley JK, Overton TR, Douglas GN. Adaptations of glucose and long-chain fatty acid metabolism in liver of dairy cows during the periparturient period. Journal of Dairy Science. 2001;**84**:E100-E112. DOI: 10.3168/jds.s0022-0302(01)70204-4

[22] Gogus U, Smith C. n-3 Omega fatty acids: A review of current knowledge. International Journal of Food Science and Technology. 2010;**45**(3):417-436. DOI: 10.1111/j.1365-2621.2009.02151.x

[23] Grummer RR, Carroll DJ. Effects of dietary fat on metabolic disorders and reproductive performance in cattle. Journal of Animal Science. 1991;**69**(9):3838-3852. DOI: 10.2527/1991.6993838x

[24] Dangour AD, Uauy R. n-3 long chain polyunsaturated fatty acids for optimal function during brain development and ageing. Asia Pacific Journal of Clinical Nutrition. 2008;**17**(Suppl. 1):185-188

[25] Bernard L, Rouel J, Leroux C, Ferlay A, Faulconnier Y, Legrand P, et al. Mammary lipid metabolism and milk fatty acid secretion in Alpine goats fed vegetable lipids. Journal of Dairy Science. 2005;**88**(4):1478-1489. DOI: 10.3168/jds.s0022-0302(05)72816-2

[26] Bagga D, Capone S, Wang HJ, Heber D, Lill M, Chap L, et al. Dietary modulation of omega-3/omega-6 polyunsaturated fatty acid ratios in patients with breast cancer. JNCI Journal of the National Cancer Institute. 1997;**89**(15):1123-1131. DOI: 10.1093/jnci/89.15.1123

[27] McFadden TB, Daniel TE, Akers RM. Effects of plane of nutrition, growth hormone and unsaturated fat on mammary growth in

prepubertal lambs. Journal of Animal Science. 1990;**68**(10):3171-3179. DOI: 10.2527/1990.68103171x

[28] Javaheri Barfourooshi H, Towhidi A, Sadeghipanah H, Zhandi M, Zeinoaldini S, Dirandeh E, et al. Effect of dietary fish oil on mammary gland development and milk production of Holstein cow. Annals of Animal Science. 2018;**18**(4):973-990. DOI: 10.2478/aoas-2018-0028

[29] Javaheri Barfourooshi H, Sadeghipanah H, Asadzadeh N, Papi N, Mousavipoor F. Effect of fat supplementation type on milk production, and composition and mammary gland morphological parameters in primiparous Saanen does. Animal Production. 2020;**22**(3):479-490. DOI: 10.22059/jap.2020.292240.623467. (In Persian)

[30] Mach N, Jacobs AAA, Kruijt L, van Baal J, Smits MA. Alteration of gene expression in mammary gland tissue of dietary cows in response to dietary unsaturated fatty acids. Animal. 2011;**5**(8):1217-1230. DOI: 10.1017/s1751731111000103

[31] Javaheri Barfourooshi H, Towhidi A, Sadeghipanah H, Zhandi M, Zeioaldini S, Banabazi MH. Evaluation of genes expression affecting mammary gland growth and development in cow fed fish oil. Iranian Journal of Animal Science. 2018;**49**(1):43-53. DOI: 10.22059/IJAS.2018.242585.653562. (In Persian)

[32] Seti H, Leikin-Frenkel A, Werner H. Effects of omega-3 and omega-6 fatty acids on IGF-I receptor signaling in colorectal cancer cells. Archives of Physiology and Biochemistry. 2009;**115**(3):127-136. DOI: 10.1080/13813450902905899

[33] Manna S, Chakraborty T, Ghosh B, Chatterjee M, Panda A, Srivastava S, et al. Dietary fish oil associated with increased apoptosis and modulated expression of Bax and Bcl-2 during 7, 12-dimethylbenz (α) anthracene-induced mammary carcinogenesis in rats. Prostaglandins, Leukotrienes and Essential Fatty Acids. 2008;**79**(1-2):5-14. DOI: 10.1016/j.plefa.2008.05.005

[34] Lennie TA, Chung ML, Habash DL, Moser DK. Dietary fat intake and proinflammatory cytokine levels in patients with heart failure. Journal of Cardiac Failure. 2005;**11**(8):613-618. DOI: 10.1016/j.cardfail.2005.06.434

[35] Huang FR, Zhan ZP, Luo J, Jiang SW, Peng J. Duration of feeding linseed diet influences peroxisome proliferator-activated receptor γ and tumor necrosis factor gene expression, and muscle mass of growing-fishing barrows. Livestock Science. 2008;**119**(1-3):194-201. DOI: 10.1016/j.livsci.2008.04.003

[36] Lin Y, Li Q. The regulation of development and lactation of the mammary gland by leptin. The Journal of American Science. 2005;**1**(1):63-67

[37] Hovey RC, McFadden TB, Akers RM. Regulation of mammary gland growth and morphogenesis by the mammary fat pad: A species comparison. Journal of Mammary Gland Biology and Neoplasia. 1999;**4**(1):53-68. DOI: 10.1023/a:1018704603426

[38] Kang JX. From fat to fat-1: A tale of omega-3 fatty acids. The Journal of Membrane Biology. 2005;**206**(2):165-172. DOI: 10.1007/s00232-005-0790-3

[39] Capuco AV, Akers RM. The origin and evolution of lactation. Journal of Biology. 2009;**8**(4):37.1-37.4. DOI: 10.1186/jbiol139

[40] Zarzynska J, Gajewska M, Motyl T. Effects of hormones and growth factors on TGF-beta1 expression in bovine mammary epithelial cells. Journal of Dairy Research. 2005;**72**(1):39-48. DOI: 10.1017/s0022029904000639

[41] Hovey RC, Davey HW, Mackenzie DDS, McFadden TB. Ontogeny and epithelial-stromal interactions regulate IGF expression in the ovine mammary gland. Molecullar Cellullar Endocrinology. 1998;**136**(2):139-144. DOI: 10.1016/s0303-7207(97)00223-2

[42] Hurley WL, Loor JJ. Mammary gland – Growth, development and involution. In: Encyclopedia of Dairy Sciences. 2011. pp. 338-345. DOI: 10.1016/b978-0-12-374407-4.00291-0

[43] Cannata D, Lann D, Wu Y, Elis S, Sun H, Yakar S, et al. Elevated circulating IGF-I promotes mammary gland development and proliferation. Endocrinology. 2010;**151**(12):5751-5761. DOI: 10.1210/en.2010-0792

[44] Sawyer MB, Field CJ. Possible mechanisms of ω-3 PUFA anti-tumour action. In: Calviello G, Serini S, editors. Dietary Omega-3 Polyunsaturated Fatty Acids and Cancer. Netherlands: Springer; 2010. pp. 3-38. DOI: 10.1007/978-90-481-3579-0_1

[45] Plath-Gabler A, Gabler C, Sinowatz F, Berisha B, Schams D. The expression of the IGF family and GH receptor in the bovine mammary gland. Journal of Endocrinology. 2001;**168**(1):39-48. DOI: 10.1677/joe.0.1680039

[46] Knight CH, Peaker M. Mammary development and regression during lactation in goats in relation to milk secretion. Quarterly Journal Experimental Physiology. 1984;**69**(2):331-338. DOI: 10.1113/expphysiol.1984.sp002809

[47] Baumrucker CR. The insulin-like growth factor (IGF) system in the mammary gland: Role of IGFBP-3 binding protein. Ruminant physiology: digestion, metabolism, growth and reproduction. 2000;**5**(1):329-351. DOI: 10.1079/9780851994635.0329

[48] Marshman E, Green KA, Flint DJ, White A, Streuli CH, Westwood M. Insulin-like growth factor binding protein 5 and apoptosis in mammary epithelial cells. Journal of Cell Science. 2003;**116**(4):675-682. DOI: 10.1242/jcs.00263

[49] Nørgaard JV, Nielsen MO, Theil PK, Sørensen MT, Safayi S, Sejrsen K. Development of mammary glands of fat sheep submitted to restricted feeding during late pregnancy. Small Ruminant Research. 2008;**76**(3):155-165. DOI: 10.1016/j.smallrumres.2007.11.001

[50] Hardman WE. Omega-3 fatty acids as an adjuvant to cancer therapy. In: Claudio PP, Niles RM, editors. Nutrition and Cancer from Epidemiology to Biology. Sharjah, United Arab Emirates: Bentham Science Publisher; 2012. pp. 26-38. DOI: 10.2174/978160805447311201010026

Chapter 3

Optimizing Transition Cow Management: Current Strategies and Future Directions

Somu Yogeshpriya, Mani Saravanan and Subramanian Sivaraman

Abstract

The transition period in dairy cows, spanning from late gestation to early lactation, is crucial due to significant physiological, metabolic, and hormonal changes that impact health and milk production efficiency. Effective management during the transition period is essential for maximizing the overall health, productivity, and profitability of dairy herds. Focus areas for effective transition cow management include nutrition (both pre- and post-calving), health monitoring, environmental factors, and management practices. Strategies such as preventing and treating metabolic disorders (e.g., hypocalcemia and ketosis), early detection of health issues, optimizing housing and facilities, and reducing stress are critical for maintaining cow welfare and performance. Future research priorities include exploring precision technologies, genomics, and innovative management approaches to further enhance transition cow health and productivity. Synthesizing current knowledge aims to provide actionable insights for dairy producers, veterinarians, and researchers to optimize transition cow management and advance the sustainability of dairy farming practices globally.

Keywords: transition period, nutrition, metabolic disorders, management practices, sustainability

1. Introduction

The transition period in dairy cows, spanning the weeks before and after calving, is a critical phase marked by significant physiological, metabolic, and hormonal changes. These changes are crucial for preparing the cow for parturition, initiating lactation, and supporting calf growth. However, this period also presents challenges, as cows become more vulnerable to metabolic disorders, infectious diseases, and reproductive issues. Effective management during this time is essential to ensure herd health, productivity, and profitability.

During the transition phase, dairy cows undergo significant metabolic adjustments in glucose, fatty acid, and mineral processes to sustain lactation and prevent metabolic issues. Nutritional management aims to support these changes. While the National Research Council addressed the nutritional needs of transition cows in [1], subsequent research has provided additional insights. Studies suggest implementing two-group nutritional strategies for dry cows to prevent nutrient overconsumption early in the dry period while enhancing nutrient provision later to support metabolic adaptation. Increasing dietary carbohydrate intake before calving generally yields positive outcomes on cow metabolism and performance [2]. Recent research indicates that the specific type of carbohydrate (e.g., starch vs. highly digestible neutral detergent fiber) may be less critical. Efforts to increase energy provision through dietary fats or to reduce energy expenditure by supplying specific fatty acids like trans-10 and cis-12 conjugated linoleic acid to decrease milk fat production during early lactation have not consistently reduced the release of non-esterified fatty acids (NEFA) from adipose tissue.

In recent years, there has been increasing interest in understanding how nutrition, management practices, environmental factors, and health outcomes interact during the transition period. This review aims to consolidate current knowledge on transition cow management, emphasize strategies for optimizing health and performance, and identify areas for future research and innovation.

2. Nutritional management

Proper nutrition plays a crucial role in supporting the health and productivity of transition cows. During late gestation, cows have increased energy requirements to support fetal growth and prepare for lactation. Postpartum, there is a rapid shift in energy metabolism to support milk production, which can lead to metabolic imbalances if not managed properly [3]. Optimal prepartum and postpartum nutrition programs, including considerations of dietary energy density, protein content, mineral supplementation, and feeding frequency, are essential for preventing metabolic disorders, such as hypocalcemia, ketosis, and fatty liver syndrome. Recent advancements in nutritional science have led to the development of tailored feeding strategies, such as precision feeding and metabolic profiling, aimed at optimizing nutrient utilization and minimizing health risks during the transition period.

Calcium regulation is critical for the body's functions, with tight control needed to maintain life. A significant drop in circulating blood calcium, up to 50%, can lead to severe calcium deficiency. The body maintains calcium levels through a precise system called homeostasis, where calcitonin and parathyroid hormone (PTH) play crucial roles. Calcitonin reduces blood calcium levels when they are high, while PTH increases active vitamin D3 production to enhance calcium absorption from the gut when calcium levels are low. PTH is the primary regulator of short-term calcium levels, while calcitonin's impact is relatively minor performance [2]. Vitamin D also plays an essential role in calcium balance, acting both as a vitamin and as a steroid hormone in the body. The transition period in dairy cattle is characterized by significant shifts in nutrient requirements, necessitating precise coordination of metabolism to meet the energy, glucose, amino acid (AA), and calcium (Ca) demands of the mammary gland post-calving. Studies estimate a substantial increase in nutrient demand by the gravid uterus at 250 days of gestation and the lactating mammary gland at 4 days postpartum, with glucose demand tripling, AA demand doubling, and fatty acid demand increasing approximately fivefold during this period [4]. Additionally, calcium demand rises approximately fourfold on the day of calving [5]. The cow utilizes homeorhetic controls to facilitate these changes in nutrient allocation efficiently.

2.1 Glucose metabolism

During lactation, a significant adjustment in glucose metabolism occurs with an increase in hepatic gluconeogenesis [6] and a decrease in glucose oxidation by peripheral tissues [7]. This metabolic shift directs glucose toward the mammary gland for lactose synthesis. Research conducted by Reynolds et al. [6] observed that the net flux of glucose across the portal-drained viscera of cows was minimal to slightly negative during the transition period and early lactation. The notable increase in total splanchnic output of glucose during this period primarily results from heightened hepatic gluconeogenesis.

The main substrates for hepatic gluconeogenesis in ruminants include propionate from ruminal fermentation, lactate from Cori cycling, amino acids (AA) from protein breakdown or absorption, and glycerol released during adipose tissue fat breakdown [8]. Studies indicate that propionate contributes approximately 50–60% to net glucose release by the liver, while lactate contributes about 15–20%, and glycerol contributes 2–4% [6]. Amino acids account for a minimum of approximately 20–30% during the transition period, with alanine playing a particularly significant role postpartum. These findings are consistent with earlier research by Overton et al. [9], which demonstrated a doubling of the hepatic capacity to convert alanine to glucose on the first day postpartum compared to 21 days of prepartum. Although amino acids may not quantitatively support milk production during early lactation, they serve as an essential substrate pool for glucose synthesis immediately after calving, facilitating the rapid adaptation of glucose metabolism in transition cows.

2.2 Lipid metabolism

During lactation, a primary adjustment in lipid metabolism involves mobilizing body fat stores to meet the cow's energy requirements, particularly during periods of negative energy balance. Body fat is mobilized and released into the bloodstream as non-esterified fatty acids (NEFA), which contribute significantly to milk fat production in the early days of lactation [4]. Skeletal muscle also utilizes NEFA for energy, reducing its reliance on glucose, especially during early lactation. Plasma NEFA concentrations typically increase when energy demands rise and feed intake is insufficient, showing an inverse correlation with dry matter intake (DMI).

While the liver uptakes NEFA proportionally to its supply, it may not fully metabolize them, leading to the accumulation of triglycerides in the liver when NEFA release from adipose tissue into circulation is high [10]. Elevated liver triglyceride levels correlate with increased peripheral ammonia concentrations during the first 2 days postpartum [11]. Research indicates that ammonium chloride can inhibit the ability of isolated hepatocytes to convert propionate into glucose *in vitro* [12], suggesting a potential inhibition of gluconeogenesis *in vivo* when liver triglyceride levels are high. This inhibition may be influenced by ammonia availability to the liver, although the exact relationship between impaired gluconeogenesis and ureagenesis in transition dairy cows requires further investigation.

Those findings underscore the importance of managing carbohydrate and protein nutrition effectively during the transition period to mitigate potential disruptions in lipid metabolism and maintain cow health and productivity.

2.3 Calcium metabolism

Calcium metabolism in dairy cows is tightly regulated by various homeostatic mechanisms involving hormones, such as parathyroid hormone (PTH), vitamin D, and calcitonin. Serum calcium and phosphate levels are maintained through processes including intestinal absorption, bone resorption or deposition, renal reabsorption and excretion, salivary recycling, fetal deposition (during pregnancy), milk secretion (during lactation), and fecal excretion. Parathyroid hormone and 1,25-dihydroxyvitamin D enhance intestinal absorption and renal reabsorption of calcium, stimulate bone resorption of calcium and phosphate, and may contribute to calcium secretion into milk during lactation via parathyroid hormone-related protein. Calcitonin, released by the thyroid gland in response to elevated serum calcium levels, promotes bone mineral deposition, reduces intestinal calcium absorption, and increases urinary calcium excretion.

Periparturient hypocalcemia (milk fever) is associated with the onset of lactation and mammary gland function, while periparturient hypophosphatemia is influenced by factors beyond milk production at parturition. Hormonal concentrations play a significant role in maintaining mineral balance, but factors such as receptor numbers, binding affinity, hormone clearance, and post-receptor signaling also affect mineral regulation.

Nutritional strategies aim to minimize periparturient hypocalcemia by manipulating these hormonal control points to enhance the cow's ability to manage the negative mineral balance associated with lactation onset. One such strategy involves adjusting the dietary cation-anion difference (DCAD), calculated as $[Na^{+} + K^{+}] - [Cl^{-} + S^{-2}]$, to prevent metabolic alkalosis and potentially induce compensated metabolic acidosis.

Research by Horst et al. [5] suggested that correcting metabolic alkalosis through a negative DCAD diet could prevent alterations in the parathyroid hormone receptor conformation on bone, facilitating calcium mobilization from bone reserves. Diets with a negative DCAD administered prepartum have consistently shown efficacy in reducing both subclinical and clinical hypocalcemia in cows prone to milk fever.

However, studies by Moore et al. [13] indicated that while anionic salts in the diet-induced a compensated metabolic acidosis, they did not significantly improve calcium metabolism. Instead, cows fed diets with anionic salts often experienced reduced prepartum dry matter intake (DMI), increased circulating non-esterified fatty acid (NEFA) concentrations, and greater liver triglyceride accumulation. Additionally, there is debate over whether solely reducing the cation content of the prepartum diet without supplementing anions through mineral- or acid-based sources can adequately prevent hypocalcemia.

In conclusion, while DCAD manipulation remains a cornerstone in preventing hypocalcemia, ongoing research is needed to optimize dietary strategies and better understand their impact on calcium metabolism and overall cow health during the critical transition period.

3. Navigating the metabolic shifts

Transitioning dairy cows through the periparturient period requires meticulous nutritional management to support metabolic adjustments and prepare cows for the demands of lactation. This phase is critical as it sets the stage for cow health, milk production, and overall productivity post-calving. Effective nutritional strategies aim to optimize metabolic adaptations and minimize the risk of metabolic disorders and immune challenges.

3.1 Nutritional regimen during the dry period

The NRC [1] recommends a phased approach to nutrition:

- *Early dry period*: Provide a diet with approximately 1.25 Mcal/kg of Net Energy for Lactation (NEL) to moderate body condition score (BCS) gain. Excessive energy intake during this phase can lead to metabolic issues in early lactation.

- *Late dry period*: Increase energy intake to 1.54–1.62 Mcal/kg of NEL in the final 3 weeks before calving to meet the rising energy demands as cows approach parturition [14].

- *Managing BCS*: BCS around 3.0 at dry off, rather than higher traditional targets, helps mitigate decreased dry matter intake associated with higher BCS, reducing the risk of metabolic disturbances [15, 16].

3.2 Mitigating NEFA and triglyceride metabolism

Additionally, besides implementing nutritional tactics aimed at reducing the availability of circulating NEFA for liver uptake, there exists the potential to employ nutritional strategies that can slow down the conversion of NEFA into triglycerides within the liver. Although ruminants have relatively limited hepatic capacities for disposing of NEFA through processes such as mitochondrial or peroxisomal β-oxidation, or export as triglycerides within VLDL compared to nonruminants [17], recent research indicates that providing specific nutrients to dairy cows during the transition period might enhance NEFA disposal rates, thereby influencing their overall performance.

3.3 Key nutrients roles

3.3.1 Choline

Choline, often described as a quasi-vitamin, plays multiple critical roles in mammalian metabolism. It serves as a key component of phospholipids in cell membranes, specifically phosphatidylcholine, participates in the formation of the neurotransmitter acetylcholine, and acts as a direct precursor to betaine in methyl metabolism. In the context of transition cow nutrition, much attention has been placed on choline's role in lipid metabolism, particularly its importance in the synthesis and secretion of VLDL (very low-density lipoprotein) by the liver, which is facilitated by phosphatidylcholine [18].

3.3.2 Amino acids (methionine and lysine)

Methionine and lysine are widely recognized as the two most crucial amino acids for milk and milk protein synthesis, according to the NRC [1]. Beyond their primary role in protein synthesis, these amino acids also play potential roles in mitochondrial beta-oxidation of fatty acids and contribute to carnitine biosynthesis in the liver.

Additionally, they are involved in the export of triglycerides as VLDL through the biosynthesis of apolipoprotein B100 [19]. Speculation regarding methionine's potential role in bovine ketosis has persisted for over three decades.

3.3.3 Essential fatty acids (linoleic and linolenic acids)

Linoleic and linolenic acids are considered essential in numerous species. Linolenic acid acts as a precursor to both docosahexaenoic acid (DHA) and eicosapentaenoic acid (EPA), collectively playing critical roles that may be vital for the secretion of apolipoprotein B100 and the stability of VLDL particles in cultured hepatocytes [20]. Consistent with these functions, *in vitro* studies using ruminant hepatocytes have shown that linolenic acid has the potential to reduce the cellular accumulation of triglycerides derived from palmitic acid [21].

3.3.4 Immune-metabolic interactions

A growing area of study in transition cow metabolism and management explores connections with the immune system. Besides the metabolic adaptations mentioned earlier, transition dairy cows undergo a phase of reduced immune function during the periparturient period. Interestingly, while leukocytes from immunosuppressed cows may show compromised function and decreased sensitivity to pathogens, they also exhibit heightened responsiveness upon activation, leading to increased production of proinflammatory cytokines [22].

3.3.5 Immunity and mastitis

In addition to the interaction between immunity and metabolism, clinical mastitis has been shown to have detrimental effects on reproductive performance in lactating dairy cows [23]. Furthermore, Schrick et al. [24] reported that subclinical mastitis similarly reduces reproductive efficiency by prolonging days to first service, increasing days open, and requiring more services per conception. Immune activation, whether through experimental manipulation or natural infection of the mammary gland, has been demonstrated to affect multiple reproductive tissues throughout various stages of the estrous cycle.

Navigating these metabolic shifts through strategic nutritional management involves balancing energy intake, optimizing nutrient composition, and supporting immune function to ensure smooth transitions and maximize cow health and productivity. Continued research and implementation of evidence-based practices are essential to refine strategies and address evolving challenges in dairy cow management during the periparturient period.

4. Prevalence of elevated biomarkers

4.1 Prepartum non-esterified fatty acids

The prevalence of elevated prepartum NEFA concentrations was assessed solely in the context of the dry-period nutritional strategy [25], as the evaluation was conducted before the fresh period in their study. The authors found no significant differences in the prevalence of elevated NEFA concentrations among the different nutritional strategies examined. However, multiparous cows in herds fed a high-forage (HF) diet exhibited a higher prevalence of elevated prepartum NEFA concentrations compared to those in low-forage (LF) fed herds.

4.2 Postpartum non-esterified fatty acids

In their study, Kerwin et al. [25] conducted separate analyzes for multiparous and primiparous cows regarding the dry and periparturient-period nutritional strategies due to differing outcomes. For multiparous cows, they did not find any significant difference in the prevalence of elevated postpartum NEFA concentrations between the dry-period or periparturient-period nutritional strategies. However, for primiparous cows, they observed that herds fed a higher forage (HF) diet had a higher prevalence of elevated postpartum NEFA concentrations compared to herds fed a lower forage (LF) diet. Furthermore, an interaction effect was noted between the close-up and fresh-period nutritional strategies for primiparous cows. Specifically, herds fed HF with high starch (HS) had a higher prevalence of elevated NEFA compared to those fed LF with HS or HF with low starch (LS). Additionally, herds fed LF with LS had a higher prevalence of elevated postpartum NEFA compared to LF with HS.

This indicates that both the level of dietary forage and the starch content interact in influencing the prevalence of elevated postpartum NEFA concentrations in primiparous cows according to their study findings [25].

4.3 Beta hydroxybutyrate

Kerwin et al. [25] analyzed the prevalence of elevated BHB concentrations during the dry period for multiparous cows. They found that high-forage (HF)-fed herds had a lower prevalence of elevated BHB concentrations during the close-up period compared to low-forage (LF)-fed herds. However, they did not find any significant difference in the prevalence of elevated BHB concentrations for the far-off nutritional strategies.

For the periparturient model, Kerwin et al. [25] combined data from both primiparous and multiparous cows due to similar results. They reported that herds fed higher forage-neutral detergent fiber (NDF) diets had a lower prevalence of elevated BHB concentrations compared to LF-fed herds. Additionally, herds fed higher starch diets had a lower prevalence of elevated BHB concentrations compared to those fed low starch diets (LS). These findings suggest that dietary factors such as forage NDF content and starch levels influence the prevalence of elevated BHB concentrations in dairy cows during the periparturient period, as observed in the study by Kerwin et al. [25].

4.4 Haptoglobin

Kerwin et al. [25] analyzed the prevalence of elevated haptoglobin (Hp) concentrations across different nutritional strategies during the dry and periparturient periods. Here are the key findings from their study:

- Dry-period nutritional strategy:
    - For the far-off nutritional strategy, there was no significant difference in the prevalence of elevated Hp concentrations observed.

  - During the close-up period, both primiparous and multiparous cows in high-forage (HF)-fed herds showed a trend toward a higher prevalence of elevated Hp concentrations compared to low-forage (LF)-fed herds.

- Periparturient-period nutritional strategy:

  - For multiparous cows, no significant difference was found in the prevalence of elevated postpartum Hp concentrations across nutritional strategies.

  - In contrast, for primiparous cows, there was a trend indicating a lower prevalence of elevated Hp concentrations in low-starch (LS)-fed herds compared to high-starch (HS)-fed herds.

Particularly forage content and starch levels may influence the prevalence of elevated haptoglobin concentrations in dairy cows during the periparturient period. The study by Kerwin et al. [25] underscores the importance of nutritional management strategies in potentially mitigating inflammatory responses indicated by Hp concentrations in transitioning dairy cows.

4.5 Oxidative biomarkers

During the transition period of dairy cows, oxidative stress plays a crucial role in their metabolic challenges. Factors such as negative energy balance (NEB), parturition, and the onset of lactation contribute to an increased production of reactive oxygen species (ROS) and reactive nitrogen species (RNS) within the organism. These oxidants target macromolecules, such as lipids, proteins, and DNA, resulting in oxidative damage. Various biomarkers of oxidative stress, particularly those associated with lipid and protein metabolism, have been identified. Carbonyl groups, formed when ROS attacks amino acid side chains, are widely utilized as biomarkers of protein oxidation. Additionally, products induced by hypochlorous acid and levels of dityrosine are indicative of oxidative damage to proteins. The ratio of advanced oxidation protein products to albumin has been suggested as a sensitive indicator of oxidative stress.

Immune cells are particularly sensitive to oxidative stress due to their high content of polyunsaturated fatty acids (PUFA) in cellular membranes, making them prone to peroxidation. Research has established connections between oxidative stress biomarkers and various physiological and pathological conditions in dairy cows, including negative energy balance (NEB), ketosis risk, inflammation, and reproductive events. Reactive oxygen metabolites (ROM) and superoxide dismutase (SOD) activity in blood have been proposed as potential indicators of oxidative stress in dairy cows.

Malondialdehyde (MDA), a marker of lipid peroxidation, has been studied in milk, showing the highest concentrations during early lactation. Milk oxidative capacity, measured by ORAC values, has also been associated with days in lactation and energy balance. While MDA has shown variability as a marker of lipid oxidation, ELISA-based isoprostanes hold promise, especially in cases of mastitis and inflammation. These biomarkers offer valuable insights into the oxidative status of dairy cows during the transition period and present opportunities for monitoring and improving their health and productivity.

5. Health monitoring and disease prevention

Detecting and addressing health issues early is crucial for mitigating the adverse effects of transition cow disorders on herd health and productivity. Routine health monitoring, encompassing physical examinations, metabolic profiling, and biomarker analysis, plays a pivotal role in identifying cows vulnerable to metabolic disorders or infections. Prompt intervention through dietary modifications, supplementation, or medical treatments can effectively prevent health complications and enhance cow welfare. Moreover, implementing vaccination programs, biosecurity measures, and stringent hygiene protocols is essential to prevent infectious diseases and limit their spread within the herd.

Evaluating nutritional strategies provides dairy nutritionists with valuable insights into optimizing cow performance on the farm, offering essential guidelines for implementation. This assessment also allows for flexibility, enabling nutritionists to customize nutrient adjustments based on individual cow needs. By continually refining and adapting these strategies with updated research and specific herd requirements, dairy nutritionists can effectively enhance cow health, productivity, and overall farm profitability.

While interaction between far-off and close-up nutritional strategies influenced the prevalence of elevated prepartum NEFA concentrations, significant differences among common nutritional strategies were not observed. However, multiparous cows in high-forage (HF)-fed herds showed a higher prevalence of elevated prepartum NEFA concentrations compared to those in low-forage (LF)-fed herds. Similar findings was reported by Mann et al. [26] who noted elevated prepartum NEFA concentrations in multiparous cows fed a controlled-energy dry-period diet compared to a high-energy dry-period diet. Additionally, Vasquez et al. [27] found high prepartum NEFA concentrations in cows fed a controlled-energy close-up diet, as observed in their study involving both primiparous and multiparous cows fed controlled-energy far-off diets with either controlled-energy or high-energy close-up diets.

5.1 Biomarkers of production-related diseases

Biomarkers are essential for detecting and managing production-related diseases in dairy cows, including mastitis, hypocalcemia, rumen acidosis, ketosis, and laminitis. Mastitis, marked by udder inflammation, is especially common and significant in dairy herds globally. The most sensitive method for identifying clinical and subclinical mastitis continues to be somatic cell count (SCC) while identifying pathogens usually involves bacteriological culture or molecular techniques such as PCR.

Besides SCC, immunoglobulins, especially IgG transferred from blood to milk during mastitis, are significant indicators of the specific immune response. Elevated IgG levels in milk, alongside SCC, can help predict the mastitis-causing pathogen. While cow-side diagnostic tests for bacterial identification are emerging, their adoption on farms remains limited. Alternative markers such as lactate dehydrogenase (LDH) and differential somatic cell count (DSCC) have demonstrated potential for early detection of mastitis.

Advancements in omics technologies have revealed insights into the components contributing to mastitis pathogenesis and the host's immune response against mastitis-causing pathogens. Techniques such as peptidomics, metabolomics, and quantitative proteomics have pinpointed specific peptides, metabolites, and proteins linked to mastitis. Notably, proteins expressed differently in milk are being explored as potential biomarkers for distinguishing between mastitis caused by gram-negative and gram-positive bacteria.

This area of research is constantly progressing, with potential applications expanding to include other species such as small ruminants and water buffalo. Biomarkers may vary in their relevance across non-bovine species, underscoring the necessity for species-specific approaches to disease detection and management. Ongoing studies in this field hold the promise of deepening our comprehension of production-related diseases and enhancing diagnostic and management techniques in dairy farming.

6. Environmental management

Environmental management during the transition period plays a crucial role in influencing cow comfort, behavior, and health outcomes. It is imperative to maintain clean, well-ventilated facilities with comfortable resting areas and sufficient space to minimize stress and enhance cow welfare. Environmental factors including temperature, humidity, and air quality can significantly affect cow physiology and immune function, underscoring the importance of optimizing housing conditions. In addition to physical facilities, management practices such as grouping strategies, social dynamics, and handling procedures also impact cow behavior and stress levels. This highlights the necessity for thoughtful and proactive management approaches to ensure optimal conditions for transition cows.

Heat stress in the environment presents a substantial challenge for dairy cows, intensifying oxidative stress and affecting their overall health and productivity. Research indicates that transition cows experiencing heat stress during the summer demonstrate elevated levels of oxidative stress markers compared to those calving during more temperate seasons.

Bernabucci et al. [28] observed increased erythrocyte activity, glutathione peroxidase activity, intracellular thiols, and malondialdehyde (MDA) levels in transition dairy cows experiencing summer heat stress, indicating oxidative stress. Similarly, Zachut et al. [29] found higher plasma concentrations of MDA in transition dairy cows calving during summer heat stress compared to those calving in winter. Harmon et al. reported a reduction in plasma antioxidant activity in mid-lactation heat-stressed cows, further underscoring the impact of heat stress on oxidative balance. However, additional research is required to fully assess the usefulness of oxidative stress biomarkers in identifying heat stress in cattle.

7. Future directions and research priorities

While significant progress has been made in transition cow management, several challenges and opportunities remain for further improvement. Future research efforts should focus on developing innovative strategies for optimizing transition cow nutrition, health monitoring, and environmental management. Precision technologies, including precision feeding systems, sensor-based monitoring devices, and predictive modeling tools, hold promise for enhancing cow health outcomes and productivity. Furthermore, genetic selection for transition cow resilience and metabolic efficiency represents a potential avenue for improving transition cow management. Collaboration between dairy producers, veterinarians, researchers, and industry stakeholders is essential for translating scientific advancements into practical solutions and promoting the sustainability of dairy farming practices.

8. Conclusion

Effective transition cow management is essential for ensuring the health, welfare, and productivity of dairy herds. The following most important conclusions can be drawn from the latest research results discussed in this chapter.

1. Implementing evidence-based strategies in nutrition, health monitoring, environmental management, and general farm practices optimizes transition cow outcomes and enhances the sustainability of dairy operations.

2. Continued research and innovation in transition cow management are crucial for addressing emerging challenges and opportunities in dairy farming practices.

3. Nutritional strategies are complex and influenced by factors, such as the cow's body condition score, interactions among dietary nutrients, and social and environmental variables.

4. This complexity contributes to variations in strategy effectiveness across farms, where what works well in one farm context may not yield the same results in another.

Adaptation and refinement of nutritional and management practices tailored to specific farm dynamics are essential for improving productivity, health outcomes, and the long-term viability of dairy farming enterprises globally.

Author details

Somu Yogeshpriya[1,2]*, Mani Saravanan[2,3] and Subramanian Sivaraman[1,2]

1 Department of Veterinary Medicine, Veterinary College and Research Institute, Orathanadu, Tamil Nadu, India

2 Tamilnadu Veterinary and Animal Sciences University (TANUVAS), India

3 Veterinary Clinical Complex, Veterinary College and Research Institute, Salem, India

*Address all correspondence to: dryogeshpriya@gmail.com

References

[1] National Research Council, Committee on Animal Nutrition, Subcommittee on Dairy Cattle Nutrition. Nutrient Requirements of Dairy Cattle: 2001. Washington, DC: National Academies Press; 2001

[2] Overton TR, Waldron MR. Nutritional management of transition dairy cows: Strategies to optimize metabolic health. Journal of Dairy Science. 2009;**87**(E. Suppl):E105-E119

[3] Burhans WS, Bell AW, Nadeau R, Knapp JR. Factors associated with transition cow ketosis incidence in selected New England herds. Journal of Dairy Science. 2003;**86**(Suppl. 1):247

[4] Bell AW. Regulation of organic nutrient metabolism during transition from late pregnancy to early lactation. Journal of Animal Science. 1995;**73**:2804-2819. DOI: 10.2527/1995.7392804x

[5] Horst RL, Goff JP, Reinhardt TA, Buxton DR. Strategies for preventing milk fever in dairy cattle. Journal of Dairy Science. 1997;**80**:1269-1280

[6] Reynolds CK, Aikman PC, Lupoli B, Humphries DJ, Beever DE. Splanchnic metabolism of dairy cows during the transition from late gestation through early lactation. Journal of Dairy Science. 2003;**86**:1201-1217

[7] Bennink MR, Mellenberger RW, Frobish RA, Bauman DE. Glucose oxidation and entry rate as affected by the initiation of lactation. Journal of Dairy Science. 1972;**55**:712

[8] Seal CJ, Reynolds CK. Nutritional implications of gastrointestinal and liver metabolism in ruminants. Nutrition Research Reviews. 1993;**6**:185-208

[9] Overton TR, Drackley JK, Douglas GN, Emmert LS, Clark JH. Hepatic gluconeogenesis and whole-body protein metabolism of periparturient dairy cows as affected by source of energy and intake of the prepartum diet. Journal of Dairy Science. 1998;**81**(Suppl. 1):295

[10] Emery RS, Liesman JS, Herdt TH. Metabolism of long-chain fatty acids by ruminant liver. The Journal of Nutrition. 1992;**122**:832-837

[11] Zhu LH, Armentano LE, Bremmer DR, Grummer RR, Bertics SJ. Plasma concentration of urea, ammonia, glutamine around calving, and the relation of hepatic triglyceride, to plasma ammonia removal and blood acid-base balance. Journal of Dairy Science. 2000;**83**:734-740

[12] Overton TR, Drackley JK, Ottemann-Abbamonte CJ, Beaulieu AD, Emmert LS, Clark JH. Substrate utilization for hepatic gluconeogenesis is altered by increased glucose demand in ruminants. Journal of Animal Science. 1999;**77**:1940-1951

[13] Moore SJ, Vande Haar MJ, Sharma BK, Pilbeam TE, Beede DK, Bucholtz HF, et al. Effects of altering dietary cation-anion difference on calcium and energy metabolism in peripartum cows. Journal of Dairy Science. 2000;**83**:2095-2104

[14] Dann HM, Litherland NB, Underwood JP, Bionaz M, Drackley JK. Prepartum nutrient intake has minimal effects on postpartum dry matter intake, serum nonesterified fatty acids, liver lipid and glycogen contents, and milk yield. Journal of Dairy Science. 2003;**86**(Suppl. 1):106

[15] Contreras LL, Ryan CM, Overton TR. Effects of dry cow grouping strategy and prepartum body condition score on performance and health of transition dairy cows. Journal of Dairy Science. 2004;**87**:517-523

[16] Hayirli A, Grummer RR, Nordheim EV, Crump PM. Animal and dietary factors affecting feed intake during the prefresh transition period in Holsteins. Journal of Dairy Science. 2002;**85**:3430-3443

[17] Grummer RR. Etiology of lipid-related metabolic disorders in periparturient dairy cows. Journal of Dairy Science. 1993;**76**:3882-3896

[18] Mashek DG, Beede DK. Peripartum responses of dairy cows fed energy-dense diets for 3 or 6 weeks prepartum. Journal of Dairy Science. 2001;**84**:115-125

[19] Bauchart D, Durand D, Gruffat D, Chilliard Y. Mechanism of liver steatosis in early lactation cows—Effects of hepatoprotector agents. In: Proceedings of the Cornell Nutrition Conference for Feed Manufacturers. Ithaca, NY: Cornell University; 1998. pp. 27-37

[20] Lang CA, Davis RA. Fish oil fatty acids impair VLDL assembly and/or secretion by cultured rat hepatocytes. Journal of Lipid Research 1990;**31**:2079-2086

[21] Mashek DG, Bertics SJ, Grummer RR. Metabolic fate of long-chain unsaturated fatty acids and their effects on palmitic acid metabolism and gluconeogenesis in bovine hepatocytes. Journal of Dairy Science. 2002;**85**:2283-2289

[22] Sordillo LM, Pighetti GM, Davis MR. Enhanced production of bovine tumor necrosis factor-alpha during the periparturient period. Veterinary Immunology and Immunopathology. 1995;**49**:263-270

[23] Barker AR, Schrick FN, Lewis MJ, Dowlen HH, Oliver SP. Influence of clinical mastitis during early lactation on reproctive performance of Jersey cows. Journal of Dairy Science. 1998;**81**:1285-1290

[24] Schrick FN, Hockett ME, Saxton AM, Lewis MJ, Dowlen HH, Oliver SP. Influence of subclinical mastitis during early lactation on reproductive parameters. Journal of Dairy Science. 2001;**84**:1407-1412

[25] Kerwin AL, Burhans WS, Nydam DV, Overton TR. Transition cow nutrition and management strategies of dairy herds in the Northeastern United States: Associations of nutritional strategies with analytes, health, milk yield, and reproduction. Animals. 2023;**13**:2701. DOI: 10.3390/ani13172701

[26] Mann S, Leal Yepes FA, Overton TR, Lock AL, Lamb SV, Wakshlag JJ, et al. Effect of dry period dietary energy level in dairy cattle on volume, concentrations of immunoglobulin G, insulin, and fatty acid composition of colostrum. Journal of Dairy Science. 2016;**99**:1515-1526. DOI: 10.3168/jds.2015-9926

[27] Vasquez A, Nydam D, Foditsch C, Warnick L, Wolfe C, Doster E, et al. Characterization and comparison of the microbiomes and resistomes of colostrum from selectively treated dry cows. Journal of Dairy Science. 2022;**105**:637-653. DOI: 10.3168/jds.2021-20675

[28] Bernabucci U et al. Markers of oxidative status in plasma and erythrocytes of transition dairy cows during hot season. Journal of Dairy Science. 2002;**85**(9):2173-2179. DOI: 10.3168/jds.S0022-0302(02)74296-3

[29] Zachut M, Kra G, Livshitz L, Portnick Y, Yakoby S, Friedlander G, et al. Seasonal heat stress affects adipose tissue proteome toward enrichment of the Nrf2-mediated oxidative stress response in late-pregnant dairy cows. Journal of Proteomics. 2017;**158**:52-61. DOI: 10.1016/j.jprot.2017.02.011

Chapter 4

Effect of Climate Change on Strategy of Forage Feeding in Cattle Farms under Dry Continental Conditions

Róbert Tóthi, Szilvia Orosz, Katalin Somfalvi-Tóth, László Babinszky and Veronika Halas

Abstract

This chapter presents the expected climate scenario in corn-producing areas and suggests alternative strategies for producing resilient forage for dairy cattle in dry continental climate zones. The consideration of irrigating corn for silage production arises due to the alterations in climate. However, it is anticipated that different crop rotations will suffice to sustain the forage supply on intensive dairy farms without requiring additional water resources in the dry season, including drought-resistant crops, early-cut whole-crop cereals, and intense annual ryegrass alongside corn and sorghum. Crop management and crop rotation strategies adapted to local and weather conditions are critical to maintaining milk production. Due to the high digestibility, digestible NDF, and undigestible NDF of the early cut, intensively growing grass silages, rye silage (harvested at the boot stage or earlier), triticale, barley, and wheat silage (harvested at boot-early heading stage) could increase dairy cows' dry matter intake and milk production under heat-stress conditions. As a result, cattle feed will contain more ingredients than it does today to cope with climate change in cattle feeding.

Keywords: climate change, double cropping, conserved forages, feeding strategies, dairy cattle

1. Introduction

An increase in average temperature during the growing season typically results in plants using more energy for respiration to sustain themselves and less for growth. An increase in average temperature of 1°C can reduce major food and cash crop species yields by 5–10 percent [1]. Extremely high temperatures of over 30°C can cause permanent physical damage to plants, and if they exceed 37°C, even seeds can be damaged during storage. The high temperatures can adversely affect photosynthesis, respiration, water relations, and membrane stability, and alter hormone levels and primary and secondary metabolite levels in the plant [2]. Due to climate change, the frequency of periods when temperatures rise above critical thresholds for corn, rice, and wheat is projected to increase worldwide [3]. The general projection is that with climate change, areas that already receive high rainfall will receive even more rainfall while dry areas will become drier [4]. As precipitation patterns become more erratic/ unpredictable, farmers may no longer be able to rely on their knowledge of the typical temporal patterns of climatic variables. Changes in planting seasons and weather patterns make it difficult for farmers to plan and manage production.

The extent of climate change can already be measured in the dry continental region of Central Europe through the example of corn silage. The whole plant corn yield range was found to be 17.0–33.5 tons per ha for Hungary during the last decades between 2012 and 2022 [5]. Silage yields exceeded 30 tons per ha in only 5 of the 11 years. Extremely low yields were observed in 2012 and 2022 (19.3 tons per ha and 17.0 tons per ha, respectively). Starch content ranged between 207 and 360 g/ kg DM (2012–2022). The whole corn plant was harvested in 2022 with the lowest starch content (207 ± 111 g/kg DM) after a sweltering and dry summer [5]. Corn silage is a common ingredient of dairy rations in most areas of the World. Climate change has increased the frequency and intensity of heat waves in dry continental areas; therefore, the safety yield and quality of corn silage are likely compromised in extensive lands in the future. Consequently, it would be important to consider how crop production and feeding strategies can be adapted to this change in the long term, considering the nutrient requirements of dairy cattle.

Winter cereals are growing during a period of potentially higher rainfall, bypassing periods of heat stress and drought (autumn sowing-early spring harvest), so can be grown with less risk than corn. Therefore, the winter cereals can be part of the climate change strategy. Additionally, the corn-whole crop rye, corn-whole crop triticale, brown midrib (BMR) sorghum-whole crop triticale, or BMR sorghum-intensive high sugar grass double cropping are new crop rotation systems to prevent yield losses due to climate change (drought and heat stress).

Silage can be made from winter whole-crop cereals, but it has a dual function as a cover crop, protecting the soil. There has been a growing interest in seeding winter cereals after corn silage harvest as cover and silage crops. This is due to the recognition by farmers and farm advisors that fall and spring ground coverage is important for erosion control after corn silage harvest. It is also due to the potential of overwintering cereals to retain end-of-season nitrogen, the need for a growing crop to improve the nutrient use efficiency of fall-applied manure, and the addition of carbon to soils through roots and crop residue [6, 7]. Winter crops prevent erosion and give good weed suppression. The rye accumulates much greater biomass than oats in the autumn, providing better winter cover to reduce runoff, erosion, and P loss potential. Rye also has a very strong positive impact on reducing nitrate leaching in the soil profile, as nitrate concentrations at 50 cm depth were extremely low according to experimental results [8].

Double cropping can provide economic and environmental advantages to dairy farmers. Winter cereals harvested early can offer a substantial quantity of extra, nourishing forage while minimally impacting the production of corn silage. Winter cereals, such as rye cultivated as dual crops in corn silage rotations, possess the capacity to enhance on-farm forage production while also offering numerous environmental, economic, and nutritional advantages to dairy farms [9].

The objective of this chapter is to present the projected climate conditions in regions where corn is grown and propose different approaches to develop a robust forage foundation for dairy cattle. We focus on field crops which could be an option for completing the forage sources of countries located in areas with a dry continental climate.

2. The current and future climate situation in dry continental areas

Agricultural production strongly depends on climate conditions. Changes in the mean temperature and precipitation, as well as weather and climate extremes, are already influencing crop yields and livestock productivity in many European regions. A projected increase in the number of extreme weather and climate events throughout Europe is expected to further increase the risk of crop losses and impose risks on livestock production. The impacts of climate change on agriculture vary across Europe. While increases in the length of the growing seasons can improve the suitability for growing crops in northern Europe, the negative effects of climate change will lead to yield losses across Europe, mostly in southern Europe. Elements of climate change affect livestock systems through direct impacts on animal physiology, behaviour production, and welfare and indirectly through water availability [10] and the quantity and quality of forage and feed crops [11, 12].

Animal production based on the use of grain crops may be less sensitive to climate change compared to ruminants that rely on conserved forage (hay and silage) and grazing.

The Intergovernmental Panel on Climate Change (IPCC) has consistently highlighted the significance of anthropogenic influences on the climate system, leading to alterations in temperature and precipitation patterns. The elevated concentrations of greenhouse gases induced by human activity, especially with the highest radiation forces, have played an unequivocal role in modifying the previously quasi-balanced

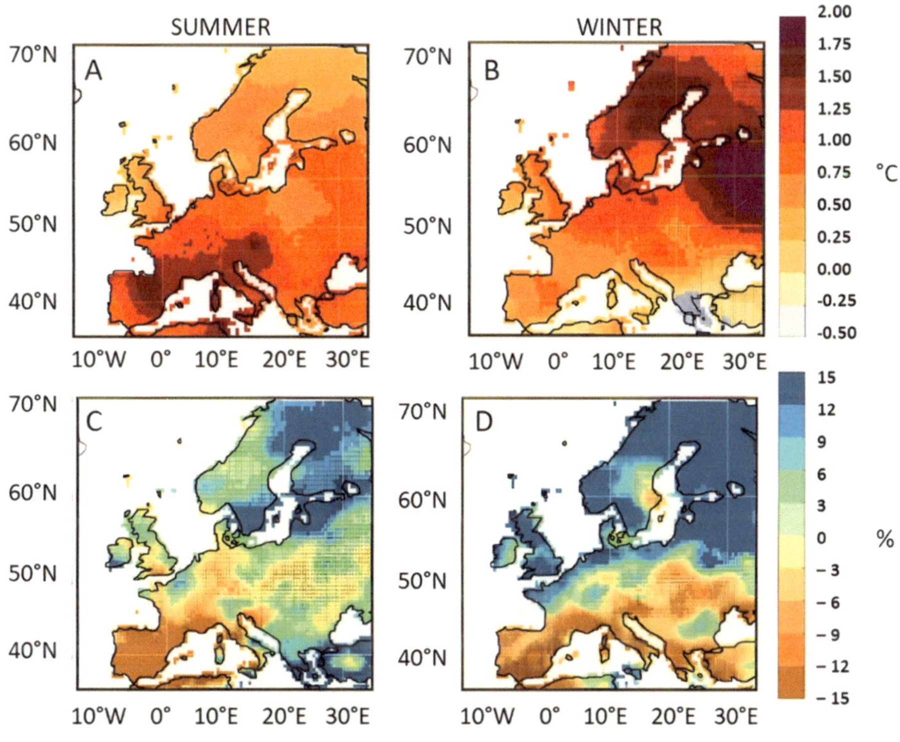

Figure 1.
Observed linear trends in mean temperature [°C] and relative precipitation change [%] between 1950 and 2016 in summer and winter (modified, based on Christensen et al. [14]).

atmospheric processes. Understanding these changes on a seasonal basis is crucial for comprehending the full scope of the impact on ecosystems, agriculture, and society.

The global mean temperature in the last 40 years was significantly warmer than in the second half of the nineteenth century. The global surface temperature was +0.99°C higher between 2001 and 2020 and + 1.09°C higher between 2011 and 2020 than it was between 1850 and 1900. The change over land is more pronounced (+1.59°C) than over the ocean (+0.88°C) [13]. Seasonal differences in Europe are also observed (**Figure 1**). In summer, the most considerable temperature change happened mostly in the lower latitudes, in the Mediterranean subregion, particularly in the surroundings of the Pirenes, Southern France, North Italy, and the Western parts of the Carpathian basin. The spatial distribution of temperature changes is the reverse in winter. The warming trend becomes more significant as latitude increases with a maximum of above 2°C in the East European Plain and the middle regions of Scandinavia.

Precipitation is the most volatile meteorological element, so analysing its trend variability is also quite difficult. However, the spatial and temporal changes indicate a more uniform pattern. The observed linear trends show a definite reduction in summer in the western basin of the Mediterranean Sea, especially over Spain and along the French and North African coasts. A less significant, but noticeable reduction has emerged in subregions in the whole of Europe. In winter, the spatial distribution of precipitation reduction is similar to those in summer, however with more remarkable changes in the eastern or southeastern parts of Europe, like the Carpathian basin, the Balkan Peninsula down to Greece, or regions around the Black Sea. Furthermore, in summer, the days of heavy rains and storms have increased and will likely further rise in the future, causing severe damage to the natural and built environment. In contrast, the northern parts of Europe can face some increase in the

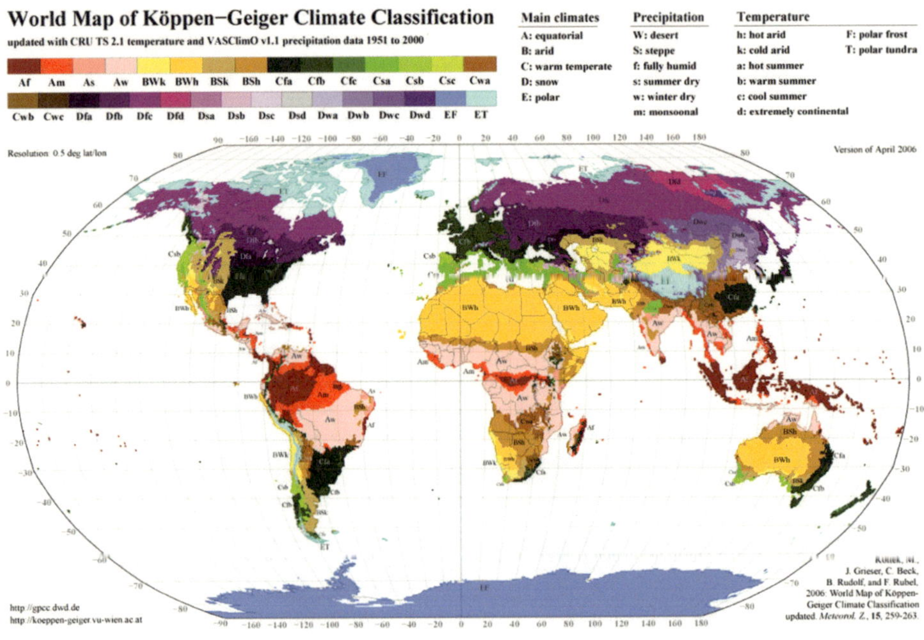

Figure 2.
Updated Köppen-Geiger climate classification by Kottek et al. [15]. Western and Central Europe are located in the Cfb, while Eastern Europe falls in the Dfb climate classification.

precipitation amount, especially in winter. The mutual effect of the increasing trends in the temperature and precipitation amount indicates a shift in the precipitation type from snow to rain during winters. Consequently, this process reduces the extension of snow-covered areas in winter, which affects the amount of water in the soils and, thereby, the speed and rate of the onset of droughts in spring or summer.

According to the updated Köppen-Geiger climate classification (**Figure 2**), there are currently large areas in the eastern half of North America and China with similar climate conditions as in Western and Central Europe (Cfa, Cfb, Dfa, Dfb). Higher

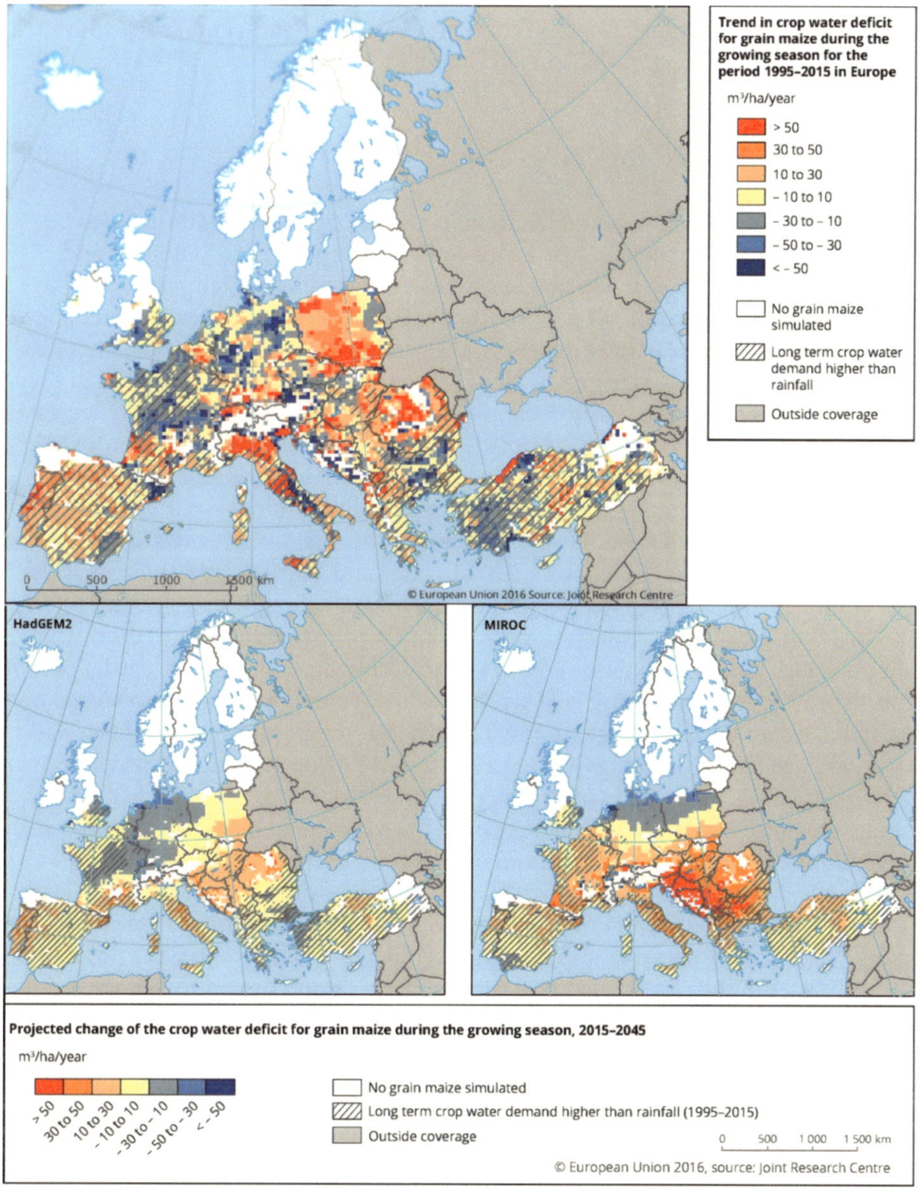

Figure 3.
Crop water demand for grain corn in the growing season based on observations between 1995 and 2015 (above), and future projections based on HadGEM2 and MIROC between 2015 and 2045.

latitude areas such as Scandinavia and areas with similar climate conditions (Dfc) are experiencing benefits from climate change.

Given the anticipated increase in frequency, intensity, and duration of drought periods in the future, it is important to investigate historical and projected patterns of soil moisture availability. The trends in water deficit for grain corn during the growing season between 1995 and 2015 show that the largest contiguous areas most affected by water scarcity are Poland, Spain, Italy, Greece, and the east part of the Carpathian basin (**Figure 3**). The results of the future projections (2015–2045) based on two different climate models (HadGEM2, MIROC) agree that the crop water deficit will extend to an even larger area; moreover, extreme water shortage is projected to the expanded areas ranging east-west from Slovenia to Bulgaria and north-south from Slovenia through the Western Balkans to Greece.

3. Reducing heat stress for dairy cows

The performance, welfare, and health of cattle are significantly influenced by climatic and meteorological factors. Dairy cows with high genetic potential and intensive metabolism are particularly sensitive to high ambient temperatures. The harmful effects of high ambient temperature in production conditions are enhanced by high humidity and insufficient airflow. If the temperature-humidity index (THI) is above 72, cows are heat-stressed, which means the cows have more heat than they can get rid of. Feed intake usually decreases and, as a result, milk yield also decreases [16, 17]. The effect of heat stress is immediate, 1 day of heat stress results in an average production loss of 1.5–2 litres per cow per day (5–10% of the daily milk yield). Genetic selection specifically aimed at increasing milk production parameters caused a decrease in the heat tolerance of cows. Recently, significant efforts have been made to identify specific genes associated with tolerance and sensitivity to thermal stress [18]. Significant advances in the environmental management of dairy cattle include improved housing and cooling systems (shading, water spraying, ventilation, and combined with fans, sprinklers, and humidification systems). In dairy cattle, part of the milk production lost during heat stress (35–50%) can potentially be restored by nutritional treatment [19]. First, the availability and temperature of drinking water may be a key tool in promoting dry matter intake (DMI) and reducing heat stress. Feed supplements can assist in improving the functionality of the rumen in cows experiencing heat stress [20–23]. Diets aimed at reducing metabolic heat gain can also contribute to enhancing feed intake and overall performance.

Energy intake is typically the primary dietary constraint for lactating dairy cows in the summer months. One commonly employed method to enhance the energy density of a diet is by decreasing the amount of forage and increasing the proportion of concentrates in the ration. However, this practice should be conducted with care, as this type of diet can be associated with a lower rumen pH. Acute and sub-acute rumen acidosis is often increased under heat-stress conditions and indirectly enhances the risk of developing negative side effects of an unhealthy rumen environment (i.e., laminitis, milk fat depression). Digestion characteristics of neutral detergent fibre (NDF) influence feeding and rumination behaviour, dry matter intake, and efficiency of milk component output [24]. Highly digestible forages can pass through the rumen at a faster rate, which in turn stimulates dry matter intake (DMI) while simultaneously decreasing the heat increment. This process ultimately assists in thermoregulation. Therefore, a rising NDF ruminal degradability not only positively impacts nutrient digestibility, but also influences feed intake and milk production. The correlation between the digestibility of forage NDF and the performance of dairy cows is widely recognised. An increase of one percentage unit in NDF digestibility leads to an additional daily intake of 0.18 kg of dry matter and a daily production of 0.25 kg of 4% fat-corrected milk [25].

When dairy cows are fed high-quality forage, they tend to produce more milk and milk components, experience fewer metabolic disorders, have healthier feet, and live longer. As a result, feeding less grain and focusing on providing quality forage can lead to a higher economic return, specifically in terms of income over feed cost [26]. The various types of whole-crop cereals are excellent sources of fermented forage for ruminants: High NDF digestibility is associated with more fast-pool NDF, less slow-pool NDF, and less undegradable NDF. During the summer months, it is possible to customise the feeding schedule by considering these factors and the NDF characteristics of forage to improve DMI efficiency, especially when animals are experiencing heat stress. Therefore, early-cut whole-crop silage as a high-quality forage type may play a role in alleviating the heat stress of dairy cows in continental areas even under climate change.

4. Possibilities for stabilisation of forage bank in dry continental regions

Climate change increased the number of heat stress days during summer in dry continental Europe. Future changes in temperature, precipitation, and atmospheric CO_2 concentration are expected to carry along an increased risk of mycotoxin contamination of cereals. Recent quantitative estimates have shown that, as a consequence of global warming, increased contamination of cereals with deoxynivalenol (DON) and aflatoxin B1 is expected in certain regions of Europe. Aflatoxins and DON are among the most critical mycotoxins affecting milk production and quality [27, 28]. Difficulties can therefore be expected in the corn silage-based diet of dairy herds; therefore, renaissance of winter whole-crop cereals cut in the early stage of maturity (in boot) is obvious in dry areas. Whole-crop cereals include wheat (*Triticum aestivum*), barley (*Hordeum vulgare*), oat (*Avena sativa*), rye (*Secale cereale*), and triticale (*x Triticosecale*) can be harvested as a forage source (silage or haylage) for ruminants, but widely used in many countries in various forms, including pasture, hay, or grain [29]. Small-grain cereals offer many advantages over forage sources, particularly alfalfa (*Medicago sativa*). They can be grown in a wide range of climatic and soil conditions. Winter cereals are also more drought and cold-resistant than alfalfa [30].

These crops were grown primarily for their grains in the past, but nowadays there are different targets in ruminant nutrition. The soft dough stage was the recommended maturity for ensiling for most small grain cereals as an alternative to corn (*Zea mays*), especially in areas with too short or too cool growing seasons for silage corn [31]. Recently, in continental regions whole-crop cereals are recommended to harvest at the flag-leaf or early-boot stage for high nutrient quality as a forage supply of high milking dairy cows in intensive systems [32–36].

Nutrient content and fibre digestibility (48 h *in vitro* digestibility of amylase treated ash corrected neutral detergent fibre, aNDFomd48) of different ensiled forages in Hungary (2013–2018) are shown in **Table 1** [36]. Digestible NDF (dNDF) and NDFD can be used to help us better determine forage quality. The dNDF is an actual nutrient that can be analysed in a lab, whereas NDFD is calculated as the percentage of NDF that is dNDF. Forage with a very high NDFD, but low NDF will not supply

	n[1]	DM[2]	CP[3]	TS[4]	aNDFom[5]	ADF[6]	ADL[7]	aNDFomd 48[8]	daNDF omd 48[9]	uNDF 240[10]
		g/kg	g/kg DM	g/kg DM	g/kg DM	g/kg DM	g/kg DM	%NDF	g/kg DM	%NDF
Alfalfa silage/haylage (medium quality)										
	1811	408	193	—	426	327	62	40.5	171	48.9
Grass silage/haylage (intensive growing on arable: *Lolium multiflorum*, *Festulolium var.*)										
	462	343	141	—	502	305	26	65.1	323	24.2
Rye silage (in boot-early heading)										
	789	294	136	—	554	330	27	66.2	363	19.3
Triticale silage										
in boot-heading	24	316	106	—	579	348	28	59.4	341	19.3
early dough stage	59	362	81	124	516	320	34	47.4	249	28.1
Barley silage										
in boot-heading	17	318	132	—	552	329	30	60.4	332	19.3
early dough	59	337	93	134	494	289	31	47.9	232	29.8
Wheat silage										
in boot-heading	10	293	118	—	571	337	34	57.9	322	19.3
early dough	32	365	92	122	499	301	34	46.6	237	26.3

[1]*Number of samples.*
[2]*Dry matter.*
[3]*Crude protein.*
[4]*Total starch.*
[5]*Amylase-treated ash-corrected NDF.*
[6]*Acid detergent fibre.*
[7]*Acid detergent lignin.*
[8]*Degradability of amylase-treated ash-corrected NDF, 48-hour in vitro incubation.*
[9]*Degradable aNDFom, 48-hour in vitro incubation, organic matter digestibility in vitro 48-hour incubation.*
[10]*Undegradable NDF, 240-hour in vitro incubation.*

Table 1.
Nutrient composition, fibre degradability, degradable, and undegradable NDF content of different ensiled forages in Hungary between 2013 and 2018 [36].

much dNDF and other sources of dNDF may be needed in the diet. The NDFD 48 (*in vitro* NDF digestibility, 48-hour incubation) values of the early dough stage were lower compared to the boot stage. These results confirm the importance of the whole crop cereal silages (harvested in boot stage) in the diet fed in the summertime to maintain the dry matter intake. We can conclude that early cut, intensive growing grass silages (*Lolium multiflorum*, *Festulolium var.*), whole crop rye silage (harvested in boot stage or earlier), triticale-, barley-, and wheat silage (harvested in boot-early heading stage) may reduce the DMI drops during the summer in cattle according to the high neutral detergent fibre digestibility (NDFD 48), high digestible NDF (dNDF 48), and low unavailable NDF (uNDF 240) results. In the context of cattle feeding in dry continental regions of Europe, we may refer to these forages as 'heat stress forages'. Because of the above-mentioned factors, there is an increasing global interest in the production and use of early-cut whole-crop cereal silages in the dairy cow diet, especially during the summer season.

4.1 Early-cut whole-crop winter rye

Winter rye is an excellent forage crop when seeded after early-fall harvested crops. It is ready for harvest in Central Europe in mid-April, which provides great opportunities for double-crop options, and can also fill the gap in years when forage supplies are short [32, 37].

The average yield of early-cut whole-crop rye was 3.63 tons of DM per ha over 3 years in New York State, USA (**Table 2**). Most cereal rye trials (70%) yielded between 2.5 and 5 t DM per ha [9]. The average yield of early-cut whole crop triticale was 4.88 tons of DM per ha [33].

The BBCH (Biologische Bundesanstalt, Bundessortenamt und Chemical Industry) scale is the main system in cereals, based on developmental phases—the principal growth stages. Orosz et al. [37] have found that the effect of three different phenological stages (boot stage: BBCH 49–51, heading: BBCH 57–58; early flowering: BBCH 61–62, respectively) was significant on DM yield of the whole-crop rye cut in very early stage (April-May 2013: 5.0–8.6 tons of DM per ha). Growth stages had a seven-times higher effect on variation of DM yield, than varieties (BBCH 49–51: 5.0–6.2 tons per ha, BBCH 57–58: 6.9–8.2 tons per ha, BBCH 61–62: 8.6–9.5 tons per ha). Therefore, cutting time is critical. Winter rye is faster growing and earlier maturing in the spring than the other winter cereals, including wheat, barley, and triticale. Rye matures rapidly at the flag-leaf, boot, and early-heading stages, with significant reductions in forage quality. This can create the challenge of a very narrow harvest window (the timeframe in which rye can be harvested), particularly if there are rain delays [32]. There can be a very large range in forage quality with only a few days

Forage	Year	Number of fields	Average t DM/ha	Min t DM/ha	Max t DM/ha	Standard deviation
Rye	2012	1	5.38			
	2013	7	3.65	2.24	5.35	1.23
	2014	11	3.47	1.64	5.40	1.16
	All	19	3.63	2.22	5.38	1.19

Table 2.
The nutrient content of rye harvested between 2012 and 2014 in New York State [33].

difference in harvest. Quality, palatability, and thus consumption reduce very quickly at the heading stage. The delayed harvest had a significant detrimental effect on nutrient content: The crude protein content at the boot stage (BBCH 49–51: 191–215 g per kg DM) reduced with maturation (BBCH 61–62:114–137 g per kg DM, $P \leq 0.01$). The NDF digestibility (aNDFomD 48) declined also with maturation (BBCH 49–51: 60–65% NDF, BBCH 57–58: 51–56% NDF, BBCH 61–62: 44–50% NDF, $P \leq 0.05$). The NDF rumen degradability decreased by 8–16% during 7 days and 18–32% during 14 days after the boot stage ($P < 0.05$) in whole crop rye silage. It can be concluded that nutrition value and digestibility drop very quickly at the heading stage of winter rye, so the optimum harvest window is very narrow. The authors concluded that the harvest window was less than 7 days in the boot stage.

According to the results of a country-wide survey in Hungary [36], the rumen degradable NDF content in corn silage was 209 g/kg DM in 2018 (n = 370). While the rye silage cut at the boot-heading stage contained 363 g/kg DM degradable NDF (2013–2018, n = 789). The degradable NDF content of the whole-crop winter rye cut at the boot-heading stage was higher by approximately 40–50% as compared to the corn silage; therefore, the early-cut whole-crop rye can be denoted as an important source of rumen degradable fibre for the high-lactating dairy cows, especially during the summer heat stress period in dry continental Europe.

Based on the experimental results we can conclude that early-cut whole-crop rye silage harvested in the boot stage (in April), in dry continental areas of Central Europe may be an alternative additional forage besides the corn silage for high-performing dairy cows.

4.2 Early cut, whole-crop winter triticale

Triticale has become more commonly used in dairy cropping strategies in recent years, in part due to the double cropping option with corn or sorghum, and environmental aspects such as the desire to capture nutrients from land-applied manure or to provide winter ground cover that improves land stewardship.

There are new triticale varieties that show promise, as they are multifunctional crops: that triticale can be harvested in the boot stage for high-producing dairy cows, or in the early-milk or dough stage for growing/beef cattle and the grain yield can also be a good commodity (for laying hens, other poultry, sheep, pigs, and cattle). This increases resilience and adaptability to environmental conditions in the face of climate change.

Furthermore, they have a much wider harvest window compared to the forage rye, so a bit more convenient to harvest because it can be harvested later and ages more slowly than rye. Mowing after early rye can open the window further, reducing the risk from weather. Finally, different triticale varieties can be cut 5–10 days later in early spring than forage rye. A week difference can be significant in terms of temperature. We are more likely to achieve successful wilting and ensiling of triticale when compared to rye, especially in regions with a longer growing season.

Experimental data confirmed that the triticale varieties can produce similar or even higher DM yields (**Table 3**) at the end of April (5.94–5.96 tons DM per ha) and in early May (7.67–7.88 tons DM per ha) as whole crop rye in the similar growth stage (BBCH 45–50, in boot) under normal growing conditions [35]. Yields of forage triticale harvested in New York State (USA) are in **Table 4** [33].

Variety	BBCH		Date	Mean
R	45	Before heading: 5–6 cm head in boot	17 April 2016	3.52^{aA}
	49	Before heading: 7–9 cm head in boot	21 April 2016	5.32^{aB}
T1	41	Before heading: 3–4 cm head in boot	21 April 2016	5.04^{A}
	45	Before heading: 5–6 cm head in boot	27 April 2016	5.96^{bB}
	50	Before heading: 6–10 cm head in boot	06 May 2016	7.88^{bC}
T2	41	Before heading: 3–4 cm head in boot	21 April 2016	4.79^{A}
	45	Before heading: 5–6 cm head in boot	27 April 2016	5.94^{bB}
	50	Before heading: 6–10 cm head in boot	06 May 2016	7.67^{bC}

$^{a–c}$Values with different letters within the BBCH 45 or 49/50 category differ statistically compared to the rye (P ≤ 0.05).
$^{A–C}$Values with different capital letters within a variety differ statistically–effect of the phenological stage (P ≤ 0.05).
Ryefood (R), triticale var. Hungaro (T1), triticale var. Dimenzio (T2) according to the different sampling dates [35].

Table 3.
Dry matter yield of rye var.

Forage	Year	Number of fields	Average DM/ha	Min. t DM/ha	Max. t DM/ha	Standard deviation
Triticale	2012	13	5.13	1.95	10.44	2.551
	2013	28	4.82	2.46	6.76	1.23
	2014	3	4.35	3.34	5.35	1.01
	All	44	4.88	2.37	7.75	1.68

Table 4.
The nutrient content of triticale harvested between 2013 and 2014 in New York State (USA), sown after corn harvest and harvested in May [33].

Orosz et al. [35] found significantly higher (P ≤ 0.05) dry matter yield with similar NDFD 48 values (**Table 5**) for the triticale varieties (BBCH 50) 2 weeks later than the rye variety at the stage of the same growth stage (BBCH 49). It can be concluded that there is a wider 'harvest window' of triticale, a longer time for harvest compared to the whole crop rye. Moreover, the optimal period of triticale harvest is later by 1–2 weeks compared to rye, when there are more favourable weather conditions for wilting.

Two triticale varieties (**Table 5**) had high NDF digestibility at the early growth stage (BBCH 45, 5–6 cm in boot: NDFD 48 76.5 and 76.7%, respectively). Nine days later there was a significant decrease in fibre digestibility (BBCH 50, 6–10 cm in boot: NDFD 48 69.6 and 70.0%, respectively). Crude protein content dropped, while the NDF, ADF, and ADL content lifted during 10 days [35]. Triticale silage harvested at an early stage (BBCH 45–50) can be an excellent forage for high-yielding dairy herds, while triticale harvested at a later stage (BBCH higher than 50) can be more suitable for beef cattle and dairy heifers.

Consequently, triticale varieties can be additional alternative forages in very early cut systems alongside the rye, but mowing can be executed (1–2 weeks later), under better weather harvesting conditions for wilting [35]. The area can be utilised in the season after triticale has been removed, as there is still time to sow corn, sorghum, and sudangrass.

Cereal		Rye	Triticale 1		Triticale 2	
BBCH code		49	45	50	45	50
Sampling time		21 April 2016	27 April 2016	06 May 2016	27 April 2016	06 May 2016
Dry matter	g/kg	157^{a}	146^{aA}	147^{aA}	169^{bA}	160^{bA}
Crude protein	g/kg DM	193^{b}	257^{cA}	196^{bB}	159^{aA}	150^{aA}
Crude fibre	g/kg DM	252^{b}	223^{aA}	247^{bB}	231^{aA}	255^{bB}
NDF	g/kg DM	545^{a}	540^{aA}	570^{c}	532^{aA}	556^{bB}
ADF	g/kg DM	274^{b}	243^{aA}	270^{bB}	245^{aA}	271^{bB}
ADL	g/kg DM	20.3^{a}	21.3^{aA}	24.7^{bB}	20.3^{aA}	23.0^{bB}
NDFD 48[1]	%NDF	68.2^{a}	76.5^{b}	69.6^{aB}	76.7^{bA}	70.0^{aB}
dNDF 48[2]	g/kg DM	372^{a}	413^{c}	396^{bB}	408^{cA}	389^{aB}
OMD[3]	%	76.4^{a}	80.5^{b}	75.3^{aB}	80.0^{bA}	75.3^{aB}

[1]*In vitro NDF digestibility, 48 hours incubation expressed as a percent of NDF. NDFD = dNDF/NDF * 100.*
[2]*Digestible NDF measured from an in vitro NDF digestion for 48 hours.*
[3]*in vitro digestibility of organic matter.*
[a–c]*Values with different letters within a row differ statistically compared to the rye (P < 0.05).*
[A–C]*Values with different capital letters within a variety differ statistically—effect of the phenological stage (P < 0.05).*
Ryefood (R), triticale var. Hungaro (T1), triticale var. Dimenzio (T2) according to the different sampling dates in fresh forage [35].

Table 5.
Nutrient content and in vivo digestibility of rye var.

4.3 Early-cut high-sugar grass (grown on arable in an intensive system)

Italian ryegrass (*Lolium multiflorum* Lam., var. italicum) evolved in the Mediterranean region, and northern Italy, its cultivation as forage for livestock dates back as far as the twelfth century [38]. Preserved Italian ryegrass is frequently used as forage for dairy cows and is known for their high energy value and highly digestible fibre [39]. Plant breeders have developed annual and perennial ryegrass cultivars with an elevated concentration of water-soluble carbohydrates (WSC) relative to conventional cultivars [40]. The new generation of intensive or sweet grasses, the so-called silage grasses, are gaining ground in arable crops. Nowadays, in addition to Italian ryegrass, the less water-intensive Festulolium, a successful cross between fescue and ryegrass, and hybrid ryegrass are also popular in the dry continental region.

This breeding has focussed on increasing the accumulation of high molecular weight storage sugars (i.e. fructans), particularly in leaf blades rather than sheath bases [41]. Research proposed that perennial ryegrass with a high WSC may improve the balance and synchrony of the nitrogen and energy supply to the rumen [42]. Italian ryegrass exhibits a higher sugar content in comparison to other varieties of grass silage provided that it is harvested in the early stages of harvesting. In this regard, Baldinger et al. [38] reported that Italian ryegrass, which is harvested at the second cut, had a significantly higher (71.87%) sugar content than corn silage.

Narasimaluhi et al. [43] reported that the apparent digestibility of DM, NDF, and ADF of Italian ryegrass were 63.6, 57.3, and 64.1%, respectively. According to Orosz [36], ryegrass silage had higher NDFD 48 values (66.2%, $P \leq 0.05$) compared to alfalfa silage (40.5%). NDF rumen degradation rate of ryegrass silages has a higher degree at the point of 12, 24, 30, 48, 120, and 240 hours *in vitro* compared to alfalfa silages, and similar to the rye silage cut in the boot (**Table 6**). It can be concluded that the intensive ryegrass silage has a significantly ($P \leq 0.05$) higher NDF degradation rate compared to alfalfa silage/haylage (at 12, 24, 30, 48, and 120 hours *in vitro* incubation time). Moreover, the undegradable NDF content was found to be 24.2% NDF in intensive grass silages (n = 462) compared to the alfalfa silage/haylage samples (48.9% NDF, n = 1811).

According to the NRC [44] and Jacobs et al.'s [45] report, the CP contents of Italian ryegrass silage were 12.8 and 12.5%, respectively, which is higher compared with other grass and cereals, including corn silage. Orosz et al. [36] have found 14.1% DM CP content, as an average between 2013 and 2018 (n = 462) in Hungary (**Table 6**).

The total-tract NDF digestibility (TTNDFD) measurement aims to assess the NDF digestibility of feed and rations in animals [46, 47]. TTNDFD can be used to compare the fibre utilisation of different feed or fibre sources. Research work at the University of Wisconsin [47] demonstrates the accuracy of TTNDFD for predicting NDF digestion *in vivo* (in dairy cows). Typical TTNDFD values for corn silage, alfalfa, and grasses are summarised in **Table 7** [48]. It can be concluded that NDF in intensive temperate annual or perennial grass silages degrade faster (kd) and potentially at a higher rate (pdNDF) compared to the corn silage and alfalfa silages. TTNDFD *in vivo* values confirmed a better NDF digestibility of grass silages.

Replacing one-third of the corn silage and alfalfa mixture with grass silage increased the NDF content of the forage and increased the TTNDFD. Partial replacement of corn silage and alfalfa fibre with more digestible fibre from grasses increased TTNDFD and improved milk fat without reducing milk production [49].

Reports regarding the positive effects on the forage intake of dairy cows are frequent [50, 51] and some researchers even reported better feed efficiency than

	Number of samples	**NDFD 12**	**NDFD 24**	**NDFD 30**	**NDFD 48**	**NDFD 120**	**NDFD 240**	**uNDF 240**
Forage		%NDF	%NDF	%NDF	%NDF	%NDF	%NDF	%NDF
Alfalfa silage/ haylage	1811	17.8	28.7	32.6	40.5	47.3	49.6	48.9
Grass silage/ haylage	462	29.2	46.8	52.9	65.1	74.8	75.7	24.2
Rye silage (in boot)	789	28.9	47.1	53.6	66.2	79.3	80.7	19.3
Triticale silage (in heading)	24	24.3	41.1	47.4	59.4	78.0	80.6	19.3
Triticale silage (milky-dough stage)	59	16.6	29.1	34.2	47.4	65.6	71.3	28.1

**NDFD 12 = NDF degradability at 12 h, NDFD 24 = NDF degradability at 24 h, NDFD 30 = NDF degradability at 30 h, NDFD 48 = NDF degradability at 48 h, NDFD 120 = NDF degradability at 120 h, NDFD 240 = NDF degradability at 240 h, uNDF 240—undegradable NDF, 240-hour in vitro incubation.*

Table 6.
The NDF rumen degradation rate of different ensiled forages in Hungary (2013–2018) [36].*

	Sample number	pdNDF[1]	kdNDF[2]	TTNDFD[3]	TTNDFD range
	(Rock River Lab.)	% NDF	%/hours	% NDF	% NDF
Corn silage	7000	75–85	2–3	42	20–60
Alfalfa silage	7000	60–65	4–6	43	30–60
Temperate grass silage	1200	80–90	6	47	20–80

[1]*pdNDF = potentially degradable NDF.*
[2]*kdNDF = rate of NDF degradation.*
[3]*TTNDFD = total-tract NDF digestibility.*

Table 7.
Typical total-tract NDF digestibility (TTNDFD) values of corn silage, alfalfa, or grass [48].

feeding corn silage [52]. The favourable nutrient digestibility of these grass silages can be attributed to their relatively low lignin content, resulting in a high concentration of energy. Therefore, new grass varieties that produce high yields offer cows a source of fibre that is both easily digestible and structurally beneficial.

Early harvesting grass silages have the potential to mitigate the negative impacts of climate change on dairy cows during the summer season. By extending the growing season beyond the summer period and avoiding the reduction in biomass harvested per hectare through double cropping with sorghum-type forage, these characteristics offer a viable solution.

4.4 Cereal-cereal and cereal-grass mixtures

The mixtures serve to complement the available forage resources within a nation, instead of replacing the current array of varieties. Italian ryegrass-cereal mixtures harvested in April and May can be an alternative feed to corn silage for high-yielding dairy cows in the dry continental areas of Central Europe. The mixtures have been formulated through extensive research and development efforts conducted by Agroteam, an esteemed company based in Italy. These mixtures possess exceptional qualities that set them apart from other feed options available in the European market. The development process relied on the careful selection of specific species and varieties, aligning their breeding periods, and establishing the appropriate germ count and germ ratio. The special mixtures of Italian ryegrass and winter cereals (triticale, oats, barley and wheat; triticale, barley, and wheat; Italian ryegrass and oats; Italian ryegrass, oats, triticale, barley, and wheat) used in practice have several feeding advantages maintain normal rumen environment, improve fibre digestibility and *in situ* rumen degradation of fibre [53–56], and fermentation processes in the rumen [9, 54, 57]. Italian ryegrass and winter cereals can be grown together [58, 59]. Legumes are excluded from special blends due to their lower fibre digestibility compared to winter cereals or Italian ryegrass. The wide harvest window results in a good quality of silage in the case of rainy weather or technical failure. The double cropping of winter cereals with Italian ryegrass and corn plants also has environmental and economic advantages, as two different fodder crops are harvested in the same season [33, 60, 61]. The silage mixtures can be successfully used in feed rations for high-production dairy cows due to their highly degradable dry matter and protein content and favourable rumen fermentability [55]. Results and experience suggest that the wider harvesting window, potential yield, multi-functionality, and flexibility make them an excellent element of a new feeding and climate strategy.

4.5 New types of sorghum

Repeated climatic challenges, such as drought, high summer temperatures, or late planting pose significant risks to corn. Therefore, more and more dairy farmers are seeking sorghum varieties suitable for silage-making, which could serve as an alternative to fully or partially replace corn silage for dairy cows. Sorghum's water usage is much more efficient than corn's, it can be planted later, it yields significant biomass, and it can still provide acceptable yields even under dry conditions, especially in areas with poor water management [62–65].

The most important modern hybrid types of sorghum (Sorghum bicolour) are as follows: brown midrib sorghum type (BMR), brachytic dwarf sorghum type, male sterile sorghum type (MS), photoperiod sensitivity sorghum type (PPS), and hybrids of sudangrass and sorghum. A summary of yield, lodging, and quality (DM basis) by sorghum forage types is given in **Table 8** [66].

4.5.1 Brown midrib sorghum type

The digestibility of silage corn in the rumen is much better than that of silage made from traditional sorghum species. Lignin, as an indigestible component of the cell wall, inhibits the breakdown of carbohydrates found in the cell wall. Corn plants contain less lignin than sorghum, and they have more easily digestible starch. Since lignin reduces the digestibility of NDF and the amount of digestible fibre [67], it slows down the ruminal passage, increasing the feeling of fullness in the rumen, which impairs dry matter intake and milk production in traditional and old types of sorghum silage [68]. In the case of BMR-type forages, both the lignin content and the chemical composition of lignin are modified [69–71]. To date, the most direct and effective way to reduce lignin content and increase the digestibility of forage sorghum is through genetic control of the lignification process via the BMR traits [72]. Both *in situ* and *in vitro* digestion studies have shown that BMR forages have better NDF digestion than traditional sorghum species [69, 73].

4.5.2 Brachytic dwarf brown midrib sorghum type

As stated earlier, the BMR trait leads to a decrease in lignin content, thereby enhancing the digestibility of the forage. However, this may increase the risk of stalk lodging. Therefore, in many cases, the BMR genotype has been further developed and combined with the dwarf, but leafy plant phenotype. The term brachytic refers to the dwarf trait, which results in fewer stems and more leaf surface area. The yield was found 18-ton silage per ha in 2020 [66]. The combination of a higher leaf-to-stem ratio and the lower lignin content from BMR brachytic dwarf sorghum results in forage quality similar to or better than corn. The NDFD 48 value (**Table 9**) was found to be 59–61% [66].

4.5.3 Male sterile sorghum type

According to Kilcer [74–76], the modern BMR forage sorghum male sterile variety provides excellent quality for silage production in dairy farming. Sorghum cultivation per hectare is cheaper than most corn varieties. The issue is that most sorghum is headed and seed-producing type, which increases the risk of lodging due to 'look-up head' and complicates harvesting. The use of MS varieties eliminates the heavy head on the thin stem. Instead of increasing starch content by filling the seeds (glassy and

Lodging	DM[1]	Yield[2]	CP[3]	aNDF[4]	Lignin	Starch	NDFD 48[5]	uNDF om 240[6]	Milk/ton[7]
%	%	t/ha				%DM			
Brown midrib forage sorghum trait									
BMR (34)									
2.3	32.5	18.2	7.8	44.9	1.5	8.4	60.8	13.9	3386
Non-BMR (37)									
4.1	32.6	18.2	7.9	46.8	2.3	8.7	58.1	15.2	3292.1
Photoperiod response forage sorghum trait									
PS (6)									
5.6	27.2	17.9	7.2	53.7	1.7	0.3	61.9	16.1	3001
Non-PS (65)									
3.0	33.1	17.9	7.9	45.2	2.0	9.3	59.2	14.4	3368
Brachytic dwarf forage sorghum trait									
0	32.8	17.9	8.4	45.5	1.8	8.0	60.7	13.9	3337
4.5	32.4	18.2	7.7	46.1	2.0	8.8	58.9	14.8	3337
Corn checks									
Corn (3)									
0	38.2	11.6	9.9	37.8	2.2	13.8	53.0	13.9	3662

[1]*Dry matter.*
[2]*Average yield (DM 35%).*
[3]*Crude protein.*
[4]*Amylase-treated ash-corrected neutral detergent fibre.*
[5]*NDF digestibility, estimated fibre digestibility after the specified length of time (48 hrs.)*
[6]*Undigested NDF after fermentation for the specified length of time (240 hrs.) expressed on an organic matter basis to account for the ash.*
[7]*A standard dairy cow to project milk produced per ton of forage.*
The number in parentheses represents the number of hybrids that make up each sorghum type in 2020 [60].

Table 8.
Summary of yield, lodging, and quality (DM basis) by forage type.

	Risk factor	First year		Second year		Third year	
		Spring	**Autumn**	**Spring**	**Autumn**	**Spring**	**Autumn**
Traditional crop rotation	+++	Silage corn[A]	Forage rye[A]	Silage corn[A]	Forage triticale[A]	BMR sorghum[B]	Forage rye[A]
Safe version	+	Sudangrass[C]	Forage rye[A]	Silage corn[A]	Forage triticale[A]	BMR sorghum[B]	Forage rye[A]
	++	Silage corn (short growing season)[A]	Italian ryegrass/ Festulollium[A]	BMR sorghum[B]	Forage rye[A]	Silage corn[A]	Triticale[A]
Irrigated area	+	Italian ryegrass[A]	Forage rye[A]	Silage corn[A]	Forage rye[A]	Silage corn[A]	Italian ryegrass[A]
Yield-focus (for heifers)	++	Silage corn[A]	Barley with pea[C]	Forage millet[A]	Forage triticale[A]	Sudangrass[C]	Forage rye[A]
	++	BMR sorghum[B]	Barley with pea[C]	Sudangrass[C]	Forage rye[A]	Silage corn[A]	Forage triticale[A]

[A]*Good for lactating dairy cows.*
[B]*only for dual-purpose cattle breeds.*
[C]*only for breeding heifers, fattening, lactating beef cows in winter.*

Table 9.
Crop rotation examples entirely for forage crop production (Németh and Fazekas, unpublished).

poorly digestible starch), it keeps the components in the cells of leaves and stems. This increases milk production capacity while simultaneously increasing the DM content of the forage. If the sorghum is harvested 1 week after heading, it shows low DM content and moderate energy content compared to corn silage. Seven weeks after heading, the sugar content increases by 500%, and the DM content increases by 18.85% [74]. The nutritive value and milk production capacity of the MS sorghum increases the longer the plant is left after heading. The longer the plant photosynthesizes after heading, the more nutrients accumulate in the stem and leaves. In one trial, non-fibre carbohydrates increased to 71% (corn silage: 82%). Non-starch carbohydrates increased by 185% by the seventh week after heading. NDF decreased by 15%. NDF digestibility, which generally decreases with maturity, decreased by only 8% over the 7 weeks and neutral detergent fibre digestibility (NDFD 30) was 64.1% [75]. During the harvest, kernel cracking should not be used as it increases the risk of effluent formation.

4.5.4 Photoperiod sensitive sorghum type

A photoperiodic sensitivity is a characteristic of sorghum species that allows for the initiation of heading for forage sorghums only when the daytime photoperiod decreases to less than 12.5 hours. The photoperiod-sensitive trait refers to sensitivity to day length, meaning long-day plants require extremely long daylight periods for flowering. This allows for a wider harvest window and ensures favourable fibre digestibility for a longer period. Under limited light conditions, they do not flower and produce seeds, thus maintaining good digestibility for a longer period. Due to this trait, their foliage is generally more abundant than non-long-day species. They can generally be harvested with high sugar content. Neutral detergent fibre digestibility (NDFD 48) was found at 61.9% and lignin content at 1.7% DM (**Table 8**) in Texas [66].

4.5.5 Hybrids of sudangrass and sorghum

Sorghum-sudangrass hybrids are intermediate in plant size between sorghum and sudangrass. Yield typically falls below that of forage sorghums but is comparable to or slightly greater than sudangrass. Larger stems make drying for hay more difficult than for sudangrasses. Sorghum-sudangrass hybrids are suitable for grazing and can be harvested with a mower-conditioner for silage. When grazed, they yield similar to sudangrass. Nevertheless, sorghum-sudangrass hybrids demonstrate superior yield performance compared to sudangrass upon harvesting the green material. The advantage of sorghum-BMR sudangrass hybrids lies in their favourable fibre digestibility, and they should be grown similarly to sorghum-sudangrass hybrids [77].

4.5.6 The impact of modern forage sorghum silage production on cattle

Feeding trials with lactating dairy cows [68, 78] have demonstrated that BMR-6 forage sorghum (BMR Gene 6 is the highest BMR level, meaning that it contains the lowest level of lignin of any sorghum) resulted in greater DMI, cell wall digestibility, and milk performance when fed to dairy cows compared with non-BMR forage sorghum (**Table 10**). Moreover, it was found that milk production was similar for cows fed the BMR-6 forage sorghum to a dual-purpose corn hybrid commonly grown in the Midwest, USA.

Similarly, the meta-analysis of nine different articles published between 1984 and 2015 by Sánchez-Duarte et al. [79] also concluded an overall improvement in lactation

Reference	Non-BMR sorghum	BMR-6	BMR-18	Corn silage
Oliver et al. [78]	29.2	33.7	31.2	33.3
Aydin et al. [68]; Study 1	20.7	23.7	—	29.0
Aydin et al. [68]; Study 2	31.4	33.8	—	32.4

Table 10.
The effect of BMR, non-BMR sorghum, and corn silage on milk production (4% FCM, kg/day).

performance when cows were fed diets containing BMR forage sorghum silage compared to those based on traditional forage sorghum silage. In the case of diets containing BMR forage sorghum silage, DMI (0.83 kg/day), milk production (1.64 kg/day), milk fat concentration (0.09%), milk fat yield (0.08 kg/day), milk protein yield (0.04 kg/day), and milk sugar yield (0.16 kg/day) improved compared to diets based on traditional forage sorghum silage. Compared to diets containing corn silage, cows fed BMR forage sorghum silage showed increased milk fat concentration (0.10%) and milk sugar yield (0.05 kg/day), but decreased milk protein concentration (0.06%).

In an experiment conducted in the warm weather of Iran, feeding forage sorghum silage (with 2.5% starch and 49.5% NDF) at 25% DM level in the diet did not result in lower milk production when completely substituting corn silage (with 20% starch and 42.3% NDF) at a milk production level of 30 kg/day [79].

BMR-6, BMR-12, and BMR-18 forage sorghum hybrids are known, depending on which allele the mutation occurred [80]. However, the different mutations cause differences in lignin biosynthesis among different hybrids. In a Nebraska experiment [78], cows fed total mixed rations containing BMR-6 or BMR-18 forage sorghum silage (at a ratio of 40% DM, respectively) and corn silage (at a ratio of 40% DM) had similar milk production levels. The apparent digestibility of NDF was similar between diets containing corn silage (54.1%) and those containing BMR-6 forage sorghum silage (54.4%), but lower for BMR-18 forage sorghum silage (47.9%), and the worst for traditional forage sorghum silage-based diets (40.8%). These data confirm that certain BMR forage sorghum hybrids (with starch contents of 14.5 and 16.8%) are capable of achieving similar results to corn silage with lower starch content (19.9%) in 30–35 kg/day milk-producing dairy cows, hence being potentially suitable for (at least) partial substitution of corn silage (**Table 10**).

4.6 Sudangrass

The brown midrib sudangrass is more palatable and significantly lower in lignin content, making it more digestible than traditional sudangrass. According to research by the University of Wisconsin Extension Forage Team, sudangrass hybrids can yield between 7.5 and 12.5 tons of DM per hectare. In several European countries (The Netherlands, Germany, and Italy), sudangrasses are harvested directly for silage at the heading stage. At this phenological stage, the DM content exceeds 30%, eliminating the need for wilting. Presumably, this technique is chosen to achieve higher yields. However, research indicates that the post-heading phenological stages of sudangrass result in a significant decrease in OM and fibre digestibility and an increase in NDF content. The heading phenological phase is not favourable for feeding silage to dairy cows. Numerous experiments conducted over an extended period have provided evidence that the most favourable period for harvesting dairy cows lies within the time-frame from the appearance of the flag leaf and the beginning of the heading. However, at this time, the DM content ranges from 20 to 27% (depending on the hybrid), which is not yet optimal for direct ensiling. The wilting as a harvesting technique is advisable at this phenological stage. However, it may increase silage ash content.

In a multi-cut forage system (early-stage harvests) 2–3 harvests can be carried out in the same area in the dry continental region. This flexible harvesting technology, combined with excellent fibre digestibility, makes the new sudangrass varieties promising plants for climate change forage strategy.

4.7 Whole crop cereal-legume mixtures (as winter crops)

The cultivation of mixtures of legumes and cereals offers several potential agronomic benefits. Coming from two different plant types, legumes and cereals complement each other in the capture of resources. Differentiation in the size and depth of the root systems of cereals and legumes allows them to utilise water and nutrients from different soil layers, resulting in the compensatory growth and development of plants. Cereal crops growing in the vicinity of legumes benefit from nitrogen assimilated by legume root nodule bacteria. Mixtures are particularly relevant to the exploitation of poorer soils that are unsuitable for the production of either component grown as a sole crop. Yielding of the mixtures is highly dependent on the species and proportions of components. Legumes tend to enhance the quality and nutritional worth of mixed forage owing to their elevated protein concentration. Researchers found that cereal/legumes (fava bean, lupin, and pea) mixed cropping resulted in a significant increase of CP of mixed forage up to 132 g/kg of DM [81].

The University of Wisconsin forage advisor suggests that the timing of harvesting pea barley, pea wheat, and pea triticale mixtures should depend on the production group intended for feeding the silage [82]. The author links the harvesting of the barley-pea mixture to the cereal's phenological phases. When the barley is in the boot, with only a few heads visible in the field within the mixture (peas not yet flowering) he recommends this excellent digestibility but lower-yielding silage for dairy cows. The starch level is below 2%, yet it possesses a notable amount of energy. At the end of the milky growth stage to the early dough stage of barley (peas in mature flowering with pod initiation), he suggests this high DM and energy-yielding, cost-effective material for heifers and dry cows [82]. Its starch content is over 10%, but its energy content is lower than younger mixes in the boot stage.

Whole crop cereal-legume mixtures harvested at the early waxy growth stage are excellent and cost-effective forages for the growing heifers due to the balanced energy-protein ratio, allowing more corn silage to be used in the dairy herd. Consequently, these silages can be important parts of climate change strategy (**Table 11**).

5. Forage growing and feeding strategy for dry continental regions under climate change situation

As is well known, crop rotation involves growing different crops in a specific order. The following tables list strategies that can be used to effectively implement crop rotation under dry continental conditions (**Tables 9** and **11–13**). These different crop rotation examples that meet the requirements of high-producing dairy cows may reduce the heat stress of the dairy cattle during the summer in continental regions, and stabilise the farm forage bank providing adequate biomass yield per ha per year, even after a dry and hot vegetation summer period.

	Growth stages of cereals			
	In boot	**Heading**	**Milk stage**	**Dough stage**
Change in the proportion of peas in the mixture				
Pea ratio	24%	28%	38%	42%
CP (% DM)				
Barley	16.6	13.3	10	6.9
Barley and pea	18.6	15.9	14.0	11.3
ADF (% DM)				
Barley	35.5	39.8	40.1	45.8
Barley and pea	36.4	38.9	38.7	42.5
NDF (% DM)				
Barley	56.1	61.0	58.8	68.8
Barley and pea	53.3	57.5	54.3	60.3

Table 11.
Changes in the nutrient content of grain and mixed silages (2-year average) [83].

6. Conclusions

Based on the large number of literary data and scientific findings, the following most important conclusions can be drawn.

- Corn silage in the dry continental region faces significant challenges due to extremely low yields, high variability in poor nutritional values, and is therefore considered a high-risk crop. Strategic crop management decisions are essential to enhance the security of the feed bank and improve the quality of silage for dairy cattle. In regions with high levels of risk, it may be deemed necessary to eliminate corn silage from the feed ration; however, there exist alternative measures to ensure the stability of the corn silage supply.

- Winter cereals, which are cultivated from autumn to early spring, have the advantage of growing in a period of increased rainfall while avoiding the adverse effects of heat stress and drought. This presents a promising opportunity to mitigate the risks and minimise yield losses of corn caused by climate change. Therefore, the whole crop winter cereals can be part of a new forage strategy.

- The implementation of novel crop rotation systems, such as corn-whole crop rye, corn-whole crop triticale, brown midrib sorghum-whole crop triticale, or brown midrib sorghum-intensive high sugar grass double cropping, has proven to be highly efficient in mitigating yield reductions caused by climate change in arid continental areas. Moreover, these innovative systems contribute to the stabilisation of the forage bank within dairy farms.

- Intensive cultivation of grass silages (*Lolium multiflorum*, Festulolium var.), whole crop rye silage (harvested in boot stage or earlier), triticale, barley, and wheat silage (harvested in boot-early heading stage) could potentially enhance

	Risk factor	First year			Second year		Third year	
		Spring	Summer	Autumn	Spring	Autumn	Spring	Autumn
Emergency situation	+++	Forage oat[A]	Forage millet[A]	Forage rye[A]	Silage corn[A]	Forage triticale[A]	Sudangrass[C]	Forage triticale[A]
	+++	Forage triticale[A] spring triticale[A]	Sudangrass[C]	Forage triticale[A]	BMR sorghum[B]	Forage rye[A]	Silage corn[A]	Forage triticale[A]
	+++	Oats with peas[C]	Forage millet[A]	Forage triticale[A]	BMR sorghum[B]	Forage rye[A]	Silage corn[A]	Forage triticale[A]

[A]*Good for lactating dairy cows.*
[B]*only for dual-purpose cattle breeds.*
[C]*only for breeding heifers, fattening, lactating beef cows in winter.*

Table 12.
Crop rotation examples in case of failure of crops in spring (Orosz, unpublished).

	Risk factor	Forages					
Forage + grain focus	++	Silage corn	Wheat (grain)		Sudangrass + legumes	Sunflower	Forage rye
	++	Rapeseed	Sudangrass/forage rye	Silage corn	Wheat (grain)		Rapeseed
Forage and seed production	+	Sudangrass	Seed production: clover		Sudangrass + legumes	Oilseed rape	Forage triticale
Forage + grain +seed production	++	Festulolium/Italian ryegrass + clover	Seed production: vetch and wheat		Sudangrass + legumes	Corn (grain)/ sunflower	Festulolium/Italian ryegrass + clover

Table 13.
Crop rotation examples for various purposes (Németh and Fazekas, unpublished).

the dry matter intake of dairy cows in hot summer conditions due to their high NDF digestibility, digestible NDF content, and low undigestible NDF levels. These forages may be classified as heat-stress forages in the context of cattle feeding in dry continental areas of Europe.

- The degradable NDF content of whole-crop winter cereals harvested at the boot stage exceeds that of corn silage by around 40–50%. Consequently, early-cut whole-crop cereals serve as significant sources of rumen degradable fibre for high-producing dairy cows, particularly in dry continental Europe during the summer heat-stress period.

- In dry continental areas, it is advisable to take into account the utilisation of summer drought-resistant crops such as sorghum and sudangrass. Provided that the NDF digestibility surpasses 60%, these particular forages can be incorporated into the diet of dairy cows.

Author details

Róbert Tóthi[1*], Szilvia Orosz[2], Katalin Somfalvi-Tóth[3], László Babinszky[4] and Veronika Halas[1]

1 Institute of Physiology and Nutrition, Hungarian University of Agriculture and Life Sciences, Kaposvár Campus, Kaposvár, Hungary

2 Livestock Performance Testing Ltd., Gödöllő, Hungary

3 Institute of Agronomy, Hungarian University of Agriculture and Life Sciences, Kaposvár Campus, Kaposvár, Hungary

4 Department of Animal Nutrition and Physiology, Hungarian University of Agriculture and Life Sciences, Kaposvár Campus, Kaposvár and University of Debrecen, Faculty of Agricultural and Food Sciences and Environmental Management, Debrecen, Hungary

*Address all correspondence to: tothi.robert@uni-mate.hu

References

[1] Lobell DB, Field CB. Global scale climate–crop yield relationships and the impacts of recent warming. Environmental Research Letters. 2007;**2**:014002. DOI: 10.1088/1748-9326/2/1/014002

[2] Wahid A, Gelani S, Ashraf M, Foolad MR. Heat tolerance in plants: An overview. Environmental and Experimental Botany. 2007;**61**:199-223. DOI: 10.1016/j.envexpbot.2007.05.011

[3] Gourdji SM, Sibley AM, Lobell DB. Global crop exposure to critical high temperatures in the reproductive period: Historical trends and future projections. Environmental Research Letters. 2013;**8**:024041. DOI: 10.1088/1748-9326/8/2/024041

[4] Liu C, Allan RP. Observed and simulated precipitation responses in wet and dry regions 1850-2100. Environmental Research Letters. 2013;**8**:034002. DOI: 10.1088/1748-9326/8/3/034002

[5] Orosz Sz, Balogh K. Corn silage 2012-2022 (dry continental region of Europe). In: Proceedings of the XIXth International Conference of Forage Conservation, Czech Republic, Brno, April 25-27, 2023. Published by Mendel University in Brno, CZ; 2023. pp. 100-101

[6] Long E, Ketterings QM, Czymmek KJ. Survey of cover crop use on New York dairy farms. Crop Management. 2013;**12**:1-5. DOI: 10.1094/CM-2013-0019-RS

[7] Long E, Van Slyke K, Kettering QM, Godwin G, Czymmek K. Triticale as a cover and double crop on a New York dairy. What's Cropping Up? 2013;**23**:3-5

[8] Graham C, Van Es H, Schindelbeck B. Rye vs. oat: Environmental benefits vary greatly. What's Cropping Up? 2012;**22**:3-4

[9] Lyons SE, Kilcer TF, Ort S, Swink S, Godwin G, Hanshar J, et al. Nutrient Management Spear Program. USA: Cornell University; 2016

[10] Henry B, Charmley E, Eckard R, Gaughan JB, Hegarty R. Livestock production in a changing climate: Adaptation and mitigation research in Australia. Crop and Pasture Science. 2012;**63**:191-202. DOI: 10.1071/CP11169

[11] Chapman SC, Chakraborty S, Dreccer MF, Howden SM. Plant adaptation to climate change: Opportunities and priorities in breeding. Crop and Pasture Science. 2012;**63**:251-268. DOI: 10.1071/CP11303

[12] Polley HW, Briske DD, Morgan JA, Wolter K, Bailey DW, Brown JR. Climate change and north American rangelands: Trends, projections, and implications. Rangeland Ecology & Management. 2013;**66**:493-511. DOI: 10.2111/REM-D-12-00068.1

[13] IPCC. Climate change 2023: Synthesis report. In: Core Writing Team, Lee H, Romero J, editors. Contribution of Working Groups I, II and III to the Sixth Assessment Report of the Intergovernmental Panel on Climate Change. Geneva, Switzerland: IPCC; 2023. pp. 35-115. DOI: 10.59327/IPCC/AR6-9789291691647

[14] Christensen JH, Larsen MAD, Christensen OB. Robustness of European climate projections from dynamical downscaling. Climate Dynamics. 2019;**53**:4857-4869. DOI: 10.1007/s00382-019-04831-z

[15] Kottek M, Grieser J, Beck C, Rudolf B, Rubel F. World map of the Köppen-Geiger climate classification updated. Meteorologische Zeitschrift. 2006;**5**:259-263. DOI: 10.1127/0941-2948/2006/0130

[16] Babinszky L, Halas V, Verstegen MWA. Impacts of climate change on animal production and quality of animal food products. In: Blanco JA, Kheradmand H, editors. Climate Change, Socioeconomic Effects. London, UK, London, UK: InTechOpen; 2011. pp. 165-190. DOI: 10.5772/23840

[17] Babinszky L, Dunkel Z, Tóthi R, Kazinczi G, Nagy J. The impacts of climate change on agricultural production. Hungarian Agricultural Research. 2011;**2**:14-20

[18] Santana ML, Bignardi AB, Pereira RJ, Stefani G, Faro LE. Genetics of heat tolerance for milk yield and quality in Holsteins. Animal The International Journal of Animal Biosciences. 2017;**11**:4-14. DOI: 10.1017/S1751731116001725

[19] Rhoads RP, Baumgard LH, Suagee JK, Sanders SR. Nutritional interventions to alleviate the negative consequences of heat stress. Advances in Nutrition. 2013;**4**:267-276. DOI: 10.3945/an.112.003376

[20] Calamari L, Petrera F, Abeni F, Bertin G. Metabolic and haematological profiles in heat-stressed lactating dairy cows fed diets supplemented with different selenium sources and doses. Livestock Science. 2011;**142**:128-137. DOI: 10.1016/j.livsci.2011.07.005

[21] Lundqvist M, Stigler J, Elia G, Lynch I, Cedervall T, Dawson KA. Nanoparticle size and surface properties determine the protein corona with possible implications for biological impacts. National Academy of Sciences of the United States of America. 2008;**105**:14265-14270. DOI: 10.1073/pnas.0805135105

[22] Callaway ES, Martin SA. Effects of a *Saccharomyces cerevisiae* culture on ruminal bacteria that utilize lactate and digest cellulose. Journal of Dairy Science. 1997;**80**:2035-2044. DOI: 10.3168/jds.S0022-0302(97)76148-4

[23] Bruno RGS, Rutigliano HM, Cerri RL, Robinson PH, Santos JEP. Effect of feeding *Saccharomyces cerevisiae* on performance of dairy cows during summer heat stress. Animal Feed Science and Technology. 2009;**150**:175-186. DOI: 10.1016/j.anifeedsci.2008.09.001

[24] Grant RJ, Contanch KW. Higher forage diets: Dynamics of passage, digestion and cow productive responses. In: Proceedings of Cornell Nutrition Conference for Feed Manufacturers, Syracuse, NY, USA. Ithaca, NY, USA: Cornell University; 2012. pp. 45-57

[25] Oba M, Allen MS. Evaluation of the importance of the digestibility of neutral detergent Fiber from forage: Effects on dry matter intake and milk yield of dairy cows. Journal of Dairy Science. 1999;**82**:589-596. DOI: 10.3168/jds.S0022-0302(99)75271-9

[26] Chase LE. Using grass forages in dairy cattle rations. In: Proceedings of the tri-State Dairy Nutrition Conference, Fort Wayne, IN, USA. Ohio State University. 2012. pp. 75-85

[27] Logrieco A, Mulè G, Moretti A, Bottalico A. Toxigenic *Fusarium* species and mycotoxins associated with maize ear rot in Europe. European Journal of Plant Pathology. 2002;**108**:597-609. DOI: 10.1023/A:1020679029993

[28] Whitlow W. Evaluation of mycotoxin binders. In: Zimmermann NG, editor. Fourth Mid-Atlantic Nutrition

Conference. College Park, MD: University of Maryland; 2006

[29] Kennelly JJ, Weinberg ZG. Small grain silage. In: Buxton DR, Muck RE, Harrison JH, editors. Silage Science and Technology. Madison, WI, USA: American Society of Agronomy. Crop Science Society of America and Soil Science Society of America; 2003. pp. 749-779

[30] Droushiotis DN. The effect of variety and harvesting stage on forage production of barley in a low-rainfall environment. The Journal of Agricultural Sciences. 1984;**102**:289-293. DOI: 10.1017/S002185960004260X

[31] Nass HG, Kunelius HT, Suzuki M. Effect of nitrogen application on barley, oats, and triticale grown as forage. Canadian Journal of Plant Sciences. 1975;**55**:49-53

[32] Bagg J, Johnson P. Double cropping fall rye for extra forage. Field Crop News. Available from: http://fieldcropnews.com/2013/08/doublecropping-fall-ryefor-extraforage [Accessed: August 28, 2023]

[33] Ketterings Q, Ort S, Swink S, Godwin G, Kilcer T, Miller J. Winter cereals as double crops in corn rotations on New York dairy farms. The Journal of Agricultural Science. 2015;**7**:18-25. DOI: 10.5539/jas.v7n2p18

[34] Auerbach H, Theobald P. Additive type affects fermentation, aerobic stability and mycotoxin formation during air exposure of early-cut rye (*Secale cereale* L.) silage. Agronomy. 2020;**10**:1432. DOI: 10.3390/agronomy10091432

[35] Orosz Sz, Kruppa J, Junior JK, Szemethy D, Fülöp EP, Futó Z, et al. Harvest window: Comparison of whole crop rye and whole crop triticale in an early cut system. In: Proceedings of the XVIIIth International Silage Conference, Bonn, Germany, 24-26 July 2018. Germany: University of Bonn; 2018. pp. 516-517

[36] Orosz Sz. Comparison of NDF degradability and degradation rate of different silages in Hungary (2013-2018). The 'heat stress diet' aspect. In: Proceedings of the XVIIIth International Conference of Forage Conservation, Czech Republic, Brno, August 13-16, 2019. Brno, Czech: Mendel University; 2019. pp. 152-153

[37] Orosz Sz, Horváthné Kovács B, Hoffmann R. Effect of 7-14 days delay in cut on yield and nutritive value of whole crop rye during the April-may harvest period. In: Proceedings of the XVIth International Conference of Forage Conservation, Czech Republic, Brno, June 3-6. Brno, Czech: Mendel University; 2014. pp. 153-154

[38] Baldinger L, Zollitsch W, Knaus WF. Corn silage and Italian ryegrass silage as high-energy forages in organic dairy cow diets: Differences in feed intake, milk yield and quality, and nitrogen efficiency. Renewable Agriculture and Food Systems. 2013;**29**:378-387. DOI: 10.1017/S1742170513000252

[39] Tamburini A, Rapetti L, Crovetto GM, Succi G. Rumen degradability of dry matter, NDF and ADF in Italian ryegrass (Lolium multiflorum) and winter cereal silages. Zootecnica e Nutrizione Animale. 1995;**21**(Suppl.):75-80

[40] Turner LB, Cairns AJ, Armstead P, Ashton J, Skøt K, Whittaker D, et al. Humphreys. Dissecting the regulation of fructan metabolism in perennial ryegrass (Lolium perenne) with quantitative trait locus mapping. New Phytologist. 2006;**169**:45-58. DOI: 10.1111/j.1469-8137.2005.01575.x

[41] Pavis N, Chatterton NJ, Harrison PA, Baumgartner S, Praznik W, Boucaud J, et al. Structure of fructans in roots and leaf tissues of Lolium perenne. New Phytologist. 2001;**150**:83-95. DOI: 10.1046/j.1469-8137.2001.00069.x

[42] Miller LA, Moorby JM, Davies DR, Humphreys MO, Scollan ND, MacRae JC, et al. Increased concentration of water-soluble carbohydrates in perennial ryegrass (*Lolium perenne* L.). Milk production from late-lactation dairy cows. Grass and Forage Science. 2001;**56**:383-394. DOI: 10.1046/j.1365-2494.2001.00288.x

[43] Narasimhalu P, Kunelius HT, McRae KB, Winter KA. Composition, intake, and digestibility of timothy and Italian and Westerwolds ryegrass silages. Canadian Journal of Plant Science. 1985;**65**:99-105. DOI: 10.4141/cjps85-014

[44] National Research Council. Nutrient Requirements of Dairy Cattle. 7th Rev ed. Washington, DC, USA: National Academy Press; 2001

[45] Jacobs JL, Hill J, Jenkin T. Effect of stage of growth and silage additives on whole crop cereal silage nutritive and fermentation characteristics. Animal Production Science. 2009;**49**:595-607. DOI: 10.1071/EA08244

[46] Lopes FDE, Cook DKC. Effects of varying ratios of corn silage to alfalfa silage on digestion of neutral detergent fiber in lactating dairy cows. Journal of Dairy Science. 2015a;**98**:6291-6303. DOI: 10.3168/jds.2014-8662

[47] Lopes F, Cook DE, Combs DK. Validation of an in vitro model for predicting rumen and total-tract fiber digestibility in dairy cows fed corn silages with different in vitro neutral detergent fiber digestibilities at 2 levels of dry matter intake. Journal of Dairy Science. 2015b;**98**:574-585. DOI: 10.3168/jds.2014-8661

[48] Combs D. Using in vitro total-tract NDF digestibility in forage evaluation. University of Wisconsin extension. Wisconsin Team Forage, Focus on Forage. 2016;**15**:1-3

[49] Verbeten WD, Combs DK, Undersander DJ. Partially replacing alfalfa and corn silage with fescue silages maintained fat-corrected milk production. Journal of Dairy Science. 2011;**94**(E-Suppl. 1):556

[50] Bernard JK, West JW, Trammell DS. Effect of replacing corn silage with annual ryegrass silage on nutrient digestibility, intake, and milk yield for lactating dairy cows. Journal of Dairy Science. 2002;**85**:2277-2282. DOI: 10.3168/jds.S0022-0302(02)74307-5

[51] Baldinger L, Baumung R, Zollitsch W, Knaus WF. Italian ryegrass silage in winter feeding of organic dairy cows: Forage intake, milk yield, and composition. Journal of the Science of Food and Agriculture. 2011;**91**:435-442. DOI: 10.1017/S1742170513000252

[52] Cooke KM, Bernard JK, West JW. Performance of dairy cows fed annual ryegrass silage and corn silage with steam-flaked or ground corn. Journal of Dairy Science. 2008;**91**:2417-2422. DOI: 10.3168/jds.2007-0715

[53] Alemayehu W, Tóthi R, Orosz Sz, Fébel H, Kacsala L, Húth B, et al. In situ ruminal degradability and fermentation characteristics of novel mixtures of winter cereals and Italian ryegrass plus winter cereal grain silages. Czech Journal of Animal Science. 2020;**66**:302-314. DOI: 10.17221/12/2021-CJAS

[54] Alemayehu W, Tóthi R, Orosz Sz, Fébel H, Tossenberger J,

Húth B, et al. Nutritive value of ensiled Italian ryegrass and winter cereal mixture. Acta Fytotechnica et Zootechnica (Monothematic Issue: Future Perspectives in Animal Production). 2020;**23**. DOI: 10.15414/afz.2020.23.mi-fpap.7-14

[55] Alemayehu W, Tóthi R, Orosz Sz, Fébel H, Kacsala L, Drew V, et al. Novel mixtures of Italian ryegrass and winter cereals: Influence of ensiling on nutritional composition, fermentation characteristics, microbial counts and ruminal degradability. Italian Journal of Animal Science. 2021;**20**:749-761. DOI: 10.1080/1828051X.2021.1924883

[56] Alemayehu W, Tóth T, Orosz Sz, Fébel H, Kacsala L, Húth B, et al. Aroma profile, microbial and chemical quality of ensiled green forage mixtures of winter cereals and Italian ryegrass. Agriculture. 2021;**11**:512. DOI: 10.3390/agriculture11060512

[57] Harper MT, Oh J, Giallongo F, Roth GW, Hristov AN. Inclusion of wheat and triticale silage in the diet of lactating dairy cows. Journal of Dairy Science. 2017;**100**:6151-6163. DOI: 10.3168/jds.2017-12553

[58] Geren H. Dry matter yield and silage quality of some winter cereals harvested at different stages under mediterranean climate conditions. Turkish Journal of Field Crops. 2012;**19**:197-202. DOI: 10.17557/tjfc.55884

[59] Baron V, Erasmus KO, Dick CA. Optimizing yield and quality of cereal silage. In: Proceedings of the 2000 Western Canadian Dairy Seminar. Vol. 12. Western Forage-Beef Group, Agriculture and Agri-Food Canada. Advanced Dairy Science and Technology. Edmonton, Canada: University of Alberta; 2000. pp. 351-367

[60] Larsen RJ, Beres BL, Blackshaw RE, Graf RJ. Extending the growing season: Winter cereals in western Canada. Candian Journal of Plant Science. 2018;**98**:267-277. DOI: 10.1139/cjps-2017-0278

[61] Ranck EJ, Holden LA, Dillon JA, Rotz CA, Soder KJ. Economic and environmental effects of double cropping winter annuals and corn using the integrated farm system model. Journal of Dairy Science. 2019;**103**:3804-3815. DOI: 10.3168/jds.2019-17525

[62] Sanderson MA, Jones RM, Ward J, Wolfe R. Silage sorghum performance trial at Stevensville: Forage research in Texas. Rep. PR-5018. Texas Agricultural Experiment Station, Stephensville, USA. 1992

[63] Peacock JM. Response and tolerance of sorghum to temperature stress. In: International Crops Research Institute for the SemiArid Tropics. Sorghum in the Eighties: Proceedings of the International Symposium on Sorghum. Patancheru, 2-7 November, International Crops Research Institute for the Semi-Arid Tropics (ICRISAT), Hyderabad, ICRISAT Patancheru P.O., Andhra Pradesh, India. 1981. pp. 143-158

[64] Jahanzad E, Jorat M, Moghadam H, Sadeghpour A, Chaichi M-R, Dashtaki M. Response of a new and commonly grown forage sorghum cultivar to limited irrigation and planting density. Agricultural Water Management. 2013;**117**:62-69. DOI: 10.1016/j.agwat.2012.11.001

[65] Blum A, Mayer J, Golan G. Agronomic and physiological assessments of genotypic variation for drought resistance in sorghum. Australian Journal of Agricultural Research. 1989;**40**:49-61. DOI: 10.1071/AR9890049

[66] Bell J, Naylor C, Heflin K, Sirmon P, Porter N, Schnell R et al. AgriLife forage sorghum silage trial. 2019. Available from https://hale.agrilife.org/files/2019/12/2019-Texas-AM-AgriLife-Forage-Sorghum-Silage-Trial-by-Jourdan-Bell.pdf [Accessed: January 12, 2021]

[67] Miron J, Zuckerman E, Sadeh D, Adin G, Nikbachat M, Yosef E, et al. Yield, composition and in vitro digestibility of new forage sorghum varieties and their ensilage characteristics. Animal Feed Science and Technology. 2005;**120**:17-32. DOI: 10.1016/j.anifeedsci.2005.01.008

[68] Aydin G, Grant RJ, O'Rear J. Brown midrib sorghum in diets for lactating dairy cows. Journal of Dairy Science. 1999;**82**:2127-2135. DOI: 10.3168/jdsS0022 -0302(99)75456-1

[69] Bucholtz DL, Cantrell RP, Axtell JD, Lechtenberg VL. Lignin biochemistry of normal and brown midrib mutant sorghum. Journal of Agricultural and Food Chemistry. 1980;**28**:1239-1245. DOI: 10.1021/ jf60232a045

[70] Cherney JH, Cherney DJR, Akin DE, Axtell JD. The potential of brown-midrib, low-lignin mutants for improving forage quality. Advances in Agronomy. 1991;**46**:157-198. DOI: 10.1016/S0065-2113(08)60580-5

[71] Vogel KP, Jung HG. Genetic modification of herbaceous plants for feed and fuel. Critical Reviews in Plant Sciences. 2001;**20**:15-49. DOI: 10.1080/20013591099173

[72] Gerhardt RL, Fritz JO, Moore KJ, Jaster EH. Digestion kinetics and composition of normal and brown midrib sorghum morphological components. Crop Science. 1994;**34**:1353-1361. DOI: 10.2135/cropsci1994.0011183X003400050039x

[73] Grant RJ, Haddad SG, Moore KJ, Pedersen JF. Brown midrib sorghum silage for mid-lactation dairy cows. Journal of Dairy Science. 1995;**78**:1970-1980. DOI: 10.3168/jds.S0022-0302(95)76823-0

[74] Kilcer T. Sorghum alternative management. In: Crop Soil News. Advanced Ag Systems's 2021. Available from https://advancedagsys.com/wp-content/uploads/2021/01/Jan-2021-Sorghum-alternative.pdf. 2021 [Accessed: January 1, 2021]

[75] Kilcer T. Sorghum management alternative part II. Crop soil news. In: Advanced Ag Systems's. 2021. Available from https://advancedagsys.com/wp-content/uploads/2021/02/Feb-2021-Sorghum-Mgt-2.pdf [Accessed: January 2, 2021]

[76] Kilcer T. Nutrient enhanced BMR forage sorghum. In: Crop Soil News. Advanced Ag Systems's. 2023. Available from: https://advancedagsys.com/wp-content/uploads/2023/03/March-2023-Nutrient-enhanced-nutrition-forage-sorghum.pdf. 2023 [Accessed: January 3, 2023]

[77] Undersander D. Sorghums, sudangrasses, and sorghum-Sudan hybrids. University Wisconsin Extension, Wisconsin Team Forage Focus on Forage. 2003;**5**(5):1-2

[78] Oliver AL, Grant RJ, Pedersen JF, O'Rear J. Comparison of brown midrib-6 and -18 forage sorghum with conventional sorghum and corn silage in diets of lactating dairy cows. Journal of Dairy Science. 2004;**87**:637-644. DOI: 10.3168/jds.S0022-0302(04)73206-3

[79] Sánchez-Duarte JI, Kalscheur KF, García AD, Contreras-Govea FE. Short communication: Meta-analysis of dairy cows fed conventional sorghum or corn silages compared with brown midrib sorghum silage. Journal of Dairy Science. 2018;**102**:1-7. DOI: 10.3168/jds.2018-14552

[80] Porter KS, Axtell JD, Lechtenberg VL, Colenbrander VF. Phenotype, fibre composition, and in vitro dry matter disappearance of the chemically induced brown midrib (BMR) mutants of sorghum. Crop Science. 1978;**18**:205-208. DOI: 10.2135/cropsci1978.0011183X0018 00020002x

[81] Strydhorst SM, King JR, Lopetinsky KJ, Harker KN. Forage potential of intercropping barley with faba bean, lupin, or field pea. Agronomy Journal. 2008;**100**:182-190. DOI: 10.2134/ agronj2007.0197

[82] Undersander D. Pea and small grain mixtures. University Wisconsin Extension, Wisconsin Team Forage Focus on Forage. 2003;**5**(7):1-2

[83] Johnston J, Wheeler B, McKinlay J. Forage production from spring cereals and cereal-pea mixtures. Ontario, Ministry of Agriculture Food & Rural Affairs (OMAF), Ontario. 1998. Available from: http://www.omafra.gov.on.ca/english/crops/facts/98-041.htm [Accessed: March 15, 2018]

Chapter 5

Heat Stress Mitigation through Feeding and Nutritional Interventions in Ruminants

Razia Kausar and Safdar Imran

Abstract

The livestock producers have been facing numerous challenges including feeding, management, diseases and environmental conditions. The changes in the environment, particularly heat stress, affect the comfort level that in turn affects production and reproduction. Heat stress in ruminants occurs due to an imbalance between heat dissipation rate and heat exposure from different sources. The external sources include environmental factors such as temperature, humidity, solar radiations, wind speed, wind direction and their indexes while internal sources of heat include metabolism. The high-producing ruminants consume more feed so higher metabolic rates produce more internal heat, which makes these animals prone to heat stress. Different heat stress mitigation strategies have been opted in the world. Nutritional interventions have been suitable and sustainable options. There are a number of nutrients/feed ingredients that may help in the mitigation of heat stress in ruminants. Supplementing ruminant feed with feed additives, minerals, vitamins, antioxidants and balancing the energy and protein level of feed and managing feeding patterns and feeding frequency have been taken as part of solution to provide relief from effects of heat stress. The nutritional interventions as a regular practice help in possible sustainable mitigation of heat stress in ruminants through regulating metabolic heat production level.

Keywords: heat stress, temperature humidity index, nutrition, ruminants, management

1. Introduction

The heat stress in livestock farming is a real factor of economic importance. The ruminants in the herd at below comfort level dispute the resources in nullifying the stress effects instead of presenting real production potential. It is necessary to mitigate the heat stress through management either by adding sprinklers and fans or through nutritional manipulation whichever fits better. The nutritional interventions present better version in term of reducing the metabolic heat production in ruminants leading to reduction in the required rate of heat dissipation and chances of heat stress. The ruminants across the globe are being reared for milk, meat and draft purposes too. Large ruminants have more requirements of food than small ruminants yet, the metabolic heat produced from fermentation and other metabolic processes both in large and small ruminants are as per the ratio of the physical structure and body capacity and the metabolic rate of these ruminants. Small ruminants have not been intensively selected for higher production at the level of genetic selection and breeding in large ruminants. The bulk of milk production in cows creates the need for a higher quantity of better composition-based feed to fulfill the protein and energy requirements of these large ruminants. These diets need higher metabolic rates for efficient conversion into valuable products, the higher metabolic rates produce more internal heat. Higher internal heat production needs more rapid dissipation of heat from the body. The external environmental temperature humidity index may influence the rate of heat dissipation. Any level of imbalance between heat exposure (from internal and external sources) and heat dissipation results in discomfort and heat stress. Heat stress in ruminants will impart negative impacts on production and reproduction, even on animal welfare. Heat stress mitigation strategies become need of hour under such conditions. These mitigation strategies have a wide range of applications starting from genetic selection to practically applying fans and cooling systems at farms. Yet, nutritional interventions for heat stress mitigation have been explored and applied for efficient and sustainable solutions. This chapter has covered various aspects of heat stress in ruminants and its mitigation through nutritional interventions.

2. Heat stress and ruminants

Animal's health, wellbeing and performance (both productive and reproductive) are affected by the climatic stressors. The ruminants in the world face environmental pressure, yet in tropics due to high environmental temperature as compared to cold regions, these animals bear more stress from the temperature extremes, particularly higher temperature combined with humidity. Heat stress in temperate areas is also a factor affecting ruminants during summer months. However, global animal production is increasing especially in tropical and subtropical areas of the world [1]. The contribution in production is also associated with the consumption of food of ruminant origin in various regions of the world. The severe heat stress causes losses at farms in terms of morbidity, sometimes even mortality, and reduced performance resulting in heavy economic losses. The rising global temperature predictions suggest a rise in the level of heat stress in ruminants in the future.

The ruminant's level of production and metabolic heat production rates are positively correlated. The genetically improved or selected animals for higher production performance may have chances of higher susceptibility to heat stress from higher ambient temperatures. Other factors include nocturnal temperatures, wind velocity, cloud cover along with air temperature and humidity which collectively or individually affect the animal's capacity to dissipate heat and maintain homeostasis [2].

However, the selection for high production is desirable for traits of economic importance including milk and meat in ruminants. The climatic condition in which ruminants are being reared is critically important. The ruminants feel heat stress when there is an imbalance between external and internal temperature and disturbance in the heat loss mechanisms due to any possible factor related to living organisms. The temperature humidity index is one of these factors used to assess the thermal comfort zone of dairy cows [3, 4]. There is a thermoneutral zone for each species at which animals generally feel comfortable without presenting any sign of thermal stress. Generally, up to 25°C ambient temperature is considered normal, above which cattle start to feel heat stress. The comfortable THI has been reported to be between 67 and 72 in different studies [5]. The THI above this level will affect the ruminants in all aspects of their welfare, production, reproduction and product quality. The threshold THI for standing cows has been used as 70 and for lying cows as 65 [6]. However, the THI levels have been categorized into severe stress conditions (THI ≥ 90), mild stress ($80 \leq$ THI ≤ 89) and mild stress ($72 \leq$ THI ≤ 79) as mentioned in [7]. Furthermore, recent studies present that these above levels underestimate the true level of heat stress and submitted that the heat stress threshold level exists under or up to 68 THI [8].

The heat stress conditions can be chronic or acute. The heat stress is generally presented in terms of indexes prepared from the data of temperature and humidity, termed as temperature humidity index [THI]. The other indexes may include various relatable variables including solar radiations and wind speed. The ruminant's capacity to cope with these acute or chronic conditions may be assessed through temperature estimations from various processes including respiration, panting, heat production and body site temperatures including skin, rectal, vaginal and cloacal temperature. Skin temperature may be recorded from different body sites. The stress's indirect indicators can also be measured including production performances. The effects of heat stress are also evident at the molecular level in living beings [9]. These parameters in turn help to estimate the capacity of animal to dissipate the heat. Heat stress also threatens the global ecological balance [10]. Animals try to maintain their body temperature within the range of ±0.5°C [11]. The effects of heat stress on animals are evident in terms of production efficiency, reproductive performance and feed consumption [12]. The animals are offered with different feed types based on composition at different physiological stages and production stages. The heat stress in ruminants is assessed from the important variables including pulse rate, respiration rate, rectal temperature, skin temperature and sweating rate, these physiological processes help in maintaining homeostasis and heat balance in ruminants. Although these variables are important, genetic differences for these variables exist in animals at species and breed levels, besides the effects of physiological stage and age of animals. Heat stress in ruminants imparts varying level of effects from cellular to physiological stages.

3. Heat stress effects

Heat stress is the most expensive factor in livestock rearing in terms of losses [13]. The three more consistent factors predisposing animals to heat stress irrespective of production level include increasing global temperature, frequent heat waves and relocating animals to unfamiliar tropical environments, yet one more factor, extended weather extremes also increase the possibility of occurrence of heat stress. The heat stress affects not only the production and reproduction but also the product quality. Animals with a rapid rate of metabolism are considered more prone to the heat stress. The acute heat stress in ruminants (beef) before slaughtering, for example, can reduce the water holding capacity of meat, softness and pale color due to glycogenolysis [14]. While the chronic heat stress on the other hand reduces the glycogen level of muscles and resulting in dark and firm meat characteristics [15]. These effects present that heat stress at different levels and durations affects product quality in different ways.

The increased animal welfare issues are the first and foremost impact of heat stress in ruminant dairy cows [16] followed by reduced production, slow growth rates and fertility, deteriorating product quality, lowering the market price of the product, inconsistent quality and also the increasing treatment costs [17]. All these factors present the importance of prevention from heat stress and heat stress mitigation strategies. The genetic selection for higher production as compared to selection for heat tolerance and climate adaptability has been prioritized in the recent past, yet the shift to the latter will help in heat stress abatement.

The ruminants (Holstein heifers) are prone to heat stress if thermodynamics changes occur, for example, the heat production contributed from feed fermentation in the rumen increased the metabolic heat and the heat excretion from the body is not balanced due to external environmental factors [18]. Sweating is the main tool in ruminants for evaporative heat loss, yet it is more in bos indicus cattle due to short and sleek hair coats and higher blood flow to the skin as compared to bos taurus cattle. Likewise, in sheep, evaporative heat loss is a major factor for cooling the animal, yet fleece length affects the rate of evaporation and below 40 mm is considered better for thermoregulation.

Catecholamines (adrenaline and noradrenaline) mediate the heat stress response along with the autonomous nervous system in animals. The responses mediated include an increase in respiration rate, pulse rate, body temperature and also the increased blood flow toward skin instead of viscera to contribute to heat loss from the body. The catecholamines act on the β2-receptors to inhibit glucogenesis and activate the glycogenolysis through a series of reactions in muscles mediated through cyclic adenosine monophosphate, resulting in inhibition of glycogen synthase and activation of glycogen phosphorylase [19]. The heat stress also increases the concentration of plasma glucocorticoids by activation of hypothalamic-pituitary-adrenal axis. These glucocorticoids increase vasodilation, and proteolysis and alter lipid metabolism, vasodilation facilitates the heat loss mechanism [20].

The decreased feed intake is another prominent effect of heat stress. The reduction in feed conversion ratio has also been observed in steers [21]. The ruminants counter the thermal stress through reduction in feed intake to keep the metabolic heat at lowest during high ambient temperature and humidity, as a natural response [22, 23]. The feed intake reduction only presents about 50% of the effects of heat stress, rest are explained through the changes in hormonal level of animals. The water intake requirements are increased twofolds during heat stress in animals. This increased water intake is important to balance the evaporative loss in ruminants (sheep) through sweating and panting [24]. It also directly increases the cooling of the rumen, so the water shortage or scarcity or lack of access to water during heat stress may trigger more harmful responses and also the dehydration in animals.

Heat stress may also induce oxidative stress through increasing reactive oxygen species and decreasing natural antioxidants. Lipid and protein oxidation, free radical mediated reactions, cytotoxicity occur due to tissue acidosis and oxidative stress which in turn result in animal health impairment, production losses and decrease in product quality [25]. Oxidative stress can even damage the cellular contents and biological molecules including carbohydrates, cholesterol, lipids, proteins and genetic material such as DNA and RNA [25]. The heat shock proteins (HSPs) also act as indicators of heat stress in ruminants. The expression of heat shock protein increases due to heat stress [26]. The heat shock proteins are important elements of living cells helping in cell repair and maintenance and cytoskeleton modulation [27]. The increased level of HSPs alters the tenderness of beef meat [28] and HSPs also play a role in proteolysis inhibition and meat toughness in sheep [29].

The thyroid gland is associated with thermogenesis in mammals. The reduced plasma concentration of triiodothyronine (T3) and tetraiodothyronine (T4) due to heat stress reduces the metabolic heat production preventing extra heat load as an adaptive mechanism and along with more actions including energy requirement reduction and reduction in lipolysis [30]. So, the reduced plasma concentration of thyroid hormone acts as an indicator of thermal tolerance in animals. The concentration of insulin increases from basal level and insulin sensitivity also increases as a result of heat stress in animals. As lipid metabolism generates more metabolic heat as compared to carbohydrates and proteins [31], the reduction in the metabolism of adipose tissues is considered heat tolerance evolutionary mechanism. The reduction in metabolism of adipose tissue is also attributed to the reduced thyroid hormones (see **Figure 1**).

Among ruminants, the feedlot cattle are more prone to heat stress [17]. There may be various factors including but not limited to rough radiant surfaces, high energy diets and less volunteering in seeking water, shade or ventilation [1]. The feed type of animals also contributes to susceptibility of heat stress, for example, increase in body temperature of cattle finished at grain is more than those fed on grasses [32]. The rapidly fermentable grains feeding to wethers (castrated male sheep) predispose them to heat stress as compared to slow-fermenting feed [33, 34]. The heat stress affects the weight gain in ruminants, two goat breeds presented different final weights after exposure to heat stress [35]. Heat stress contributes to altering the physiological mechanisms of the rumen, which may lead to metabolic disorders and related health problems [36, 37]. Changes in the metabolic mechanism in the rumen may alter the microbial population and pH, decrease rumination and rumen motility and decrease feed intake and salivary production [37]. To better understand the effects

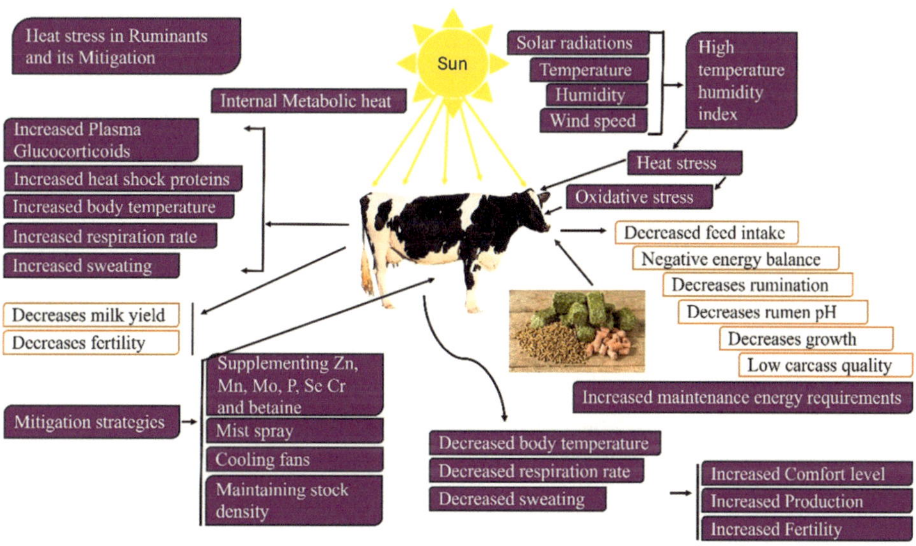

Figure 1.
Heat stress effects in cattle and its modulations.

of heat stress on metabolism, it is necessary to understand the metabolism in animals at comfort level. The metabolic adaptation to heat stress in dairy cows is attributed to the endocrine system and signaling proteins associated with these systems that may alter the endocrine status and target tissue responses if there is a heat stress challenge [31]. The effects of heat stress on feeding behavior are evident in dairy animals [38]. The exposure of cattle to heat stress during early lactation has negative impacts on the biochemical indices in blood, fertility and production [39].

4. Heat stress mitigation

The heat stress mitigation strategies are based on the basic reasons of heat stress. The thermal stress may be due to factors, alone or in combination, including high THI values, higher internal heat production (due to varying feed ingredients), feeding patterns, water intake frequency, animal's physiology, production level and farm management practices. Accordingly, mitigation strategies are devised to be implemented for efficient solutions. A basic understanding of the source of heat stress is of vital importance. The cooling aids or systems can be one of the approaches that can be applied on different production levels. The permanent solution for avoiding negative effects of heat stress, can be the genetic selection for thermo-tolerance, yet it may take time to bring in the final results and altering the genetic makeup of billions of animals particularly ruminants, however, once genetic changes have been achieved, there will be the availability of base population for future breeding and production of thermo-tolerant ruminants. As in the future, the effect of thermal stress seems to increase as a result of increasing global warming. It can be done by identification of thermotolerant animals from among the high-producing cows [40] so as to not reducing production when selecting for thermotolerance. However, it is established that selection for higher production has increased the chances of heat stress in highly producing animals. The high-yielding dairy cows, due to high energy requirement in transition period, undergo various physiological and metabolic adaptations [41]. These changes involve the increased lipolysis of adipose tissues and release of non-esterified fatty acids during third week before and up to 5th week after calving [42]. These are used for β-oxidation and in tricarboxylic acid cycle for generating energy, resulting in hepatic gluconeogenesis. However, in ruminants (dairy cattle), non-esterified fatty acids could be incompletely oxidized or re-esterified to triglycerides, resulting in a negative energy balance [43]. Different phenotypic markers, phenotypes and *omic* techniques may be implicated to identify the heat tolerant animals [44]. The anatomical and physiological differences of animals across the species or within species, including coat colors in animals, sweat gland density and sleek hair coat, can also be used for the selection of animals with thermotolerance or adaptability. Nutritional interventions are also of prime importance in animals for the heat stress mitigation. These interventions include different versions including balancing of energy in animal feed intake, changing the composition of the feed, energy and fiber contents of the feed offered, feeding time and feeding frequency, supplementation of vitamins and minerals and addition of yeasts and other feed additives to improve the provision of nutrients and at the same time to prevent the animal from internal metabolic impacts that possibly may contribute to the thermal stress. Such interventions lonely or in combination with managemental strategies including cooling aids and sprinkler systems may help in alleviating the negative effects of heat stress in feedlot cattle [45]. The interest in nutritional interventions to ameliorate the heat stress effects on production and health is rising [46]. The rumen degradable proteins and ruminal undegradable protein reduction in feed results in increased use of amino acid in synthesis of milk and also helps limit the catabolism in warm climate exposed cattle [47].

Supplementation of Ionophores in dairy cattle during heat stress improved the feed intake and feed efficiency [48]. Ionophores and monensin feeding also have beneficial effects in cattle experiencing heat stress [48]. The dietary cation-anion differences and bicarbonates by their buffering nature also contribute to relief from the heat stress in animals. Supplementing dietary yeast improves the condition of heat-stressed animals. Cows in summers fed with a diet containing ruminal by-pass fats and good crude protein contents maintain the production level and also have cooling effects by less metabolic heat production. Lactating dairy cows fed on a palm oil-supplemented diet have better dry matter intake and fewer signs of heat stress [49]. The heat stress has affected the nitrogen utilization, rumen function and digestibility in buffalo [50]. The negative energy balance has been improved in animals during heat stress when fed on a diet containing conjugated linoleic acids, yet it reduces the milk fat percentage. Supplementation of lipoic acid could be beneficial for alleviating heat stress in animals due to its effects on metabolism. The heat stress may also disrupt the metabolism along with effects on other physiological parameters.

The minerals, including Mn, Mo, P, Se and Zn, in animal feed improve the metabolism and health of animals. The supplementation of Zn in ruminants (dairy cows) during heat stress and mist sprays help in reducing effects of heat stress and maintaining the production level [51]. The dietary supplementation of Zn improves the intestinal health and has potent antioxidant effects. The dietary antioxidants mitigate the heat stress.

Vitamin A, which comprises retinol, retinal, and retinoic acid, presents a vital role in body functions including vision, growth and reproduction and possesses powerful antioxidant property [52]. This vitamin helps in mitigating the oxidative stress created by heat exposure. The supplementation of vitamin D_3 and Ca reduced hyperthermia in heat-stressed Holstein cows and also reduced markers of leaky gut and inflammation [53]. Vitamins including ascorbic acid, Vitamin B, Vitamin E, protected Niacin and Nicotinic acid are beneficial in thermotolerance in Holstein cows [54]. Niacin supplementation improves the metabolism and reduces the thermal stress effects in lactating dairy cows. Vitamin B has anti-heat stress effects and anti-inflammatory effects. The nicotinic acid has protective effects on intestinal integrity against negative impacts of heat stress [55]. The dietary niacin improves the immune function of beef cattle during heat stress and provides relief from heat stress [56]. The supplementation of Vitamin C and niacin, either in combination or alone, alleviates the effects of heat stress and improves the feed conversion efficiency, digestibility, rumen fermentation, feed intake and milk yield in lactating Friesian cows [57].

The supplementation of dietary betaine helps in mitigating the negative effects incurred by the heat stress in Karan Fries heifers [58]. Dietary betaine and chromium supplementation improves the betterment of heat-stressed dairy cows and Girolando cows, improving energy metabolism and production [59–61]. Chromium (Cr) has potential antioxidant effects and prevents lipid peroxidation in heat-stressed animals as heat stress primarily may cause lipid peroxidation due to oxidative stress [60]. The Cr also improves the humeral and cellular immunity in buffalo calves under heat stress. The Cr also improves the function of insulin in insulin-sensitive tissues, resulting in better growth, improved feed intake, fertility parameters, carcass quality and immune functions [60]. Chromium propionate has potential heat stress mitigating effects in animals by reducing metabolic heat production. The supplementation of Chromium propionate in mid-lactation dairy cows increases the milk yield by improving dry matter intake, antioxidant status and by decreasing rectal temperature and respiration rate in Holstein cows [62]. Propionate supplementation also yields better results as its conversion into glucose is around 30%. Chromium propionate (Cr-Pro) and calcium propionate (Ca-Pro) supplementation provide relief from heat stress in Holstein dairy cows [63].

The dietary intake of substrates as an evolutionary mechanism of adaptation produces less insulin during summer in ruminants (Holstein) as compared to spring and winter [64]. The reduction in RDP and RUP resulted in lowering insulin levels in the body which has an association with fatty acid mobilization and utilization in lactating dairy cows [47]. Nutritional interventions are recommended to effectively mitigate the heat stress effects [51]. The diet containing higher dietary fiber contents was better taken by the heat stressed Holstein calves, as compared to particle size, resulting in increased intake of dietary fibers that increases the longer lying behavior, digestion, feed intake, growth and final body weight [65]. The effects of heat stress on rumen microbiota were observed [66]. The dietary curcumin nano-micelles benefited the rumen microbiota and increased the rumen function in heat-stress animals [67]. The exploration of further products and byproducts of plant origin, microbial origin and mineral and vitamins may contribute more to mitigating the unwanted effects of heat stress.

5. Conclusion

The ruminants reared in grazing or feedlot systems have been exposed to environmental conditions. The environmental conditions in temperate and tropical climates are different. During heat stress, animal welfare, production, reproduction and behavior are affected. The mitigation of the condition through nutritional interventions becomes the need of time. The nutrients in the rumen have different fates and different metabolic activities including regulation of metabolism, enriching ruminal microbiota, improving rumen function, maintenance of pH, improving digestibility and reducing metabolic heat production. Based on scientific studies, following conclusions were drawn:

1. The supplementation of vitamins, minerals, fatty acids, yeasts, products of microbial origin, probiotics and plant extracts helps in regulating the internal heat production level.

2. The nutritional interventions bring changes in cellular response in terms of heat shock proteins, favoring suitable microbiota in the rumen.

3. The nutritional interventions improve the physiological condition in ruminants including respiration rate, lowering body temperature and reducing the need for sweating.

These responses create comfort in ruminants and help in maintaining production too. Thus, the heat stress mitigation through nutritional intervention needs to be explored more at molecular, cellular and organism levels in ruminants to improve welfare, comfort and productivity and to reduce losses. The future prediction of global warming creates the need to pay more attention to explore and provide alternative sustainable nutritional solutions for heat stress mitigation.

Conflict of interest

The authors declare no conflict of interest.

Author details

Razia Kausar[1]* and Safdar Imran[2]

1 Department of Anatomy and Histology, Faculty of Veterinary Science, University of Agriculture, Faisalabad, Pakistan

2 Faculty of Veterinary and Animal Sciences, The Islamia University of Bahawalpur, Pakistan

*Address all correspondence to: razia.kausar@uaf.edu.pk

References

[1] Renaudeau D, Collin A, Yahav S, de Basilio V, Gourdine JL, Collier RJ. Adaptation to hot climate and strategies to alleviate heat stress in livestock production. Animal. 2012;**6**(5):707-728

[2] Edwards-Callaway LN, Cramer MC, Cadaret CN, Bigler EJ, Engle TE, Wagner JJ, et al. Impacts of shade on cattle well-being in the beef supply chain. Journal of Animal Science. 2021;**99**(2):skaa375

[3] Ammer S, Lambertz C, Von Soosten D, Zimmer K, Meyer U, Dänicke S, et al. Impact of diet composition and temperature–humidity index on water and dry matter intake of high-yielding dairy cows. Journal of Animal Physiology and Animal Nutrition. 2018;**102**(1):103-113

[4] Wildridge AM, Thomson PC, Garcia SC, John AJ, Jongman EC, Clark CE, et al. The effect of temperature-humidity index on milk yield and milking frequency of dairy cows in pasture-based automatic milking systems. Journal of Dairy Science. 2018;**101**(5):4479-4482

[5] Sammad A, Wang YJ, Umer S, Lirong H, Khan I, Khan A, et al. Nutritional physiology and biochemistry of dairy cattle under the influence of heat stress: Consequences and opportunities. Animals. 2020;**10**(5):793

[6] Pinto S, Hoffmann G, Ammon C, Amon T. Critical THI thresholds based on the physiological parameters of lactating dairy cows. Journal of Thermal Biology. 2020;**88**:102523

[7] Armstrong D. Heat stress interaction with shade and cooling. Journal of Dairy Science. 1994;77(7):2044-2050

[8] Pinto S, Hoffmann G, Ammon C, Amon B, Heuwieser W, Halachmi I, et al. Influence of barn climate, body postures and milk yield on the respiration rate of dairy cows. Annals of Animal Science. 2019;**19**(2):469-481

[9] Belhadj Slimen I, Najar T, Ghram A, Abdrrabba M. Heat stress effects on livestock: Molecular, cellular and metabolic aspects, a review. Journal of Animal Physiology and Animal Nutrition. 2016;**100**(3):401-412

[10] Rashamol VP, Sejian V, Bagath M, Krishnan G, Archana PR, Bhatta R. Physiological adaptability of livestock to heat stress: An updated review. Journal of Animal Behaviour and Biometeorology. 2020;**6**(3):62-71

[11] Henry B, Charmley E, Eckard R, Gaughan JB, Hegarty R. Livestock production in a changing climate: Adaptation and mitigation research in Australia. Crop & Pasture Science. 2012;**63**(3):191-202

[12] Daramola JO, Abioja MO, Onagbesan OM. Heat stress impact on livestock production. In: Sejian V, Naqvi S, Ezeji T, Lakritz J, Lal R, editors. Environmental Stress and Amelioration in Livestock Production. Berlin, Heidelberg: Springer; 2012. DOI: 10.1007/978-3-642-29205-7_3

[13] Babinszky L, Halas V, Verstegen MW. Impacts of Climate Change on Animal Production and Quality of Animal Food Products. Climate Change Socioeconomic Effects. Rijeka: IntechOpen; 2011

[14] Warner R, Dunshea F, Gutzke D, Lau J, Kearney G. Factors influencing the incidence of high rigor temperature in beef carcasses in Australia. Animal Production Science. 2014;**54**(4):363-374

[15] Adzitey F, Nurul H. Pale soft exudative (PSE) and dark firm dry (DFD) meats: Causes and measures to reduce these incidences-a mini review. International Food Research Journal. 2011;**18**(1):11-20

[16] Becker C, Collier R, Stone A. Invited review: Physiological and behavioral effects of heat stress in dairy cows. Journal of Dairy Science. 2020;**103**(8):6751-6770

[17] Gonzalez-Rivas PA, Chauhan SS, Ha M, Fegan N, Dunshea FR, Warner RD. Effects of heat stress on animal physiology, metabolism, and meat quality: A review. Meat Science. 2020;**162**:108025

[18] Tajima K, Nonaka I, Higuchi K, Takusari N, Kurihara M, Takenaka A, et al. Influence of high temperature and humidity on rumen bacterial diversity in Holstein heifers. Anaerobe. 2007;**13**(2):57-64

[19] Franch J, Aslesen R, Jensen J. Regulation of glycogen synthesis in rat skeletal muscle after glycogen-depleting contractile activity: Effects of adrenaline on glycogen synthesis and activation of glycogen synthase and glycogen phosphorylase. The Biochemical Journal. 1999;**344**(1):231-235

[20] Kuo T, Harris CA, Wang J-C. Metabolic functions of glucocorticoid receptor in skeletal muscle. Molecular and Cellular Endocrinology. 2013;**380**(1-2):79-88

[21] Canozzi M, Clariget J, Roig G, Pérez E, Aznárez V, Banchero G, et al. Shade effect on behaviour, physiology, performance, and carcass weight of heat-stressed feedlot steers in humid subtropical area. Animal Production Science. 2022;**62**(17):1692-1705

[22] Russell JB. Can the heat of ruminal fermentation be manipulated to decrease heat stress. In: Proceedings of the 22nd Annual Southwest Nutrition and Management Conference. Vol. 22. Ithaca, New York; 2007. pp. 109-115

[23] Odongo N, AlZahal O, Lindinger M, Duffield T, Valdes E, Terrell S, et al. Effects of mild heat stress and grain challenge on acid-base balance and rumen tissue histology in lambs. Journal of Animal Science. 2006;**84**(2):447-455

[24] Marai I, El-Darawany A, Fadiel A, Abdel-Hafez M. Physiological traits as affected by heat stress in sheep—a review. Small Ruminant Research. 2007;**71**(1-3):1-12

[25] Celi P, Gabai G. Oxidant/antioxidant balance in animal nutrition and health: The role of protein oxidation. Frontiers in Veterinary Science. 2015;**2**:48

[26] Cruzen S, Pearce S, Baumgard L, Gabler N, Huff-Lonergan E, Lonergan S. Proteomic changes to the sarcoplasmic fraction of predominantly red or white muscle following acute heat stress. Journal of Proteomics. 2015;**128**:141-153

[27] Carra S, Alberti S, Arrigo PA, Benesch JL, Benjamin IJ, Boelens W, et al. The growing world of small heat shock proteins: From structure to functions. Cell Stress & Chaperones. 2017;**22**(4):601-611

[28] Bernard C, Cassar-Malek I, Le Cunff M, Dubroeucq H, Renand G, Hocquette J-F. New indicators of beef sensory quality revealed by expression of specific genes. Journal of Agricultural and Food Chemistry. 2007;**55**(13):5229-5237

[29] Cramer T, Penick ML, Waddell JN, Bidwell CA, Kim YHB. A new insight into meat toughness of callipyge lamb

loins-the relevance of anti-apoptotic systems to decreased proteolysis. Meat Science. 2018;**140**:66-71

[30] Collin A, Cassy S, Buyse J, Decuypere E, Damon M. Potential involvement of mammalian and avian uncoupling proteins in the thermogenic effect of thyroid hormones. Domestic Animal Endocrinology. 2005;**29**(1):78-87

[31] Min L, Zhao S, Tian H, Zhou X, Zhang Y, Li S, et al. Metabolic responses and "omics" technologies for elucidating the effects of heat stress in dairy cows. International Journal of Biometeorology. 2017;**61**:1149-1158

[32] Jacob R, Surridge V, Beatty D, Gardner G, Warner R. Grain feeding increases core body temperature of beef cattle. Animal Production Science. 2014;**54**(4):444-449

[33] Gonzalez-Rivas P, DiGiacomo K, Russo V, Leury B, Cottrell J, Dunshea F. Feeding slowly fermentable grains has the potential to ameliorate heat stress in grain-fed wethers. Journal of Animal Science. 2016;**94**(7):2981-2991

[34] Gonzalez-Rivas P, DiGiacomo K, Giraldo P, Leury B, Cottrell J, Dunshea F. Reducing rumen starch fermentation of wheat with three percent sodium hydroxide has the potential to ameliorate the effect of heat stress in grain-fed wethers. Journal of Animal Science. 2017;**95**(12):5547-5562

[35] Archana P, Sejian V, Ruban W, Bagath M, Krishnan G, Aleena J, et al. Comparative assessment of heat stress induced changes in carcass traits, plasma leptin profile and skeletal muscle myostatin and HSP70 gene expression patterns between indigenous Osmanabadi and Salem Black goat breeds. Meat Science. 2018;**141**:66-80

[36] Nardone A, Ronchi B, Lacetera N, Ranieri MS, Bernabucci U. Effects of climate changes on animal production and sustainability of livestock systems. Livestock Science. 2010;**130**(1-3):57-69

[37] Soriani N, Panella G, Calamari L. Rumination time during the summer season and its relationships with metabolic conditions and milk production. Journal of Dairy Science. 2013;**96**(8):5082-5094

[38] West JW. Effects of heat-stress on production in dairy cattle. Journal of Dairy Science. 2003;**86**(6):2131-2144

[39] Stefanska B, Sobolewska P, Fievez V, Pruszynska-Oszmałek E, Purwin C, Nowak W. The effect of heat stress on performance, fertility, and adipokines involved in regulating systemic immune response during lipolysis of early lactating dairy cows. Journal of Dairy Science. 2024;**107**(4):2111-2128

[40] Amamou H, Beckers Y, Mahouachi M, Hammami H. Thermotolerance indicators related to production and physiological responses to heat stress of holstein cows. Journal of Thermal Biology. 2019;**82**:90-98

[41] Heirbaut S, Jing X, Stefańska B, Pruszyńska-Oszmałek E, Buysse L, Lutakome P, et al. Diagnostic milk biomarkers for predicting the metabolic health status of dairy cattle during early lactation. Journal of Dairy Science. 2023;**106**(1):690-702

[42] Contreras GA, Strieder-Barboza C, De Koster J. Symposium review: Modulating adipose tissue lipolysis and remodeling to improve immune function during the transition period and early lactation of dairy cows. Journal of Dairy Science. 2018;**101**(3):2737-2752

[43] Mann S. Symposium review: The role of adipose tissue in transition dairy

cows: Current knowledge and future opportunities. Journal of Dairy Science. 2022;**105**(4):3687-3701

[44] Carabaño MJ, Ramón M, Menéndez-Buxadera A, Molina A, Díaz C. Selecting for heat tolerance. Animal Frontiers. 2019;**9**(1):62-68

[45] Castro-Pérez BI, Estrada-Angulo A, Ríos-Rincón FG, Núñez-Benítez VH, Rivera-Méndez CR, Urías-Estrada JD, et al. The influence of shade allocation or total shade plus overhead fan on growth performance, efficiency of dietary energy utilization, and carcass characteristics of feedlot cattle under tropical ambient conditions. Asian-Australasian Journal of Animal Sciences. 2020;**33**(6):1034

[46] Khafaga AF, Noreldin AE, Taha AE. The adaptogenic anti-ageing potential of resveratrol against heat stress-mediated liver injury in aged rats: Role of HSP70 and NF-kB signalling. Journal of Thermal Biology. 2019;**83**:8-21

[47] Kaufman J, Pohler K, Mulliniks J, Ríus A. Lowering rumen-degradable and rumen-undegradable protein improved amino acid metabolism and energy utilization in lactating dairy cows exposed to heat stress. Journal of Dairy Science. 2018;**101**(1):386-395

[48] Barreras A, Castro-Pérez B, López-Soto M, Torrentera N, Montaño M, Estrada-Angulo A, et al. Influence of ionophore supplementation on growth performance, dietary energetics and carcass characteristics in finishing cattle during period of heat stress. Asian-Australasian Journal of Animal Sciences. 2013;**26**(11):1553

[49] Melo R, Castro L, Cardoso F, Barbosa E, Melo L, Silva R, et al. Supplementation of palm oil to lactating dairy cows fed a high fat diet during summer. Journal of Animal Science. 2016;**94**:640-641

[50] Yadav B, Yadav P, Kumar M, Vasvani S, Anand M, Kumar A, et al. Effect of heat stress on Rumen microbial diversity and fermentation pattern in Buffalo. Advanced Gut and Microbiome Research. 2022;**2022**:1-14

[51] Molaee Berneti P, Mahdavi A, Chashnidel Y, Yousefi MH, Narenji Sani R, Farhadi I. The effect of management and nutrition strategies on the function and expression of HSP70 gene in dairy cows under heat stress. Iranian Journal of Veterinary Medicine. 2024;**18**:44

[52] Shastak Y, Gordillo A, Pelletier W. The relationship between vitamin A status and oxidative stress in animal production. Journal of Applied Animal Research. 2023;**51**(1):546-553

[53] Ruiz-González A, Suissi W, Baumgard L, Martel-Kennes Y, Chouinard P, Gervais R, et al. Increased dietary vitamin D3 and calcium partially alleviate heat stress symptoms and inflammation in lactating Holstein cows independent of dietary concentrations of vitamin E and selenium. Journal of Dairy Science. 2023;**106**(6):3984-4001

[54] Rungruang S, Collier J, Rhoads R, Baumgard L, De Veth M, Collier R. A dose-response evaluation of rumen-protected niacin in thermoneutral or heat-stressed lactating Holstein cows. Journal of Dairy Science. 2014;**97**(8):5023-5034

[55] Zou B, Long F, Xue F, Chen C, Zhang X, Qu M, et al. Protective effects of niacin on rumen epithelial cell barrier integrity in heat-stressed Beef Cattle. Animals. 2024;**14**(2):313

[56] Long F, Zou B, Wang L, Qu M, Chen C, Yang J, et al. Effects of Dietary Niacin on Serum Biochemical, Immune and Antioxidant Indexes of Beef Cattle under Heat Stress. Beijing, China:

Chinese Association of Animal Science and Veterinary Medicine; 2023

[57] Eweedah N, Salem A, Gaafar H, Shams A, Mahmoud A-A, Mesbah R, et al. Effect of Rumen-Protected Niacin and Vitamin C Supplements on Productive Performance of Lactating Friesian Cows under Heat Stress Condition. Pakistan: Pakistan Journal of Zoology; 2023

[58] Lakhani P, Kumar P, Alhussien MN, Lakhani N, Grewal S, Vats A. Effect of betaine supplementation on growth performance, nutrient intake and expression of IGF-1 in Karan Fries heifers during thermal stress. Theriogenology. 2020;**142**:433-440

[59] Wang B, Wang C, Guan R, Shi K, Wei Z, Liu J, et al. Effects of dietary rumen-protected betaine supplementation on performance of postpartum dairy cows and immunity of newborn calves. Animals. 2019;**9**(4):167

[60] Bin-Jumah M, Abd El-Hack ME, Abdelnour SA, Hendy YA, Ghanem HA, Alsafy SA, et al. Potential use of chromium to combat thermal stress in animals: A review. The Science of the Total Environment. 2020;**707**:135996

[61] Ribeiro LS, Brandão FZ, Carvalheira LR, Goes TJF, Torres Filho RA, Quintão CCR, et al. Chromium supplementation improves glucose metabolism and vaginal temperature regulation in Girolando cows under heat stress conditions in a climatic chamber. Tropical Animal Health and Production. 2020;**52**:1661-1668

[62] Wang M, Yang J, Shen Y, Chen P, Li Y, Cao Y, et al. Effects of chromium propionate supplementation on lactation performance, nutrient digestibility, rumen fermentation patterns, and antioxidant status in Holstein cows under heat stress. Animal Feed Science and Technology. 2023;**305**:115765

[63] Zhao C, Shen B, Huang Y, Kong Y, Tan P, Zhou Y, et al. Effects of chromium propionate and calcium propionate on lactation performance and Rumen microbiota in postpartum heat-stressed Holstein Dairy Cows. Microorganisms. 2023;**11**(7):1625

[64] Abdelnour SA, Abd El-Hack ME, Khafaga AF, Arif M, Taha AE, Noreldin AE. Stress biomarkers and proteomics alteration to thermal stress in ruminants: A review. Journal of Thermal Biology. 2019;**79**:120-134

[65] Izadbakhsh M-H, Hashemzadeh F, Alikhani M, Ghorbani G-R, Khorvash M, Heidari M, et al. Effects of dietary fiber level and forage particle size on growth, nutrient digestion, Ruminal fermentation, and behavior of Weaned Holstein Calves under heat stress. Animals. 2024;**14**(2):275

[66] Patra AK, Kar I. Heat stress on microbiota composition, barrier integrity, and nutrient transport in gut, production performance, and its amelioration in farm animals. Journal of Animal Science and Technology. 2021;**63**(2):211

[67] Bokharaeian M, Toghdory A, Ghoorchi T. Evaluating the dose-dependent effects of curcumin nano-micelles on rumen fermentation, nitrogen metabolism, and nutrient digestibility in heat-stressed fattening lambs: Implications for climate change and sustainable animal production. Journal of Animal Physiology and Animal Nutrition. 2024;**108**

Chapter 6

Advances in Managing Nitrogen and Phosphorus Emissions in Ruminants: A Holistic Approach

Zulfqarul Haq, Snober Irshad, Azmat Alam Khan, Syed Mudasir Ahmad and Showkeen Muzamil

Abstract

"Balancing Nutrition and Environmental Sustainability: Advances in Managing Nitrogen and Phosphorus Emissions in Ruminants" explores the intricate relationship between ruminant nutrition and environmental stewardship. It delves into the dynamics of nitrogen and phosphorus metabolism in ruminants, addressing the environmental repercussions of their emissions. These emissions, primarily in the form of ammonia and phosphates, pose significant environmental challenges, contributing to air and water pollution, soil degradation, and climate change. The chapter highlights innovative strategies and technological breakthroughs aimed at mitigating nitrogen and phosphorus excretion, crucial for reducing environmental pollution. It offers insights into dietary adjustments, feed additives, and best practices for sustainable ruminant production. Key areas of focus include dietary adjustments tailored to optimize nutrient utilization and reduce waste, the utilization of feed additives to enhance nutrient absorption and minimize excretion, and the implementation of best management practices to promote sustainable ruminant production. By integrating scientific findings with practical applications, this review underscores the importance of achieving harmony between nutrition optimization and environmental responsibility in modern agriculture. Through this comprehensive analysis, the chapter aims for balancing the dual goals of optimizing ruminant nutrition and minimizing environmental impact, thereby contributing to more sustainable and resilient agricultural systems.

Keywords: ruminants, reduction of nitrogen and phosphorus emissions, nutrition, water bodies, soil, crop production

1. Introduction

Nitrogen in ruminant systems primarily originates from protein in the feed. During digestion, protein is broken down into amino acids, which are either utilized for growth and milk production or deaminated, resulting in the production of ammonia (NH_3). Excess ammonia is converted into urea in the liver and excreted in urine.

When urine is excreted onto the soil, urea is rapidly hydrolyzed to ammonia, which can volatilize into the atmosphere or undergo nitrification and denitrification processes, leading to the formation of nitrous oxide (N_2O), a potent greenhouse gas [1]. Excess nitrogen can be converted to nitrate (NO_3-) and leach into groundwater, contributing to water pollution and eutrophication. Nitrogen emissions in ruminant production primarily stem from the metabolism of dietary protein by the animals, resulting in the excretion of nitrogen-rich compounds such as urea and ammonia. These emissions can lead to air and water pollution, contributing to acidification, eutrophication, and greenhouse gas emissions [2]. The environmental consequences underscore the urgent need to optimize nitrogen utilization within livestock systems. Phosphorus in ruminant diets is essential for various physiological functions, including bone formation and energy metabolism. However, ruminants typically have low efficiency in utilizing dietary phosphorus, leading to substantial amounts being excreted in feces [3]. When phosphorus-rich manure is applied to land, it can contribute to soil phosphorus accumulation and subsequent runoff into water bodies, causing eutrophication and harmful algal blooms. The environmental impacts of nitrogen and phosphorus emissions extend beyond localized pollution, affecting regional and global ecosystems [4].

Sustainable management of these nutrients in ruminant agriculture necessitates holistic strategies that consider animal nutrition, feed management, and manure handling practices. Ruminant agriculture plays a pivotal role in global food production, providing essential proteins and nutrients through the rearing of cattle, sheep, and goats. However, the environmental footprint associated with this sector, particularly in terms of nitrogen and phosphorus emissions, poses significant challenges to sustainability [5]. In recent decades, the intensification of ruminant production has led to heightened concerns about environmental pollution, driven largely by the excessive excretion of nitrogen and phosphorus from livestock operations. These nutrients, crucial for animal growth and metabolism, can become environmental pollutants when not efficiently utilized by the animals. Therefore, developing strategies to enhance nutrient utilization while reducing waste is essential for mitigating the environmental impact of ruminant agriculture [6]. Balancing nutrition in ruminant diets involves optimizing the intake and utilization of key nutrients such as protein and phosphorus. Achieving this balance not only enhances animal performance but also minimizes the release of excess nutrients into the environment.

Ruminant agriculture significantly contributes to N and P emissions, primarily through manure. These emissions can lead to environmental issues such as eutrophication and greenhouse gas emissions. Optimizing dietary formulations is a key strategy to improve nutrient efficiency and reduce these ecological footprints. According to Pell *et al.* [7], precise diet formulations can enhance nutrient efficiency, thereby reducing the environmental impact of ruminant farming. By tailoring diets to meet the exact nutritional needs of ruminants, it is possible to minimize excess nutrient excretion. Innovative dietary interventions and management practices are crucial for reducing N and P excretion while supporting animal health and welfare. These approaches include using feed additives, optimizing protein intake, and incorporating more digestible feed components to improve nutrient uptake and reduce waste.

The efficient utilization of nitrogen and phosphorus in ruminant diets is multifaceted and involves various aspects of animal nutrition, feed management, and waste handling. Moreover, the environmental impacts associated with nitrogen and phosphorus losses from ruminant production systems necessitate integrated solutions that consider both ecological and agronomic factors. By fostering a deeper understanding of the intricate relationship between ruminant nutrition and environmental sustainability, this chapter aims about promising avenues for achieving sustainable intensification in livestock production.

Management of nitrogen and phosphorus in agroecosystems.

- *Nitrogen and phosphorus* are both crucial for plant growth and are obtained through various organic and inorganic sources.

- Both nutrients face significant losses through crop harvest, erosion, and runoff, with nitrogen additionally lost through gaseous emissions.

- Management challenges include inefficiencies in nutrient use, environmental issues like eutrophication and GHG emissions for nitrogen, and soil fixation and loss of phosphorus.

- There are several management strategies available to mitigate these challenges, including conservation tillage, intercropping, mixed cropping-livestock systems, recycling organic matter, and landscape management (**Table 1**).

This table is useful for understanding the dynamics of nutrient management in agriculture and highlights the importance of integrated [8].

	Role in plants	Major sources into agroecosystems	Major losses from agroecosystems	Management challenges	Management opportunities
Nitrogen	Component of chlorophyll, amino acids, and nucleic acids	N-fixing plants, plant residue organic fertilizers, inorganic fertilizers, manure	Crop harvest Runoff & leaching Gaseous emissions	~50% N use efficiency Eutrophication GHGs	Conservation tillage, Covers and residues, Mixed cropping-livestock, Intercropping, Recycling organic matter Landscape design and management
Phosphorus	Component of DNA, RNA, ATP, and cell membranes	Organic fertilizers, inorganic fertilizers, manure	Crop harvest Erosion Runoff & leaching	P fixation in soil Peak P Soil loss Eutrophication	Conservation tillage, mycorrhizal interactions, Covers and residues, Mixed cropping-livestock, Recycling organic matter, pH management

Table 1.
Strategies to enhance nutrient use efficiency and minimize environmental impacts.

2. Nitrogen and phosphorus dynamics in ruminants

2.1 Nitrogen metabolism in ruminant animals

Nitrogen is an essential nutrient for ruminants, integral to their productivity and overall health. It is a key component of amino acids, the building blocks of proteins, which are crucial for growth, milk production, and other physiological functions. However, when excreted in excess, nitrogen becomes a significant environmental pollutant. It contributes to various environmental issues such as acid deposition, which can damage ecosystems, and eutrophication, which leads to excessive growth of algae in water bodies. This, in turn, can cause oxygen depletion and harm aquatic life. Nitrogen emissions also contribute to human respiratory problems and climate change through the release of nitrous oxide, a potent greenhouse gas. Understanding the intricacies of nitrogen metabolism in ruminants is essential to devise strategies to mitigate these environmental impacts while maintaining animal productivity.

In ruminants, the digestion of dietary proteins begins in the rumen, a specialized stomach chamber hosting a complex community of microbes. These microbes play a crucial role in breaking down plant proteins into smaller peptides and amino acids through enzymatic action [9]. The fermentation process in the rumen not only aids in protein breakdown but also facilitates the synthesis of microbial protein from non-protein nitrogen sources like ammonia. This microbial protein becomes a significant source of amino acids for the host animal, contributing substantially to its nutritional needs [10]. The efficiency of this process can be influenced by various factors, including the composition of the diet and the balance of nutrients provided.

One of the critical aspects of nitrogen metabolism in ruminants is the absorption and utilization of ammonia. Ammonia, released from the breakdown of amino acids and urea, is absorbed from the rumen into the bloodstream and transported to the liver, where it can be converted back into urea or used for microbial protein synthesis in the rumen [11]. This recycling of urea is a unique feature of ruminant metabolism, allowing the animal to conserve nitrogen and optimize its use. Urea is secreted in the saliva and returned to the rumen, where it is hydrolyzed back to ammonia, providing a continual source of nitrogen for microbial protein synthesis. This efficient recycling mechanism helps reduce the overall nitrogen excretion, though any imbalance can still lead to significant nitrogen losses.

Despite these efficient processes, some nitrogen is inevitably excreted. Excess nitrogen, not utilized for microbial protein synthesis or other physiological functions, is primarily excreted as urea in urine. This excretion helps maintain nitrogen balance within the animal but poses environmental challenges when managed poorly. The regulation of nitrogen metabolism in ruminants is a finely tuned process influenced by dietary protein intake, the activity of rumen microbes, and hormonal signals. Achieving a balance that maximizes nitrogen utilization while minimizing environmental impact requires a comprehensive understanding of these processes and the implementation of appropriate dietary and management strategies. The complexity of microbial metabolic activity in the rumen and its subsequent effects on intestinal and bodily processes underscore the challenge of studying nitrogen metabolism in ruminants compared to non-ruminants. This complexity necessitates ongoing research to develop sustainable practices that align ruminant productivity with environmental stewardship.

2.2 Ruminal degradation of protein

The ruminal degradation of protein begins with the attachment of bacteria to feed particles, followed by the activity of cell-bound microbial proteases [12]. Approximately 70 to 80% of ruminal microorganisms attach to undigested feed particles in the rumen [13], and 30 to 50% of these attached microbes exhibit proteolytic activity. A diverse consortium of microbial species forms a symbiotic association on each feed particle, working together to degrade and ferment nutrients, including proteins. The initial products of this microbial degradation are peptides and amino acids (AAs). The rate and extent of protein degradation depend on the proteolytic activity of the ruminal microflora and the type of protein, particularly the susceptibility and accessibility of peptide bonds. Peptides and AAs produced by extracellular proteolytic activity are then transported inside microbial cells, where they can be further utilized for microbial protein synthesis.

Protozoa, although present in lower numbers in continuous culture fermenters, play a significant role in protein degradation in vivo. These large, single-celled organisms have a remarkable ability to engulf substantial molecules, including proteins, carbohydrates (CHO), and even ruminal bacteria [14]. This engulfment process is crucial because protozoa can regulate bacterial nitrogen (N) turnover in the rumen and provide soluble protein to sustain microbial growth. Protozoa themselves cannot utilize ammonia nitrogen (NH3-N); instead, they contribute to the nitrogen cycle in the rumen by later returning a fraction of the previously engulfed insoluble protein to the rumen fluid as soluble protein. This re-release of soluble protein helps maintain a balance in nitrogen availability, which is essential for microbial growth and overall rumen function.

The dynamic interaction between bacteria and protozoa in the rumen highlights the complexity of protein degradation in ruminants. Protozoa play a regulatory role by modulating bacterial activity and contributing to the pool of soluble protein in the rumen. This interaction is vital for maintaining ammonia nitrogen concentrations at optimal levels, which is why defaunation, or removing protozoa, can lead to decreased ammonia nitrogen concentrations in the rumen [15]. The collaborative efforts of bacteria and protozoa ensure efficient protein degradation and utilization, underscoring the importance of these microorganisms in the overall nitrogen metabolism of ruminants. Understanding these processes is essential for optimizing protein use in ruminant diets and minimizing environmental nitrogen losses (**Figure 1**).

2.3 Factors affecting ruminal protein degradation

Ruminal protein degradation is influenced by several key factors, including the type of protein, interactions with other nutrients (mainly carbohydrates within the same feedstuff and the rumen contents), the predominant microbial population, the ruminal passage rate, and ruminal pH. Understanding these factors is crucial for optimizing protein utilization and improving the nutritional efficiency of ruminants.

- *Type of Protein*

The solubility of proteins is a fundamental factor determining their susceptibility to microbial proteases and thus their degradability. For instance, proteins such as

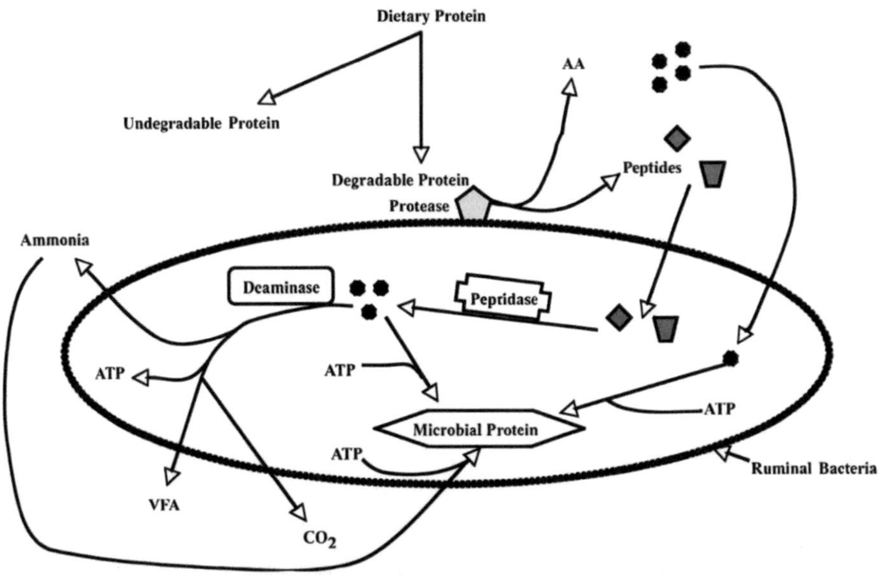

Figure 1.
Nitrogen metabolism in ruminants [16].

prolamins and glutelins are insoluble and degrade slowly, whereas globulins are soluble and highly degradable in the rumen [17]. However, the solubility of a protein alone does not fully dictate its degradation rate. The structural complexity of proteins, including the presence of disulfide bonds in some soluble albumins, can make them slowly degradable despite their solubility. The tertiary and quaternary structures, characterized by the bonds within and between protein chains, also significantly impact degradability. These structural features influence how accessible the proteins are to microbial enzymes. Consequently, proteins with complex structures may resist degradation despite their solubility, illustrating that multiple factors contribute to the overall degradability of proteins in the rumen.

- *Ruminal Dilution Rate*

Protein degradation is inversely related to the passage rate of digesta through the rumen. As the passage rate increases, the time proteins spend in the rumen decreases, leading to reduced degradation. According to NRC [18], a cow consuming 18 kg of dry matter (DM) of a 70:30 forage-to-concentrate ration would have a digesta passage rate of 0.049 to 0.057/h for wet forages, 0.040 to 0.046/h for dry forages, and 0.056 to 0.068/h for concentrates. If the same cow consumes 26 kg of DM of a 40:60 forage-to-concentrate ration, the passage rate increases, resulting in less time for ruminal microbes to act on the proteins. This can lead to modest reductions in protein degradation: 1.2 percentage units for standard ryegrass silage, 2.1 for alfalfa hay, and 3.5 for soybean meal [19]. Although these reductions are small, they represent a modest increase in the flow of undegraded dietary protein to the small intestine, thus enhancing the overall protein efficiency of dairy cows. Adjusting the forage-to-concentrate ratio to manage passage rates can be a strategic approach to improving protein utilization in ruminants.

- *Ruminal pH, substrate, and nutrient interaction*

The optimal pH range for rumen proteolytic enzymes is between 5.5 and 7.0 [20]. Within this range, protein degradation is most efficient. However, protein degradation decreases significantly when the ruminal pH falls below this optimal range. Low pH can affect the activity of proteolytic enzymes and alter the microbial population in the rumen. The type of substrate available in the rumen also plays a critical role in protein degradation. Nutrient interactions, such as the presence of carbohydrates, can influence the degradation process. Assoumani et al. [21] demonstrated that starch interferes with protein degradation, noting that the addition of amylase increased the total ruminal protein degradation of cereal grains by 6 to 20 percentage units. The combined effect of pH and substrate availability can modify the predominant microbial population, impacting overall protein degradation. For example, low pH can reduce the population of cellulolytic bacteria, which are essential for fiber degradation. This reduction in fiber degradation can limit the access of proteolytic bacteria to proteins, indirectly diminishing protein degradation.

2.4 Phosphorus (P) in ruminants: functionality and distribution

Phosphorus (P) is an essential macromineral for all forms of life, playing a crucial role in numerous biological processes. Phosphorus, combined with oxygen to form phosphate (PO4), exists in both organic (PO) and inorganic (PI) forms, making its biological presence ubiquitous. This macromineral is integral to many essential molecules and structures, including nucleic acids (DNA and RNA), where it forms part of the backbone structure, and cell membranes, where it is a component of phospholipids. Additionally, phosphorus is vital in bone composition as calcium phosphate, contributing to skeletal integrity. It also plays a critical role in metabolic activities through protein phosphorylation, which affects enzyme functionality and post-translational modifications impacting gene expression. Furthermore, phosphorus is essential for energy transmission within cells, being a key component of adenosine triphosphate (ATP), the primary energy carrier in biological systems (**Figure 2**).

Phosphorus distribution within the animal body is predominantly in the skeleton. Grünberg [24] reported that approximately 80–85% of total phosphorus in the animal body is present as insoluble salts in the bones, mainly in the form of calcium phosphate compounds such as Ca3(PO4)2 and Ca10(PO4)6(OH)2. These compounds provide structural strength and rigidity to the skeletal system. The remaining 15–20% of total body phosphorus constitutes a more readily available pool present in soft tissues and body fluids. This pool includes both inorganic phosphorus (PI) and organic phosphorus (PO), which is bound to carbon-containing components. Intracellularly, phosphorus is predominantly present (>99%) and is estimated to be approximately 100 mmol/L, with only 1 mmol/L existing as inorganic phosphate while the rest is incorporated into organic molecules such as ATP, phospholipids, and nucleic acids.

In the extracellular space, phosphorus is found in both inorganic and organic forms. Inorganic phosphorus exists as free ions, bound to carrier proteins, or complexed with cations. Organic phosphorus, on the other hand, is present in molecules like lipoproteins. The serum inorganic phosphate concentration in dairy cattle is on average 1.5 mmol/L and is maintained in close equilibrium with the extracellular phosphorus status. This equilibrium is crucial for numerous physiological functions, including energy metabolism, cell signaling, and structural integrity.

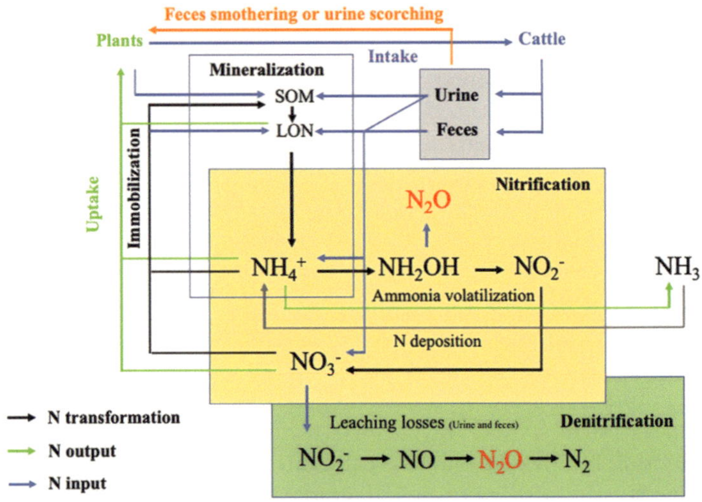

Figure 2.
Pathways of microbial driven nitrogen transformations in excreta patches in grassland ecosystems [22]. The N_2O can also be produced by nitrifier denitrification, chemodenitrification, and dissimilatory nitrate reduction to ammonium. The SOM and LON are soil organic matter and labile organic nitrogen, respectively [23].

The role of phosphorus in energy metabolism is particularly significant in ruminants, where it is involved in the synthesis and utilization of ATP. ATP is essential for numerous cellular processes, including muscle contraction, protein synthesis, and maintenance of cell membrane integrity. Phosphorus also contributes to cell signaling mechanisms through phosphorylation and dephosphorylation processes that regulate enzyme activity and gene expression. These processes are critical for the adaptation of metabolic pathways to changing physiological conditions and dietary intake. Therefore, adequate phosphorus nutrition is essential for maintaining optimal health, productivity, and reproductive performance in ruminants.

2.5 Phosphorus metabolism in ruminants

Phosphorus metabolism in ruminants is a complex and dynamic process that involves multiple stages, including the digestion, absorption, utilization, and excretion of phosphorus [25].

1. *Dietary phosphorus intake*: Ruminants primarily obtain phosphorus from their diet, which includes both organic phosphates (phytates) and inorganic phosphates. Phosphorus in plant material predominantly exists as phytate, a form that is not readily bioavailable to ruminants due to their limited ability to produce phytase, the enzyme required to break down phytate. This limitation presents a challenge since phytase activity in the ruminant digestive tract is relatively low [25]. Therefore, the bioavailability of dietary phosphorus from plant sources is significantly influenced by the ruminant's ability to digest phytates, necessitating dietary strategies to ensure adequate phosphorus intake.

2. *Digestion in the rumen*: In the rumen, microbes play a crucial role in the breakdown of plant material, including phytates, thereby releasing some phosphorus.

However, the extent of phytate degradation in the rumen is limited because rumen microbes produce low levels of phytase. Consequently, a significant portion of phytate-bound phosphorus remains undigested and continues through the digestive system. This limited degradation poses a challenge in optimizing phosphorus utilization from plant-based diets. Despite this, the microbial action in the rumen still contributes to the release of some free phosphorus, which can be absorbed and utilized by the animal. Understanding the microbial ecology and enhancing phytase activity in the rumen are areas of ongoing research aimed at improving phosphorus availability from dietary sources. Wang and Shang [26] found out the benefits of phytase that are its double effects on reducing the use of expensive inorganic phosphorus in animal diets and the environment pollution from excessive manure phosphorus runoff. Guerrand [27] showed through his experimental findings that the addition of phytase to feed results in a lower excretion of the phosphorous content in manure, contributing to a lower environmental impact of livestock farming. Phytase for feed application is produced by fermentation of microbial strains.

3. *Absorption*: As phytate-bound phosphorus that escapes rumen degradation enters the lower digestive tract, particularly the small intestine, it encounters pancreatic enzymes, including pancreatic phytase. This enzyme hydrolyzes phytate into inositol and orthophosphate (free phosphate), making phosphorus available for absorption. The majority of phosphorus absorption occurs in the small intestine, especially in the jejunum. This process involves active transport mechanisms facilitated by specific carriers in the intestinal epithelial cells. These carriers ensure efficient uptake of phosphate into the bloodstream. Phosphorus absorbed from the intestine is then distributed throughout the body, playing vital roles in various metabolic processes, including bone formation, energy metabolism through ATP, and cellular signaling. The effective absorption of phosphorus is critical for maintaining the mineral's balance and supporting the overall health and productivity of ruminants.

4. *Phosphate Utilization and Regulation*: Once absorbed, phosphorus is utilized in multiple metabolic functions. It is crucial for the formation and maintenance of bones, as it combines with calcium to form calcium phosphate, the primary mineral in bone structure. Additionally, phosphorus is integral to energy metabolism, as it is a key component of ATP, which is essential for energy transfer within cells. It also plays a significant role in cellular signaling pathways, affecting various physiological processes. The regulation of phosphorus metabolism involves hormonal control, primarily through parathyroid hormone (PTH) and vitamin D. PTH increases the release of phosphorus from bones and enhances its reabsorption in the kidneys, while vitamin D promotes the absorption of calcium and phosphorus in the intestine. The kidneys play a pivotal role in excreting excess phosphorus, thereby maintaining homeostasis. Ruminants efficiently regulate phosphorus excretion based on dietary intake and physiological demands, ensuring that excess phosphorus is eliminated to prevent toxicity.

5. *Strategies for Phosphorus Supplementation*: To meet the phosphorus requirements of ruminants, dietary supplements are often necessary. Inorganic phosphorus sources, such as dicalcium phosphate, and organic phosphorus sources, like phytase, are commonly added to ruminant diets. These supplements help to ensure

that the animals receive sufficient phosphorus to support their metabolic needs. Feed management practices, including balancing the dietary calcium-to-phosphorus ratio, are essential for optimizing phosphorus utilization and preventing metabolic disorders. Proper supplementation and management strategies are critical to enhancing the efficiency of phosphorus use in ruminant nutrition, thereby improving animal health and productivity while minimizing environmental impacts.

3. Environmental consequences of nitrogen and phosphorus emissions

Nitrogen and phosphorus are vital nutrients essential for plant growth and are widely utilized in agriculture as fertilizers. However, their excessive use and resultant emissions have profound environmental consequences, particularly eutrophication and water pollution. Understanding these impacts is crucial for devising strategies to mitigate their negative effects on ecosystems.

3.1 Eutrophication

Eutrophication is a process wherein a water body becomes overly enriched with nutrients, especially nitrogen and phosphorus, resulting in excessive growth of plants and algae. This phenomenon significantly disrupts aquatic ecosystems and diminishes water quality. The primary culprits of eutrophication are the over-enrichment of water bodies with nutrients, principally phosphorus, which leads to uncontrolled growth of primary producers like algae and aquatic plants (**Figure 3**). This overgrowth often leads to episodes of oxygen depletion when the algal blooms die and decompose. The decomposition process consumes oxygen, leading to hypoxic or anoxic conditions, which can cause massive die-offs of fish and other aquatic organisms, thereby disrupting the entire ecosystem [29].

Excess phosphorus typically enters water bodies from both point sources, such as sewage and industrial discharges, and nonpoint sources, such as agricultural runoff.

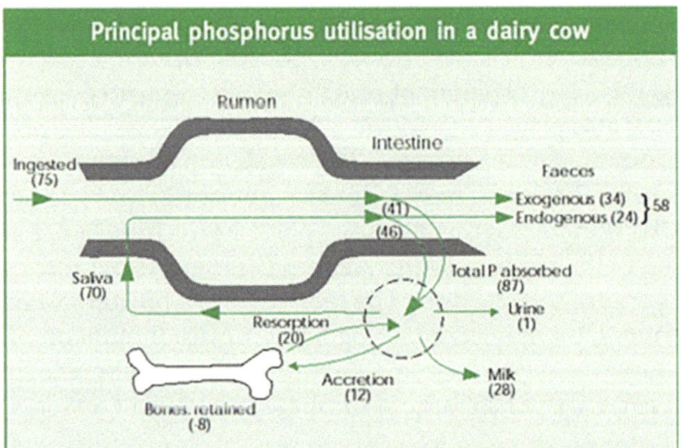

Principal paths of phosphorus utilisation in a 600kg dairy cow producing 30kg milk per day. (Bracketed figures represents numerical values in grams per day.)

Figure 3.
Principal paths of phosphorus utilization in dairy cows per day producing 30 kg milk per day [28].

In many regions, nonpoint sources have become the primary contributors to eutrophication. The over-application of fertilizers or manure in agriculture causes phosphorus to accumulate in soils, which is then washed into lakes and rivers during rainfall. This phosphorus stimulates the growth of phytoplankton and aquatic plants, leading to dense algal blooms. Historically, eutrophication due to anthropogenic nutrient inputs has become a significant environmental problem, especially from the mid-twentieth century onward. Recovering from such eutrophication, particularly in regions heavily impacted by agricultural runoff, could take centuries or more [30, 31].

Animal production systems contribute significantly to nitrogen pollution, affecting both groundwater and air quality. Managing these impacts requires an integrated approach involving better manure management practices, dietary adjustments for livestock, improved application techniques, and effective monitoring and regulatory frameworks (**Figure 4**).

3.1.1 Causes of nutrient overload

Excess nitrogen and phosphorus from agricultural runoff, sewage discharges, and fertilizers are primary contributors to nutrient overload in water bodies such as lakes, rivers, and coastal areas. Numerous activities within a drainage basin influence the water quality of these bodies. For instance, a lake or reservoir might naturally experience eutrophication if it is located in a fertile region with nutrient-rich soils. However, human activities significantly exacerbate this process. In many lakes and

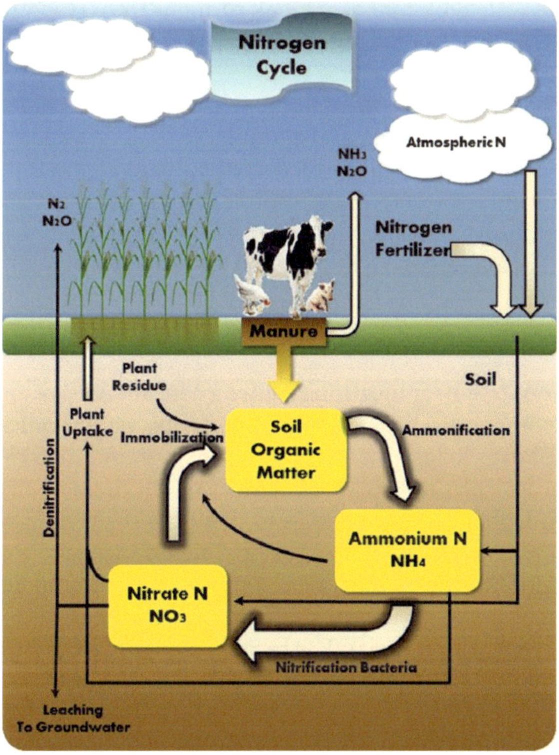

Figure 4.
The flow of nitrogen associated with animal production. Potential impacts include effects on groundwater and air quality.

reservoirs, untreated or inadequately treated wastewater remains a major source of nutrient input. Conventional mechanical-biological wastewater treatments do not fully remove nitrogen (25–40 mg/L) and phosphorus (6–10 mg/L), leading to their continued presence in the effluent [31].

Agriculture, including livestock farming, is the largest source of nonpoint water pollution. Runoff from agricultural lands carries both phosphorus and nitrogen, with nitrogen being more prevalent due to its solubility. The extensive use of fertilizers results in high concentrations of these nutrients in runoff. When eroded soil reaches water bodies, both phosphorus and nitrogen contribute to eutrophication. Deforestation, often a result of poor land management, exacerbates soil erosion and nutrient runoff. Nitrates, due to their water-soluble nature, easily move with surface runoff into rivers or percolate through the soil into groundwater. A 1998 assessment by the Ecological Society of America found that only about 18% of the nitrogen applied as fertilizer is taken up by crops, with the remaining 82% is left in the soil. This residual nitrogen either accumulates, erodes with the soil, leaches into groundwater, or volatilizes into the atmosphere [32].

3.1.2 Consequences of nutrient enrichment

Nutrient enrichment from nitrogen and phosphorus runoff promotes rapid growth of algae and aquatic plants, leading to dense algal blooms. As these organisms die and decompose, oxygen is consumed by bacteria, resulting in hypoxic (low-oxygen) conditions. These conditions can cause massive fish kills and the decline of other aquatic species. Algal blooms also block sunlight from reaching deeper waters, affecting the growth of submerged aquatic vegetation, which is crucial for maintaining healthy aquatic ecosystems.

Eutrophication poses a serious threat to the environment, heavily degrading freshwater systems by reducing water quality and altering the structure and function of ecosystems globally. The root causes of this problem are population growth, industrialization, and the excessive use of fertilizers, which result in disproportionate amounts of nutrients stimulating the overgrowth of plants and algae. Addressing eutrophication is urgent, as nutrient accumulation makes controlling it more difficult over time.

3.1.3 Mitigation strategies

Effective solutions to eutrophication require a comprehensive approach. The first and most obvious step toward protecting and restoring water bodies is to reduce the nitrogen and phosphorus loads entering freshwater systems. This can be achieved through changes in agricultural practices, such as restricting fertilizer use, optimizing nutrient use to match crop requirements, and planning the timing and methods of fertilizer application. Establishing more sustainable agricultural practices is crucial.

Moreover, reducing atmospheric sources of nitrogen, improving sewage and wastewater treatment, and controlling diffuse urban nutrient sources, such as runoff from streets and storm sewers, are essential. The introduction of wetlands as nutrient sinks can help absorb and filter excess nutrients before they reach water bodies. However, these measures alone are insufficient for immediate and long-lasting effects.

Modern strategies must consider various aspects, including phosphorus enrichment and food web structures, to understand the changes that occur after nutrient load alterations. An improved understanding of the interactive effects between grazers, nutrients, and algal production is necessary for successful eutrophication management. Governments must implement more effective policies to regulate industrial and agricultural activities that contribute to nutrient pollution. By promoting sustainable agricultural practices, enhancing wastewater treatment, and restoring natural ecosystems like wetlands, we can mitigate the adverse impacts of nitrogen and phosphorus emissions on our water bodies and ensure healthier aquatic environments for future generations [33].

3.1.4 Phases of eutrophication

Eutrophication is the process by which water bodies become enriched with nutrients, particularly phosphorus (P) and nitrogen (N), leading to excessive plant and algal growth. This process can be broken down into three phases, each influenced by the increasing difference in P and N emissions. Here is a detailed explanation of these phases:

3.1.4.1 Phase 1: Oligotrophic to mesotrophic transition

1. *Nutrient Input Increase*

    - *Phosphorus and Nitrogen Sources*: Initial nutrient inputs come from agricultural runoff, wastewater discharge, and atmospheric deposition. Both phosphorus and nitrogen levels begin to increase.

    - *Difference in Emissions*: Initially, the increase in phosphorus and nitrogen emissions might be relatively balanced.

2. *Primary Productivity Increase*

    - *Algal Growth*: Enhanced nutrient availability promotes the growth of algae and aquatic plants.

    - *Oxygen Levels*: During this phase, primary productivity increases, which can lead to higher oxygen production during the day but potentially lower levels at night due to respiration.

3. *Water Quality Changes*

    - *Clarity and Algal Blooms*: Water clarity may decrease slightly due to the initial algal blooms. However, this phase is often still characterized by relatively good water quality.

    - *Biodiversity*: The ecosystem might still support a diverse range of aquatic organisms, including fish and invertebrates.

3.1.4.2 Phase 2: Mesotrophic to eutrophic transition

1. *Nutrient Imbalance*

    - *Phosphorus vs. Nitrogen*: As agricultural practices intensify and urbanization increases, phosphorus inputs (e.g., from fertilizers and detergents) often exceed those of nitrogen. This imbalance can drive significant changes in water chemistry and ecosystem dynamics.

2. *Algal Bloom Intensification*

- *Cyanobacteria Dominance*: Excess phosphorus can lead to the dominance of cyanobacteria (blue-green algae), which can outcompete other algae and aquatic plants. These blooms can be toxic and harmful to aquatic life.

- *Hypoxia*: The decomposition of large algal blooms consumes oxygen, leading to hypoxic (low oxygen) or anoxic (no oxygen) conditions, particularly in deeper waters.

3. *Water Quality Deterioration*

- *Decreased Clarity*: Water clarity significantly decreases due to dense algal growth.

- *Odors and Toxins*: Cyanobacterial blooms can produce unpleasant odors and release toxins that are harmful to fish, wildlife, pets, and humans.

4. *Biodiversity Decline*

- *Fish Kills*: Hypoxic conditions can lead to fish kills and the loss of other aquatic organisms, reducing biodiversity.

Phase 3: Eutrophic to Hypereutrophic Transition

1. *Severe Nutrient Overload*

- *Extreme Nutrient Levels*: Continued and excessive inputs of phosphorus and nitrogen lead to hypereutrophic conditions, where nutrient levels are extremely high.

- *Nitrogen Saturation*: At this stage, nitrogen inputs might also become excessive, compounding the eutrophication problem.

2. *Massive Algal Blooms*

- *Algae and Cyanobacteria*: Algal and cyanobacterial blooms become more frequent, intense, and persistent.

- *Light Limitation*: Dense algal mats limit light penetration, severely affecting submerged aquatic vegetation.

3. *Chronic Hypoxia and Anoxia*

- *Dead Zones*: Large areas of the water body may become dead zones, where oxygen levels are too low to support most aquatic life.

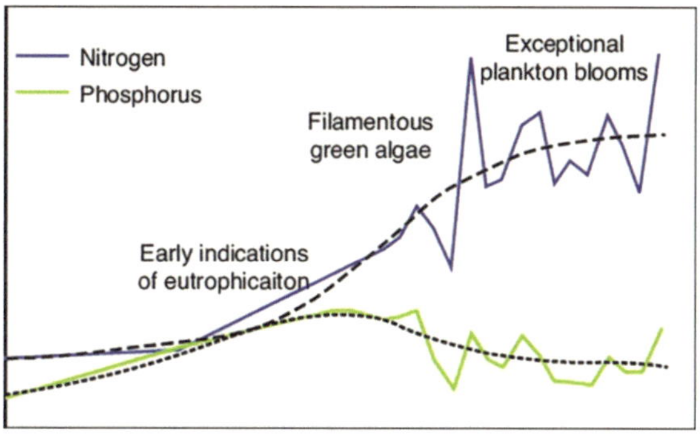

Figure 5.
Note the increasing difference in P and N emission. Three phases of eutrophication are indicated: Early indications of eutrophication (color and visibility), filamentous green algae, and exceptional plankton blooms [34].

- *Sediment Accumulation*: Accumulated organic matter from dying algae settles on the bottom, creating thick layers of sediment that further consume oxygen during decomposition.

4. *Ecosystem Collapse*

- *Loss of Biodiversity*: The ecosystem can collapse, with the loss of most fish and invertebrate species, leaving a community dominated by a few tolerant species.

- *Economic and Health Impacts*: The collapse of the ecosystem can have severe economic impacts on fisheries, tourism, and water treatment costs. Health risks also increase due to toxins from harmful algal blooms (**Figure 5**).

4. Water pollution

4.1 Source

Agricultural activities, particularly the extensive use of synthetic fertilizers and manure, are major contributors to nitrogen and phosphorus pollution in water bodies. Water pollution occurs when these excess nutrients enter water systems, leading to significant environmental degradation. This pollution primarily results from agricultural runoff, septic tank discharges, feedlot effluents, and combustion emissions. Raw sewage is also a significant contributor to cultural eutrophication, where untreated or partially treated sewage is released into large water bodies, introducing high levels of nutrients that stimulate algal growth. Despite regulations, sewage dumping still occurs globally, exacerbating the issue.

The agricultural boom, particularly since the 1910s and again in the 1940s to meet increased food demand, has heavily relied on fertilizers. These substances, whether natural or chemically modified, enhance soil fertility but also lead to an influx of nutrients into the environment. Commercial fertilizers primarily—contain nitrogen, phosphorus, and potassium—referred to as the "Big 3" essential nutrients for plant growth. However, when these nutrients are not fully absorbed by crops, they can leach into the soil and eventually find their way into water systems. This runoff from farm fields and pastures is a significant source of water pollution, contributing to the eutrophication of surface waters.

4.2 Consequences

Excessive nutrient pollution has several detrimental effects on water quality and aquatic ecosystems. When nitrogen and phosphorus levels rise, they disrupt the natural balance of aquatic systems. One of the most visible consequences is the formation of dense algal blooms. These blooms, often comprising harmful algae, can produce toxins such as microcystins that pose severe risks to human and animal health. The decomposition of these algal blooms by bacteria consumes large amounts of oxygen in the water, leading to hypoxic conditions or "dead zones," where oxygen levels are too low to support most marine life.

Furthermore, nitrogen and phosphorus pollution can cause harmful algal blooms (HABs) that not only deplete oxygen but also release toxins that contaminate drinking water sources and harm aquatic life. HABs can lead to fish kills, loss of biodiversity, and disruption of food webs. In coastal areas, these blooms can also affect tourism and fishing industries, causing economic losses. The excessive presence of nutrients in water bodies can lead to long-term ecological imbalances, making recovery difficult and slow.

4.3 Runoff

Rainwater and irrigation play a significant role in transporting excess nutrients from agricultural fields into nearby water bodies. When rain falls on fertilized fields, it dissolves the nitrogen and phosphorus present in the soil, creating nutrient-rich runoff. This runoff flows into streams and rivers, eventually reaching larger water bodies such as lakes, estuaries, and oceans. The cumulative effect of nutrient runoff can be profound, causing widespread eutrophication and water quality degradation across entire watersheds.

In addition to agricultural runoff, urban runoff also contributes to nutrient pollution. Stormwater runoff from streets, lawns, and industrial areas can carry nutrients into storm sewers and directly into water bodies. This urban runoff often contains fertilizers from residential lawns, pet waste, and other sources of nitrogen and phosphorus. Combined with agricultural sources, urban runoff exacerbates the problem of nutrient pollution, making comprehensive management strategies essential.

4.4 Mitigation approaches

Addressing nutrient pollution requires a multifaceted approach. Effective mitigation strategies include nutrient remediation, nutrient trading, and nutrient source apportionment. Nutrient remediation involves techniques to remove or neutralize excess nutrients in water bodies, such as using constructed wetlands to absorb nutrients or applying chemical treatments to bind phosphorus.

Nutrient trading is an innovative market-based approach where sources of nutrient pollution can buy and sell pollution credits. This system encourages reductions in nutrient emissions by allowing entities that reduce their nutrient outputs below a certain threshold to sell their excess reduction capacity to others struggling to meet regulatory limits. This creates a financial incentive for pollution reduction.

Nutrient source apportionment involves identifying and quantifying the various sources of nutrient pollution within a watershed. By understanding the specific contributions of agriculture, urban runoff, and other sources, targeted interventions can be implemented. For example, best management practices (BMPs) in agriculture, such as precision farming, buffer strips, and cover crops, can significantly reduce nutrient runoff. Urban areas can improve stormwater management through green infrastructure, such as rain gardens and permeable pavements, which help absorb and filter runoff before it reaches water bodies.

Ultimately, addressing nitrogen and phosphorus pollution requires coordinated efforts across multiple sectors, including agriculture, urban planning, and wastewater management. Governments must enforce stricter regulations on nutrient emissions, promote sustainable agricultural practices, and invest in infrastructure improvements to mitigate urban runoff. Public awareness campaigns can also play a crucial role in encouraging responsible fertilizer use and reducing pollution at the source. By implementing these comprehensive strategies, we can protect our water bodies from nutrient pollution and ensure the health of aquatic ecosystems for future generations [35].

5. Impact on biodiversity

5.1 Loss of diversity

Eutrophication caused by excessive nitrogen and phosphorus pollution significantly impacts biodiversity in aquatic ecosystems. The over-enrichment of water bodies with these nutrients leads to the rapid proliferation of certain algae and aquatic plants, often at the expense of other species. This shift in species composition favors fast-growing, nutrient-loving species such as cyanobacteria and some types of algae, which can outcompete and displace more diverse and less tolerant species. Consequently, the overall biodiversity of the ecosystem declines. For example, clear-water ecosystems that supported a wide variety of fish, plants, and invertebrates can become dominated by a few species of algae and cyanobacteria, leading to a loss of ecological complexity and resilience. These changes can disrupt food webs and reduce the habitat availability for many aquatic organisms, from microscopic zooplankton to larger fish species [36].

5.2 Fisheries decline

The depletion of oxygen in water bodies due to eutrophication, known as hypoxia, severely affects fish populations and other aquatic organisms. As algal blooms die and decompose, the decomposition process consumes large amounts of dissolved oxygen, creating hypoxic conditions. Fish and other aerobic organisms struggle to survive in such low-oxygen environments, leading to mass die-offs and significant declines in fish populations. This not only disrupts local ecosystems but also impacts human communities that rely on fisheries for their livelihoods. The economic impact can be profound, particularly in regions where fishing is a primary source of income and food. The decline in fish populations can also have cascading effects throughout the ecosystem, affecting species that depend on fish for food and altering the balance of aquatic communities [36].

6. Human health

6.1 Toxin exposure

Harmful algal blooms (HABs), driven by excess nitrogen and phosphorus, produce toxins that pose serious risks to human health. These toxins, such as microcystins and saxitoxins, can contaminate drinking water supplies and accumulate in seafood, posing health risks to humans who consume contaminated water or seafood. Exposure to these toxins can lead to a range of health issues, including gastrointestinal illnesses, liver damage, and neurological symptoms. In severe cases, exposure can be fatal. Recreational water bodies affected by HABs also pose direct health risks to swimmers and other water users. The economic costs associated with HABs are significant, including healthcare costs, loss of tourism revenue, and the expense of water treatment and mitigation efforts [37].

6.2 Drinking water contamination

The proliferation of algae and cyanobacteria in nutrient-enriched waters can lead to the contamination of drinking water sources. Algal blooms can clog water intake pipes and filters, complicating the water treatment process. Moreover, the toxins produced by some algal species can survive conventional water treatment processes, necessitating additional and often costly treatment steps to ensure water safety. The presence of high nutrient levels can also foster the growth of pathogenic bacteria, further compromising water quality. Communities relying on affected water sources face increased costs and potential health risks, underscoring the importance of controlling nutrient inputs to protect drinking water supplies.

7. Mitigation strategies

7.1 Sustainable agricultural practices

To mitigate nitrogen and phosphorus emissions, adopting sustainable agricultural practices is crucial. Precision farming techniques, which optimize fertilizer application based on crop needs and soil conditions, can significantly reduce nutrient runoff. Proper fertilizer management involves timing applications to coincide with crop uptake periods and using the appropriate amounts to avoid excess. Establishing buffer zones along waterways can trap nutrient runoff before it reaches water bodies. Utilizing alternative nutrient sources, such as organic fertilizers, can also help reduce the reliance on synthetic fertilizers. These practices not only improve water quality but also enhance soil health and agricultural productivity.

7.2 Effective wastewater treatment and regulations

Advanced wastewater treatment technologies are essential for removing nutrients from sewage before it is discharged into water bodies. Implementing stringent regulations to control nutrient runoff from agricultural and urban areas can also reduce nutrient pollution. Policies that promote the use of cover crops, conservation tillage, and other best management practices (BMPs) can mitigate runoff. Urban stormwater management practices, such as green infrastructure, rain gardens, and permeable pavements, can help reduce nutrient loads from urban areas. Together, these measures can significantly reduce the environmental impact of nitrogen and phosphorus emissions.

8. Innovative approaches to managing nitrogen and phosphorus emissions

Innovative approaches to managing nitrogen and phosphorus emissions include precision agriculture techniques, such as using GPS and soil sensors to apply fertilizers more efficiently and accurately, reducing excess application. Advanced manure management practices, like anaerobic digestion and composting, can stabilize nutrients and reduce emissions. Constructed wetlands and buffer strips can capture and filter runoff, preventing nutrient leaching into water bodies. Bioreactors and microbial treatments can enhance the breakdown and removal of excess nutrients in agricultural and wastewater systems. Additionally, policy measures, including nutrient trading schemes and stricter regulations, can incentivize better management practices and reduce overall nutrient loads (**Table 2**).

Management practice	Description	Impact on emissions	References
Dietary modification	Adjusting the diet to optimize nutrient utilization and reduce excess nitrogen and phosphorus excretion.	Decreases nitrogen and phosphorus emissions by improving feed efficiency.	[38]
Precision feeding	Feeding animals according to their specific nutrient requirements.	Reduces nutrient excretion by matching intake with requirements.	[39]
Use of feed additives	Incorporating additives such as enzymes, probiotics, or nitrification inhibitors to enhance nutrient absorption.	Can significantly reduce nitrogen emissions and improve phosphorus utilization.	[40]
Manure management	Proper storage, treatment, and application of manure to minimize nutrient losses.	Decreases nitrogen volatilization and phosphorus runoff.	[41]
Pasture management	Rotational grazing, appropriate stocking rates, and maintaining pasture health.	Reduces nitrogen and phosphorus losses through leaching and runoff.	[42]
Use of forage crops	Incorporating high-quality forage crops to improve nutrient uptake.	Enhances nutrient efficiency and reduces emissions by providing balanced nutrition.	[43]
Supplementation with amino acids	Adding specific amino acids to the diet to balance protein intake.	Decreases nitrogen excretion by improving protein utilization.	[44]
Water management	Ensuring adequate water supply and quality to support metabolic processes.	Improves overall nutrient utilization and reduces environmental impact.	[45]
Integrated crop-livestock systems	Combining crop and livestock production to recycle nutrients efficiently.	Reduces reliance on external inputs and decreases nutrient losses.	[46]

Table 2.
Management practices to control nitrogen and phosphorus emissions in ruminants.

8.1 Improved feeding strategies

In ruminant production systems, optimizing feeding strategies is essential to reduce nitrogen (N) and phosphorus (P) emissions. Formulating balanced diets that match the protein supply with the animals' requirements can minimize excess nitrogen excretion. This involves precise feeding practices tailored to the specific needs of ruminants at different stages of life and production cycles. For instance, using rumen-protected amino acids can reduce the total crude protein needed while still meeting the animals' amino acid requirements, thereby lowering nitrogen excretion. Implementing precision feeding techniques, such as automated feeders and real-time monitoring systems, can adjust diets based on individual animal needs, further reducing nitrogen waste [2, 47].

8.2 Improved forage quality

Utilizing high-quality forages that are more digestible and have better protein efficiency can reduce the need for supplementary protein sources and decrease nitrogen excretion in ruminant production systems. High-quality forages typically have lower fiber content and higher digestibility, allowing ruminants to extract more nutrients from the feed. These forages also have a balanced ratio of rumen-degradable and rumen-undegradable proteins, ensuring a steady supply of amino acids for microbial protein synthesis and direct absorption. By improving forage quality, farmers can enhance nutrient uptake and minimize environmental impact [48].

8.3 Feed additives

The use of feed additives such as nitrification inhibitors, tannins, and saponins can effectively reduce nitrogen emissions in ruminant production. Nitrification inhibitors slow down the conversion of ammonium to nitrate in the soil, reducing ammonia volatilization and nitrate leaching. This keeps nitrogen in a less leachable form, minimizing groundwater contamination and nutrient runoff into surface waters. Tannins and saponins in the diet can bind to proteins, reducing protein degradation in the rumen and lowering nitrogen emissions. These additives can be included in ruminant diets as feed additives or applied directly to soils [49].

By adopting these innovative approaches and implementing effective management strategies, it is possible to mitigate the environmental impacts of nitrogen and phosphorus emissions, ensuring the protection and restoration of aquatic ecosystems and the preservation of biodiversity.

8.4 Phosphorus emissions mitigation strategies

8.4.1 Phosphorus optimization

One of the effective strategies to mitigate phosphorus emissions in ruminant production systems involves optimizing phosphorus utilization through the use of phytase enzymes. In many plant-based feeds, phosphorus is stored in the form of phytic acid or phytate, which is largely indigestible by ruminants because they lack sufficient endogenous phytase enzymes. As a result, phytate-bound phosphorus passes through the digestive system without being absorbed, leading to lower phosphorus bioavailability and higher excretion in manure.

Phytase is an enzyme that catalyzes the hydrolysis of phytate, releasing inorganic phosphorus that can be readily absorbed by the animal. By incorporating phytase into ruminant diets, the bioavailability of phosphorus is significantly increased, allowing for better utilization of this essential nutrient. Improved phosphorus utilization means that less phosphorus is excreted in manure, thereby decreasing the environmental impact associated with phosphorus runoff and eutrophication. Studies have shown that phytase supplementation in animal feeds can reduce the need for inorganic phosphorus supplements, thus lowering overall phosphorus emissions from agricultural operations [50].

8.4.2 Manure management

Effective manure management is crucial for reducing phosphorus runoff and its associated environmental impacts. This involves applying manure at appropriate rates and times to match crop nutrient requirements and minimize losses. Precision application technologies, such as GPS-guided manure spreaders and variable-rate technology (VRT), ensure uniform distribution of manure across fields, thereby reducing the risk of phosphorus runoff. By implementing these technologies, farmers can apply manure more efficiently, targeting specific areas of the field that need nutrients and avoiding over-application that can lead to runoff and leaching [51].

Additionally, advanced manure processing technologies such as composting, anaerobic digestion, and chemical treatment can be used to reduce the phosphorus content in manure before it is applied to fields. Composting and anaerobic digestion not only reduce the volume of manure but also stabilize nutrients, making them less prone to runoff. Chemical treatments can precipitate phosphorus, making it less soluble and thus less likely to leach into waterways. The rate of manure application should be based on comprehensive soil testing to determine existing nutrient levels and manure testing to ascertain its nutrient composition. Adhering to recommended application rates prevents the buildup of excess phosphorus in the soil, further mitigating the risk of nutrient runoff.

8.4.3 Erosion control and buffer strips

Erosion control measures are also essential in managing phosphorus emissions. Implementing practices such as conservation tillage, cover cropping, and the establishment of buffer strips along waterways can significantly reduce soil erosion and phosphorus runoff. Buffer strips, which are vegetated areas between agricultural fields and water bodies, act as filters, trapping sediment and phosphorus before they reach streams and rivers. These vegetative barriers can absorb and utilize nutrients, reducing the amount of phosphorus that enters aquatic ecosystems.

8.4.4 Nutrient management planning

Developing comprehensive nutrient management plans that include regular soil testing, crop nutrient needs assessment, and careful timing of fertilizer applications can optimize phosphorus use and reduce environmental impacts. These plans should be tailored to the specific conditions of each farm, considering factors such as soil type, crop rotation, and weather patterns. By implementing precision agriculture techniques, farmers can apply fertilizers more efficiently, ensuring that crops receive the necessary nutrients without excess application that can lead to runoff and pollution.

By adopting these innovative approaches and implementing effective management strategies, it is possible to mitigate the environmental impacts of nitrogen and phosphorus emissions, ensuring the protection and restoration of aquatic ecosystems and the preservation of biodiversity. Improved phosphorus management not only enhances environmental sustainability but also contributes to the long-term productivity and resilience of agricultural systems.

8.5 Integrated approaches

8.5.1 Crop-livestock integration

Integrated crop-livestock systems (ICLS) are a sustainable agricultural practice that fosters synergistic relationships between crop production and livestock farming. In these systems, crop residues serve as animal feed, and manure is utilized as fertilizer, thereby enhancing nutrient recycling and reducing the reliance on external inputs. Applying manure to croplands recycles essential nutrients, such as nitrogen (N), phosphorus (P), and potassium (K) and provides organic matter that improves soil structure and microbial activity. This practice enhances soil fertility and reduces the need for synthetic fertilizers. Properly managed manure application also minimizes nutrient runoff into water bodies, thus mitigating water pollution and eutrophication [52]. By integrating crops and livestock, farmers can create a closed-loop system that maximizes resource efficiency and environmental sustainability.

8.5.2 Cover crops

The use of cover crops is a key strategy to capture excess nitrogen (N) and phosphorus (P), preventing them from leaching into waterways and improving soil health. Cover crops, such as clover, vetch, and peas, are planted during off-season periods when main crops are not cultivated. These plants provide multiple agronomic and environmental benefits, including reducing soil erosion, enhancing soil structure, and increasing organic matter content. Cover crops contribute to carbon sequestration by incorporating organic carbon into the soil, which helps mitigate climate change. Leguminous cover crops can fix atmospheric nitrogen, thereby adding to the soil nitrogen content and reducing the need for chemical fertilizers [53]. This practice not only improves soil fertility but also promotes biodiversity and ecosystem health.

8.5.3 Monitoring and management tools

Effective nutrient management in agricultural systems involves the use of advanced monitoring and management tools to optimize nutrient use and minimize environmental impacts.

By adopting these innovative approaches and implementing effective management strategies, it is possible to mitigate the environmental impacts of nitrogen and phosphorus emissions. Integrated crop-livestock systems, the use of cover crops, nutrient management plans, and decision support systems collectively enhance the efficiency and sustainability of agricultural production. These practices not only reduce the environmental footprint of farming but also contribute to the resilience and productivity of agricultural systems, ensuring long-term food security and environmental health.

9. Dietary interventions, feed additives, and management practices designed to reduce nitrogen and phosphorus excretion

Reducing nitrogen (N) and phosphorus (P) excretion in livestock production is a complex challenge that can be addressed through a combination of dietary interventions, feed additives, and advanced management practices. Each strategy aims to optimize nutrient utilization by the animals, thereby minimizing the environmental footprint of livestock farming.

9.1 Dietary interventions

Precision Feeding: One of the most effective dietary interventions is precision feeding, which involves closely tailoring the diet to meet the specific nutritional needs of the animal. This approach reduces excess N and P excretion by ensuring that animals receive the exact amounts of nutrients they require for their growth stage, production level, and health status [54]. Formulating diets that match the animals' specific nutrient requirements can significantly reduce nutrient wastage. For example, adjusting dietary protein levels to just meet, but not exceed, the animal's needs can decrease urinary nitrogen output. Lower protein diets that still maintain productivity have been shown to reduce nitrogen excretion substantially.

Balanced Rations and Fiber: Providing balanced rations that include the right ratios of protein, energy, and other essential nutrients can improve overall nutrient utilization. This balance minimizes the excess N and P that would otherwise be excreted. Additionally, increasing dietary fiber can enhance rumen microbial activity, promoting better nitrogen utilization and reducing ammonia emissions. High-fiber diets improve the efficiency of nutrient uptake and decrease the environmental impact of livestock operations. However, dietary interventions require careful formulation to avoid compromising animal health and performance, and they need to be tailored to specific animal types and production systems.

9.1.1 Feed additives

Ionophores and Urease Inhibitors: Feed additives such as ionophores and urease inhibitors play a crucial role in improving nitrogen utilization efficiency in the rumen, thereby reducing ammonia emissions [55]. Ionophores alter the rumen microbial population, decreasing the deamination of amino acids and the subsequent production of ammonia. This ensures that more nitrogen from the protein remains as amino acids and peptides, which can be absorbed and utilized by the animal.

Phytase and Phosphorus Binders: Phytase enzymes are particularly beneficial for enhancing phosphorus digestibility. Many plant-based feeds contain phosphorus in the form of phytate, which is indigestible by ruminants. Phytase breaks down phytate, releasing phosphorus in a form that can be absorbed by the animal, thereby lowering phosphorus excretion in manure [56]. Other phosphorus binders can also be included in feed to reduce phosphorus waste. Feed additives are cost-effective and practical solutions, although their effectiveness can vary based on the feed composition and the animal's physiology.

9.2 Management practices

Manure Management: Effective manure management strategies are essential to reduce nutrient losses and environmental impacts. Techniques such as composting, anaerobic digestion, and solid-liquid separation can stabilize nutrients in manure, making them easier to handle and apply appropriately. Composting, for example, stabilizes nitrogen and reduces the volume of manure, facilitating better nutrient management [57]. Covered storage systems can also minimize ammonia volatilization from manure.

Precision Feeding Technologies: Utilizing precision feeding technologies allows farmers to match nutrient supply with animal requirements more accurately, minimizing excess nutrient intake and subsequent excretion. Feed analysis and ration formulation software can optimize the levels of protein and phosphorus in the diet, thereby minimizing nutrient excretion. These technologies ensure that animals receive only what they need, reducing wastage and environmental impact [58].

Grazing Management: Grazing management practices such as rotational grazing and managed intensive grazing systems can optimize nutrient cycling and reduce the need for supplemental feed. By rotating livestock through different paddocks, pasture growth is optimized, and nutrient distribution from manure is more even. This reduces nutrient excretion and improves the sustainability of the farming system [59]. These management practices are critical for overall nutrient management but may require infrastructure investment and operational changes.

10. Innovative approaches

Biochar and Nutrient Recovery: Biochar, a type of charcoal produced from biomass, is emerging as a promising feed additive that can improve nutrient retention and reduce nutrient excretion in manure. Biochar has a high surface area and porosity, allowing it to adsorb and retain nutrients. When included in animal feed, biochar can bind to nutrients in the gastrointestinal tract, enhancing nutrient retention by the animal and reducing nutrient excretion [60].

Nutrient recovery technologies, such as phosphorus extraction from manure, aim to recycle nutrients and minimize their loss to the environment. These technologies involve processes that capture and reuse nutrients from manure, thus preventing them from entering and polluting water bodies. While these emerging technologies show significant promise, they require further research and development to assess their scalability and economic feasibility.

By integrating these dietary interventions, feed additives, and management practices, livestock producers can significantly reduce nitrogen and phosphorus excretion, thereby mitigating the environmental impacts of livestock farming. These strategies not only enhance the sustainability of livestock production systems but also contribute to improved environmental health and long-term agricultural productivity.

11. Nutritional strategies for reducing nitrogen and phosphorus excretion

To effectively reduce nitrogen and phosphorus excretion from ruminants, strategic dietary manipulation and formulation are essential.

11.1 Reduction of nitrogen excretion

Ruminants often excrete a significant portion of ingested nitrogen, primarily as urea in urine, which can contribute to environmental pollution through ammonia volatilization and nitrate leaching. Providing a balanced ratio of rumen-degradable protein (RDP) and rumen-undegradable protein (RUP) can improve nitrogen utilization. RDP is broken down by microbes in the rumen, while RUP bypasses the rumen and is digested in the intestines. Specific feed additives such as amino acids, protected proteins, and enzymes can enhance the efficiency of nitrogen utilization [61]. Apelo et al. [62] found out in his experimental findings that dairy cows consume an excess of N, resulting in approximately 75% of dietary N being lost to the environment as urine and feces. Reductions in environmental N release could be attained through an improvement in N efficiency. The reduction in milk yield associated with feeding a low-protein diet to lactating dairy cows could be avoided by dietary supplementation with 1 or more ruminally protected (RP) AA.

11.2 Balanced protein and energy ratio

Ensure diets are formulated with a balanced ratio of protein to energy. This helps optimize microbial protein synthesis in the rumen and reduces excess nitrogen excretion. Use high-quality protein sources that are efficiently utilized by rumen microbes, such as soybean meal, canola meal, or alfalfa hay. The microbes in the rumen convert ingested feedstuffs into volatile fatty acids (VFAs) and microbial protein, which the ruminant then uses for growth and production. Adequate energy from carbohydrates is necessary for the microbes to synthesize amino acids from ammonia and other nitrogen sources. Insufficient energy or excess protein can lead to imbalances, affecting microbial growth and activity. The efficiency of nitrogen utilization is influenced by the dietary balance of protein and energy. Misra *et al.* [63] found that diets with high protein but low energy levels led to increased nitrogen excretion, while balanced diets reduced nitrogen losses. A balanced protein-to-energy ratio minimizes the nitrogen load in manure, thereby reducing ammonia emissions and nitrate leaching into water bodies. Castillo et al. [64] emphasized that improved nitrogen utilization through balanced diets can significantly lower the environmental impact of dairy farming.

11.3 Rumen-protected protein supplements

Incorporate rumen-protected protein supplements into diets to deliver protein directly to the intestines, thereby reducing the amount of protein degraded in the rumen and subsequently excreted as urea [65]. Rumen-protected proteins are coated or treated with substances that protect them from ruminal degradation. Common methods include heat treatment, chemical treatments (e.g., formaldehyde), and encapsulation with fat or polymers. In Mazinani et al.'s [66] experiment, essential amino acid (Methionine) and two chemical compounds were used to make ligands that produce pH-sensitive amino acids that are stable in the rumen and absorbable in the post-rumen part of the digestive tract. Result shows that this chemical method increased retention time in rumen and the bond is reversible in lower pHs, similar to the abomasum. This protection ensures that the protein remains intact through the rumen and becomes available for enzymatic digestion in the small intestine. By protecting protein from ruminal degradation, RPPs increase the amount of amino acids available for absorption in the small intestine, thus enhancing protein utilization efficiency [18]. RPPs reduce the amount of protein degraded into ammonia in the rumen, which is then excreted as urea. This results in lower nitrogen losses and reduced environmental pollution from nitrogen excretion [67].

11.4 Alternative feed ingredients

Explore alternative feed ingredients that are lower in nitrogen and phosphorus content while still meeting nutritional needs. Utilize by-products from food processing industries (e.g., brewers' grains, citrus pulp) that have lower nitrogen and phosphorus concentrations compared to traditional feedstuffs. Lower N content in alternative feeds like brewers' grains and citrus pulp reduces the overall dietary N, leading to lower ammonia production in the rumen and decreased urinary N excretion. This can significantly reduce the environmental impact associated with ammonia volatilization from manure [68]. By using ingredients with lower P content, such as citrus pulp, the dietary P level can be controlled, minimizing the risk of P runoff from manure, which is a major environmental concern [69]. These by-products can enhance nutrient efficiency, lower feeding costs, and mitigate environmental impacts associated with traditional feedstuffs. Careful formulation and monitoring are essential to maximize the benefits of these alternative ingredients.

11.5 Rumen microbial manipulation

Modify the rumen microbial population through diet to improve nitrogen utilization efficiency and incorporate dietary fiber sources that promote the growth of microbes involved in nitrogen recycling and synthesis of microbial protein. Fibrolytic bacteria, such as *Ruminococcus and Fibrobacter*, specialize in breaking down cellulose and hemicellulose. Dietary fibers enhance their growth, leading to improved fiber digestion and VFA production, which provides energy for nitrogen-recycling microbes [70]. Certain fibers can increase the population of microbes that recycle nitrogen, such as the *Prevotella* genus. These microbes utilize ammonia to synthesize amino acids, which are then used by other bacteria for growth and microbial protein production [71].

11.6 Mineral supplementation

Provide targeted mineral supplementation based on soil and forage analysis to ensure adequate but not excessive intake of phosphorus. Consider the use of slow-release mineral supplements to enhance phosphorus utilization and reduce excretion. Slow-release phosphorus supplements provide a consistent supply of phosphorus over an extended period, aligning with the animals' metabolic needs and reducing the risk of phosphorus peaks and troughs in the diet [72]. Minerals are coated with substances that slow down their dissolution rate, ensuring a gradual release in the digestive tract. Phosphorus is embedded in a matrix of slowly digestible material, which controls the release rate as the matrix is broken down [73].

By integrating these strategies, ruminant producers can optimize nutrient utilization, improve animal performance, and reduce the environmental impact associated with nitrogen and phosphorus excretion.

12. Role of balanced diets and nutrient management in minimizing environmental pollution

The role of balanced diets and nutrient management in minimizing environmental pollution, particularly concerning the reduction of nitrogen and phosphorus excretion from livestock, is essential for sustainable agriculture. Addressing these issues effectively can lead to significant environmental benefits, including the prevention of water pollution and the enhancement of soil health.

12.1 Balanced diets for optimal nutrient utilization

Balanced diets are crucial for ensuring that ruminants receive the correct proportion of essential nutrients without an excess intake of nitrogen and phosphorus. Tailoring diets to match the specific nutritional requirements of animals at different production stages (e.g., growth, lactation) optimizes nutrient utilization and minimizes excess excretion. A well-balanced diet maintains efficient rumen fermentation, promotes microbial activity, and supports overall digestive health, thereby reducing the need for excessive protein and phosphorus supplementation.

For instance, providing diets that match the animals' requirements based on precise feeding practices can help in reducing nitrogen excretion. Lower protein diets, supplemented with essential amino acids, can decrease urinary nitrogen output without compromising productivity. Similarly, the inclusion of high-quality forages that are more digestible can enhance nitrogen use efficiency, reducing the amount of nitrogen excreted.

12.2 Phosphorus management

Phosphorus excretion from livestock is a significant contributor to the eutrophication of water bodies, leading to harmful algal blooms and oxygen depletion. Managing phosphorus intake through dietary adjustments is vital. Utilizing phytase enzymes in animal diets improves phosphorus utilization by breaking down phytic acid (the form in which phosphorus is stored in plants) into a bioavailable form. This reduces the need for excessive phosphorus supplementation and minimizes phosphorus excretion.

Feeding diets with balanced phosphorus levels tailored to the animal's needs and using alternative phosphorus sources that are more bioavailable can significantly lower the environmental impact. For example, formulating diets that incorporate more bioavailable phosphorus sources ensures that more of the nutrient is absorbed by the animal, reducing the amount excreted in manure.

12.3 Manure management

Proper management of livestock manure is essential for reducing nutrient runoff and pollution. Implementing nutrient management plans that focus on utilizing manure as a valuable resource rather than a waste product can help recycle nitrogen and phosphorus back into the soil. Techniques such as composting, anaerobic digestion, and precision application of manure to fields help retain nutrients and prevent leaching into water bodies.

Composting stabilizes nitrogen in manure, reducing the risk of nitrogen volatilization and runoff. Anaerobic digestion processes manure to produce biogas and nutrient-rich digestate, which can be used as a soil amendment. Precision application methods ensure that manure is applied at rates that match crop nutrient needs, reducing the risk of over-application and subsequent nutrient runoff.

12.4 Environmental regulations and best practices

Compliance with environmental regulations and the adoption of best management practices (BMPs) are crucial for minimizing environmental pollution from livestock operations. Educating farmers on nutrient stewardship, including proper feed management and manure handling practices, promotes sustainable agriculture and reduces environmental impact. BMPs include regular soil and manure testing to determine nutrient content and appropriate application rates, thus preventing nutrient overload in the soil.

Investing in research and innovation to develop advanced feed technologies and nutritional strategies that optimize nutrient utilization while minimizing waste contributes to long-term environmental sustainability. For example, the development of feed additives that enhance nutrient absorption or reduce nutrient excretion can significantly lower the environmental footprint of livestock production.

Balanced diets and effective nutrient management play a fundamental role in reducing nitrogen and phosphorus excretion from ruminants, thereby mitigating environmental pollution associated with agriculture. By adopting these strategies alongside responsible manure management and adherence to environmental standards, livestock producers can contribute to a more sustainable and environmentally friendly food production system. Implementing these practices not only benefits the environment but also enhances the efficiency and productivity of agricultural operations, ensuring a sustainable future for food production.

13. Practical implementation and adoption

13.1 Guidance for farmers and stakeholders on implementing sustainable practices to manage nitrogen and phosphorus emissions

Implementing sustainable practices to manage nitrogen and phosphorus emissions requires a comprehensive approach that involves farmers, stakeholders, and agricultural advisors.

13.1.1 Nutrient management planning

Development and implementation of a nutrient management plan tailored to the specific needs and conditions of the farm. Conducting soil testing to determine nutrient levels and pH, which helps optimize fertilizer and manure application to match crop requirements. Use tools and resources provided by agricultural extension services or government agencies to create and maintain effective nutrient management plans. Collect soil samples from various locations and depths within the field to get a representative sample. Submit the samples to a certified laboratory where they are analyzed for macro- and micro-nutrients (e.g., nitrogen, phosphorus, potassium, calcium, magnesium, and sulfur) and pH level. The results from the soil tests are interpreted using established guidelines to determine nutrient deficiencies, excesses, and soil pH adjustments needed. These guidelines are often provided by agricultural extension services or research institutions [74]. Strategies for applying nutrients at the right time and using the right methods to maximize uptake and minimize losses. Applying manure at rates that meets the crop needs, using methods that minimize nutrient losses e.g., incorporation into soil.

13.1.2 Optimized feed formulation

Working with nutritionists and feed suppliers to formulate balanced diets for livestock that optimize nutrient utilization and minimize excess nitrogen and phosphorus excretion. Also by incorporating alternative feed ingredients that are lower in nitrogen and phosphorus content without compromising animal health and performance. Precision feeding involves tailoring diets to meet the exact nutrient needs of animals at different growth stages. This reduces waste and improves nutrient utilization efficiency. Optimized diets ensure the correct balance of amino acids, particularly lysine and methionine, which are essential and often limiting in typical feed ingredients. An imbalance can lead to excess nitrogen excretion. Dietary phosphorus must be carefully managed to meet animal requirements without excess. This involves balancing available phosphorus with phytase enzyme supplementation to improve phosphorus availability from plant sources [75].

13.2 Education and training

It involves providing training and educational resources to farmers and agricultural advisors on sustainable nutrient management practices and encouraging participation in workshops, field days, and extension programs focused on nutrient stewardship and environmental conservation. Providing training helps bridge the gap between research findings and practical applications on farms. Education fosters awareness and encourages the adoption of sustainable practices, leading to behavioral changes that benefit the environment. Well-informed farmers can make better decisions regarding nutrient management, improving both crop yields and environmental outcomes. Field demonstrations showcase real-world applications of nutrient management practices, such as precision farming techniques, cover cropping, and integrated pest management. Many agricultural universities offer extension programs that provide ongoing education and support to farmers. These programs often include seminars, online courses, and printed materials. Extension agents work directly with farmers to implement nutrient management plans. Creating networks of farmers who share a commitment to sustainability can foster a supportive community. Peer learning and mentorship are powerful tools for spreading knowledge [76].

13.3 Monitoring and evaluation

It involves regularly monitoring nutrient levels in soil, water, and crops to assess the effectiveness of nutrient management practices and using monitoring data to make informed decisions and adjustments to nutrient management strategies over time. It ensures that nutrients are applied at appropriate levels to meet crop needs without causing excess that could lead to environmental pollution; helps in identifying nutrient deficiencies or surpluses, allowing for timely corrective measures; minimizes the risk of nutrient runoff and leaching into water bodies, thus protecting water quality; and reduces greenhouse gas emissions associated with excessive fertilizer application.

13.4 Collaboration and networking

Collaborating with local agricultural organizations, conservation groups, and government agencies to access technical support, funding opportunities, and incentives for adopting sustainable practices. Participate in farmer networks and peer-to-peer learning groups to share experiences and learn from successful case studies.

By embracing these practical strategies and fostering a culture of continuous improvement and innovation, farmers and stakeholders can contribute to reducing nitrogen and phosphorus emissions while promoting sustainable agriculture practices that benefit both the environment and agricultural productivity.

14. Considerations for integrating environmental sustainability into ruminant production systems

Integrating environmental sustainability into ruminant production systems requires thoughtful consideration of various factors and practices aimed at minimizing environmental impact while maintaining or improving productivity. Some of the key considerations and practical approaches for implementing sustainable practices in ruminant production are as follows:

14.1 Pasture management

It involves utilizing rotational grazing systems to optimize pasture utilization and prevent overgrazing, which can lead to soil erosion and degradation and implementing managed intensive grazing practices that mimic natural grazing patterns, promoting soil health, biodiversity, and carbon sequestration.

Key strategies include rotational grazing, proper stocking rates, forage diversification, soil health management, and water conservation. Rotational grazing involves dividing pastureland into smaller paddocks and rotating livestock through them. This allows for periods of grazing followed by rest, which promotes regrowth and reduces overgrazing. It enhances pasture productivity, increases plant diversity, improves soil structure, and reduces soil erosion [77]. Maintaining appropriate stocking rates ensures that the number of animals matches the carrying capacity of the land. Overgrazing can lead to soil degradation and loss of plant species, while undergrazing can result in underutilization of forage. Introducing a variety of plant species in pastures increases resilience against pests, diseases, and extreme weather conditions. It improves nutrient cycling, enhances forage availability throughout the year, and promotes animal health. Practices such as maintaining ground cover, minimizing soil disturbance, and adding organic matter (e.g., compost, manure) are essential for soil health. It implements efficient water management practices, such as constructing ponds, maintaining riparian buffers, and using controlled grazing to protect water sources; reduces water wastage; prevents water pollution from runoff; and ensures adequate water supply for livestock [78].

14.2 Feed management

It optimizes feed efficiency by formulating balanced diets that meet nutritional requirements of ruminants while minimizing waste and nutrient excretion and incorporates locally sourced and sustainable feed ingredients to reduce carbon footprint associated with feed production and transportation. Integrating environmental sustainability into ruminant production systems through feed management is a critical approach to mitigating the ecological impact of livestock farming. Effective feed management strategies can help reduce these emissions, improve animal health, and enhance overall farm sustainability. Effective feed management is a cornerstone of sustainable ruminant production. By formulating balanced diets that meet nutritional requirements while minimizing waste and nutrient excretion, incorporating locally sourced and sustainable feed ingredients, and implementing practices that enhance environmental sustainability, farmers can significantly reduce the ecological impact of livestock farming. These strategies not only help mitigate greenhouse gas emissions but also promote animal health and farm sustainability [79].

14.3 Water management

It implements water conservation practices to minimize water use and prevent contamination of water sources from nutrient runoff and provides clean and adequate water supply for ruminants to support optimal health and productivity. Providing clean and adequate water supply ensures animal health and productivity. These practices not only conserve water resources but also enhance the sustainability and profitability of livestock farming. Efficient irrigation systems, such as drip or sprinkler systems, minimize water wastage and ensure that crops grown for fodder receive adequate moisture without excessive runoff [80]. Drip Irrigation: This system delivers water directly to the plant roots through a network of valves, pipes, tubing, and emitters, reducing evaporation and runoff. Drip irrigation is highly efficient and can save up to 60% more water compared to traditional irrigation methods. Sprinkler Systems: Sprinkler systems distribute water evenly across the crop field, simulating natural rainfall. They are suitable for various terrains and can be automated to optimize water use, ensuring that crops receive adequate moisture without excessive runoff. Using soil moisture sensors helps monitor soil water content in real-time, allowing farmers to apply water only when necessary. This prevents over-irrigation and reduces water waste. Applying organic or synthetic mulches helps retain soil moisture by reducing evaporation, moderating soil temperature, and suppressing weed growth. Planting buffer strips of grasses, trees, and shrubs between agricultural fields and water bodies helps filter out nutrients and sediments from runoff before they reach water sources. Plowing along the contour lines of a field reduces soil erosion and water runoff, helping to retain soil moisture and nutrients. Constructing well-designed manure storage facilities with impermeable linings prevents leachate from contaminating groundwater and surface water. Ensuring that water troughs and tanks are appropriately sized and positioned to allow easy access for all animals in the herd is essential. Regular cleaning and maintenance prevent contamination and ensure a continuous supply of clean water. Automatic waterers can provide a consistent and clean water supply while reducing waste. They are particularly useful in larger operations where manual watering would be labor-intensive [81].

14.4 Energy efficiency

Adopt energy-efficient practices on the farm, such as using renewable energy sources (solar and wind) for electricity and heating. Implement energy-saving technologies in facilities and equipment used for feeding, milking, and manure handling. Biogas production from manure digestion is another viable option. The Penn State digester project showed that biogas could replace conventional fuels for heating and electricity generation. The biogas system, which uses manure to produce methane, can reduce overall energy costs and enhance farm sustainability by utilizing waste products efficiently. Biogas can be used to power generators, producing electricity for farm use, or for sale back to the grid. This reduces the farm's dependence on external energy sources. The heat generated from biogas combustion can be used for space heating, water heating, and other thermal applications on the farm. The by-product of anaerobic digestion is a nutrient-rich digestate that can be used as a fertilizer, reducing the need for synthetic fertilizers and enhancing soil health. Utilizing energy-efficient manure scrapers and pumps reduces the electricity required for manure management. These systems can be automated to operate during off-peak hours to save on energy costs [82].

14.5 Biodiversity conservation

It involves preserving and enhancing biodiversity on the farm by maintaining natural habitats, planting native vegetation, and creating wildlife corridors; avoiding the usage of pesticides and herbicides that can harm beneficial insects and pollinators essential for ecosystem health; and allocating and protecting specific areas of land within ruminant production systems to preserve natural habitats such as forests, wetlands, and grasslands. These areas can serve as biodiversity reservoirs, supporting native flora and fauna.

14.6 Soil health and carbon sequestration

It involves implementing soil conservation practices, such as reduced tillage and cover cropping, to improve soil structure, fertility, and water retention. Reduced tillage minimizes soil disturbance, which helps maintain soil structure and promotes the formation of soil aggregates. This enhances soil porosity, water infiltration, and root penetration. By leaving crop residues on the soil surface, reduced tillage protects the soil from erosion caused by wind and water. This practice also decreases the loss of organic matter and nutrients from the soil. Promote carbon sequestration through agroforestry, silvopasture, and perennial grassland systems that capture and store carbon in soils and vegetation. Agroforestry integrates trees and shrubs into crop and livestock systems. Trees capture carbon dioxide through photosynthesis and store it in biomass and soil. The deep roots of trees also help in nutrient cycling and improving soil structure. Agroforestry systems increase biodiversity, providing habitat for various species and enhancing ecosystem resilience. This diversity can lead to more stable and productive agricultural systems [83].

14.7 Compliance with regulations and standards

Stay informed about environmental regulations and voluntary sustainability certifications relevant to ruminant production. Strive to exceed minimum requirements and adopt voluntary standards to demonstrate commitment to environmental stewardship. Farms must comply with regulations on nutrient management to prevent water contamination from runoff. Regulations like the Clean Air Act in the United States set limits on emissions of pollutants from agricultural operations, including ammonia and particulate matter from livestock facilities (USEPA). Compliance involves managing emissions through practices like proper manure storage and handling. Proper disposal and management of animal waste are regulated to prevent environmental contamination. Regulations may require farms to have waste management plans that include manure storage, treatment, and application to fields. The USDA Organic certification requires farms to adhere to organic farming practices, including avoiding synthetic fertilizers and pesticides, implementing crop rotations, and maintaining soil health. For livestock, it includes requirements for organic feed, access to the outdoors, and prohibition of antibiotics and growth hormones. Staying informed about relevant regulations and adopting voluntary standards can help farms not only meet legal requirements but also gain market advantages and improve their sustainability practices. By exceeding minimum requirements and embracing best practices, farms can contribute to a more sustainable agricultural sector and ensure their long-term viability.

15. Future directions and challenges

15.1 Exploration of emerging trends and areas for further research in managing nitrogen and phosphorus emissions

15.1.1 Precision agriculture technologies

Utilizing precision agriculture tools such as remote sensing, GPS, and data analytics can help optimize nutrient application, reducing nitrogen and phosphorus runoff. Real-time monitoring of soil conditions and crop needs allows for targeted and efficient fertilizer application. Sensor technologies are advancing rapidly in precision agriculture, offering real-time data on soil nutrient status, crop growth, and environmental conditions. These technologies enable farmers to apply nitrogen and phosphorus fertilizers precisely where and when they are needed, reducing over-application and subsequent emissions [84]. VRA (Variable Rate Application) technologies allow farmers to adjust fertilizer application rates based on spatial variability within fields. By mapping soil nutrient levels and crop requirements, VRA optimizes nutrient application efficiency, reducing nitrogen and phosphorus losses to the environment [85]. Remote sensing techniques, including satellite imagery and unmanned aerial vehicles (UAVs), provide valuable insights into crop health and nutrient stress. This information can guide targeted nutrient applications, optimizing fertilizer use efficiency, and minimizing nutrient runoff. Advancements in nutrient management models facilitate predictive modeling of nitrogen and phosphorus dynamics in agroecosystems. These models integrate soil data, weather conditions, and crop characteristics to optimize nutrient applications and reduce environmental impacts.

15.2 Cover crops and crop rotation

Research focuses on the effectiveness of cover crops and diverse crop rotations in reducing nutrient leaching and erosion. Understanding which cover crops and rotations work best in different regions and climates is an area of ongoing investigation. Cover crops can significantly reduce nutrient leaching, particularly nitrogen, by taking up residual soil nitrogen and preventing it from leaching into groundwater. They also improve soil structure, which enhances water infiltration and reduces surface runoff [86].

15.3 Nutrient recovery and recycling

Technologies to recover and recycle nitrogen and phosphorus from waste streams (such as manure, food waste, or wastewater) are advancing. These recovered nutrients can then be used as fertilizers, reducing the reliance on synthetic inputs. Technologies like struvite precipitation, ion exchange, and membrane filtration are used to extract and concentrate nutrients (nitrogen and phosphorus) from waste streams such as livestock manure and wastewater [87]. Technologies like thermal conversion (e.g., pyrolysis, gasification) can convert organic waste materials into biochar or ash, which can be used as nutrient-rich soil amendments. Algae-based technologies utilize microalgae to capture and assimilate nutrients (particularly nitrogen and phosphorus) from wastewater, producing biomass that can be used as organic fertilizer. The adoption of advanced nutrient recovery and recycling technologies is crucial for sustainable agriculture. Struvite precipitation, ion exchange, and membrane filtration are effective methods for extracting and concentrating nitrogen and phosphorus from waste streams. These technologies not only provide valuable fertilizers, reducing reliance on synthetic inputs but also contribute to environmental protection and economic efficiency in farming operations.

15.4 Biological nitrogen fixation

Exploring and optimizing biological nitrogen fixation through plants and microbes can reduce the need for synthetic nitrogen fertilizers. This includes breeding crops with enhanced nitrogen-fixing abilities or engineering microbial communities to enhance nutrient availability. Biological nitrogen fixation (BNF) is a vital process that converts atmospheric nitrogen (N_2) into ammonia (NH_3) by certain microorganisms, predominantly bacteria known as diazotrophs. This process plays a crucial role in supplying nitrogen to plants, reducing the dependency on synthetic nitrogen fertilizers, which can have environmental impacts [88].

15.5 Advanced nutrient management models

Developing sophisticated models that integrate soil health data, weather patterns, and crop needs can help predict nutrient requirements more accurately. This leads to more targeted and efficient fertilizer applications, reducing nutrient runoff.

15.6 Climate-smart agriculture approaches

Understanding the interaction between nutrient management practices and climate change is critical. Research is needed to develop strategies that mitigate greenhouse gas emissions associated with nitrogen and phosphorus use while maintaining agricultural productivity.

15.7 Policy and socio-economic research

Exploring policy interventions and economic incentives that promote sustainable nutrient management practices is essential. Understanding the socio-economic factors influencing farmer decisions around nutrient management can inform effective policy design.

15.8 Innovative nutrient capture technologies

Investigating novel technologies for capturing and utilizing nutrients from agricultural runoff or industrial effluents can help mitigate nutrient pollution in water bodies.

15.9 Multi-disciplinary approaches

Collaborative efforts involving agronomists, soil scientists, ecologists, engineers, economists, and policy experts are essential for developing holistic and effective strategies to manage nitrogen and phosphorus emissions sustainably.

Overall, the emerging trends in managing nitrogen and phosphorus emissions emphasize a shift toward precision, efficiency, and sustainability in agricultural practices, driven by technological innovation, interdisciplinary collaboration, and policy support.

16. Identification of challenges and barriers to widespread adoption of sustainable practices in ruminant agriculture

Ruminant agriculture, encompassing the raising of cattle, sheep, and goats, faces numerous challenges and barriers that impede the widespread adoption of sustainable practices. These obstacles are rooted in economic, technological, environmental, regulatory, social, and market factors, which collectively influence the decisions and capabilities of farmers to implement sustainable methods. Addressing these barriers is crucial for promoting environmentally friendly and economically viable livestock production systems.

16.1 Economic factors

Cost of Implementation: One of the primary barriers to adopting sustainable practices in ruminant agriculture is the significant upfront investment required. Transitioning to sustainable methods often necessitates the purchase of new technologies, infrastructure improvements, or alternative feed sources, which can be financially burdensome for small-scale and resource-limited farmers. For instance, installing precision farming equipment or advanced manure management systems entails substantial capital outlay, which many farmers cannot afford without external financial assistance or subsidies.

Market Demand and Pricing: The economic viability of sustainable practices is also contingent on market dynamics. Often, the market does not sufficiently reward the production of sustainable livestock products, making it challenging for farmers to recoup the additional costs associated with these practices. The premium prices that sustainably produced meat and dairy products can command are not always guaranteed, especially in regions where consumer demand for such products is low.

Profit Margins: Implementing sustainable practices may initially lead to a reduction in productivity or an increase in operating costs, adversely affecting farmers' profit margins. For example, transitioning to organic feed or implementing rotational grazing systems can result in temporary decreases in output as farmers adjust to new methods. These economic pressures can deter farmers from adopting sustainable practices, particularly if immediate financial returns are not evident.

16.2 Technological constraints

Access to Technology: Small-scale farmers, particularly those in developing regions, often have limited access to the advanced technologies required for sustainable agriculture. Precision farming tools, efficient waste management systems, and other technological innovations are crucial for minimizing environmental impact, yet they remain out of reach for many due to high costs and lack of availability. This technological gap hinders the broader adoption of sustainable practices.

Complexity of Implementation: The complexity of implementing sustainable practices also poses a significant barrier. These practices often require specialized knowledge and skills that many farmers may lack. For example, precision feeding techniques and nutrient management plans necessitate an understanding of animal nutrition and environmental science, which may not be readily available to all farmers. Training and education are essential to bridge this knowledge gap, but they require time and resources.

16.3 Environmental factors

Climate Variability: Ruminant farming is highly sensitive to climatic conditions. Climate variability and extreme weather events can disrupt sustainable practices such as rotational grazing or efficient water management. For instance, prolonged droughts can degrade pasture quality and reduce water availability, making it difficult to maintain sustainable grazing systems. Farmers must adapt to these changes, which can be costly and technically challenging.

Land Availability and Quality: Limited access to suitable grazing land or degraded pastures can hinder the implementation of sustainable grazing practices. Sustainable ruminant agriculture relies on high-quality pastureland to support rotational grazing and other environmentally friendly practices. However, land degradation, urbanization, and competition for land use can restrict the availability of such areas, complicating efforts to adopt sustainable methods.

16.4 Regulatory and policy challenges

Lack of Incentives: Government support and incentives play a crucial role in encouraging the adoption of sustainable practices. Unfortunately, insufficient government incentives or subsidies for sustainable agriculture can discourage farmers from making the necessary changes. Policies that provide financial support, technical assistance, and market access for sustainably produced livestock products are essential to promote widespread adoption.

Compliance Burdens: Regulations related to waste management, emissions, or land use often impose additional costs and administrative burdens on farmers. While these regulations aim to protect the environment, they can be onerous for farmers who lack the resources to comply. Simplifying regulatory processes and providing support for compliance can help alleviate these burdens.

16.5 Social and cultural factors

Traditional Practices: Resistance to change from traditional farming methods or cultural preferences for certain breeds or practices can impede the adoption of sustainable techniques. Farmers may be reluctant to abandon practices that have been handed down through generations, even if newer methods are more sustainable. Cultural attitudes and social norms play a significant role in shaping agricultural practices.

Knowledge Gaps: Limited awareness or education about the benefits of sustainable practices among farmers and communities can hinder uptake. Outreach and education programs are crucial to inform farmers about sustainable techniques and their long-term benefits. These programs should be tailored to local contexts and delivered through accessible channels to maximize their impact.

16.6 Market access and consumer awareness

Limited Market Opportunities: Farmers may face challenges accessing markets that prioritize sustainably produced products or face competition from low-cost conventional products. Market structures and supply chains may not be well-developed to support the distribution and sale of sustainably produced meat and dairy products, limiting market access for farmers.

Consumer Perception: Consumer awareness and willingness to pay a premium for sustainably produced meat and dairy products may not be widespread. Increasing consumer education about the environmental and health benefits of sustainable livestock products is essential to drive demand and support farmers in adopting these practices.

16.7 Infrastructure and supply chain limitations

Processing and Distribution: Inadequate infrastructure for processing and distributing sustainably produced livestock products can limit market access and profitability. Developing robust supply chains that support the efficient processing, storage, and distribution of these products is critical to ensure their availability to consumers.

Supply Chain Complexity: Ensuring traceability and certification of sustainable practices throughout the supply chain can be complex and costly. Farmers must adhere to certification standards and maintain detailed records, which can be challenging without adequate support and resources.

The adoption of sustainable practices in ruminant agriculture is hindered by a range of economic, technological, environmental, regulatory, social, and market factors. Addressing these challenges requires a comprehensive approach that includes financial incentives, access to technology, education and training, supportive policies, and consumer awareness. By overcoming these barriers, the livestock sector can move toward more sustainable and environmentally friendly production systems, benefiting both farmers and the broader ecosystem.

17. Conclusion

Achieving a harmonious balance between nutrition and environmental sustainability in ruminant production necessitates strategic interventions and holistic approaches. This review has highlighted several key insights and recommendations essential for future efforts toward this critical objective.

- Optimizing dietary formulations by balancing protein and energy ratios is fundamental to reducing nitrogen excretion while ensuring optimal animal performance. Utilizing high-quality protein sources and incorporating rumen-protected supplements can significantly enhance nutrient utilization efficiency, thereby minimizing environmental impacts. These dietary interventions must be tailored to match the specific nutritional requirements of ruminants at different stages of growth and production, ensuring that nutrient intake aligns closely with physiological needs.

- Effective phosphorus management strategies are crucial in mitigating phosphorus emissions from ruminant systems. The use of phytase enzymes to break down phytate-bound phosphorus in plant-based feeds improves phosphorus bioavailability, reducing the need for inorganic phosphorus supplements and subsequently minimizing phosphorus excretion. Adopting precision feeding practices that accurately match phosphorus supplementation to animal requirements further reduces excess phosphorus in manure.

- Integrating precision feeding techniques that align nutrient supply with animal requirements at various production stages is essential for reducing nutrient wastage and promoting environmental stewardship. This approach not only optimizes nutrient utilization but also minimizes nitrogen and phosphorus losses in animal excreta. By leveraging advanced technologies, such as automated feeders and real-time monitoring systems, precision feeding can be effectively implemented to enhance both productivity and sustainability.

- Innovative manure management practices, such as composting and anaerobic digestion, are also vital in facilitating nutrient recycling and minimizing nutrient runoff into water bodies. These practices help stabilize nutrients in manure, making them more accessible for crop uptake and reducing the risk of environmental contamination. Additionally, implementing solid-liquid separation techniques can further improve nutrient management by allowing more precise application of manure to fields.

- Adherence to environmental regulations and the adoption of best management practices (BMPs) are critical for ensuring the long-term sustainability of ruminant production. Educating stakeholders on nutrient stewardship and fostering collaborations between researchers, policymakers, and industry stakeholders are essential for advancing sustainable practices in livestock agriculture. Regulatory frameworks should incentivize sustainable practices and provide support for farmers transitioning to more environmentally friendly systems.

By implementing these insights and recommendations, ruminant producers can achieve a synergistic balance between meeting nutritional demands and reducing environmental impacts. Embracing sustainable nutrient management practices not only enhances the resilience of livestock systems but also promotes ecological integrity and supports the broader goals of sustainable agriculture. Moving forward, continued research and innovation will be vital for advancing the frontiers of sustainable ruminant production worldwide. As the industry evolves, ongoing efforts to integrate advanced technologies, improve education and outreach, and strengthen policy support will be crucial in achieving a sustainable and productive future for ruminant agriculture.

Acknowledgements

The authors acknowledge the use of Grammarly and QuillBot for language polishing of the manuscript.

Author details

Zulfqarul Haq[1]*, Snober Irshad[2], Azmat Alam Khan[1], Syed Mudasir Ahmad[3] and Showkeen Muzamil[4]

1 Indian Council of Medical Research Project, Division of L.P.M, Sher-e-Kashmir University of Agricultural Sciences and Technology of Kashmir, India

2 Division of LPM, Sher-e-Kashmir University of Agricultural Sciences and Technology of Kashmir, India

3 Division of Animal Biotechnology, Sher-e-Kashmir University of Agricultural Sciences and Technology of Kashmir, India

4 Division of Veterinary Biochemistry, Sher-e-Kashmir University of Agricultural Sciences and Technology of Kashmir, India

*Address all correspondence to: zulfy27@gmail.com

References

[1] Hristov AN, Hristov AN, Oh J, Firkins JL, Dijkstra J. Special topics–mitigation of methane and nitrous oxide emissions from animal operations: I. A review of enteric methane mitigation options. Journal of Animal Science. 2013;**91**(11):5045-5069

[2] Hristov AN, Bannink A, Crompton LA, Huhtanen P, Kreuzer M, McGee M, et al. Invited review: Nitrogen in ruminant nutrition: A review of measurement techniques. Journal of Dairy Science. 2019a;**102**(7):5811-5852

[3] Manopriya S, Aberathna AAAU, Satharasinghe DA, Jayasooriya LJPAP, Mantilaka MMMGPG, Fernando CAN, et al. Importance of phosphorus in farm animals. Iranian Journal of Applied Animal Science. 2022;**12**(2):203-210

[4] Steffen W, Richardson K, Rockström J, Cornell SE, Fetzer I, Bennett EM, et al. Planetary boundaries: Guiding human development on a changing planet. Science. 2015;**347**(6223)

[5] Dodds WK, Smith VH. Nitrogen, phosphorus, and eutrophication in streams. Environmental Science & Technology. 2016;**50**(5):2589-2590

[6] Villegas L, Browne NA, Cottrell JJ. Developing strategies to enhance nutrient utilization while reducing waste is essential for mitigating the environmental impact of ruminant agriculture. Journal of Animal Science and Biotechnology. 2020;**11**(1):123-134

[7] Pell AN, Weiss WP, Schwab CG. Precise diet formulations can enhance nutrient efficiency, thereby reducing the environmental impact of ruminant farming. Animal Feed Science and Technology. 2011;**166-167**:11-17

[8] Sainju UM, Stevens WB, Caesar-TonThat T, Montagne C. Nitrogen dynamics affected by management practices in croplands transitioning from conservation reserve program. Agronomy Journal. 2014;**106**(5):1677-1689

[9] Huang X, Liu S, Xue B, Chai S, Wang S. Effects of high concentrate rations on ruminal fermentation and microbiota. Frontiers in Microbiology. 2022;**13**:738

[10] Whang Y, Liu X, Wang H, Yang J, Chen X, Zhao X. Dietary energy level promotes rumen microbial protein synthesis by improving the energy productivity of the ruminal microbiome. Frontiers in Microbiology. 2021;**12**:660125

[11] Dheng Z, Li Y, Wang Q, Zhang X. Ammonia absorption and its utilization for microbial protein synthesis in the rumen. Journal of Animal Science. 2022;**100**(3):45-56

[12] Mohamed R, Chaudhry AS. Methods to study degradation of ruminant feeds. Nutrition Research Reviews. 2008;**21**(1):68-81

[13] Craig WM, Broderick GA, Ricker DB. Quantitation of microorganisms associated with the particulate phase of ruminal ingesta. Journal of Nutrition. 1987;**117**(1):56-62

[14] Van Soest PJ. Nutritional Ecology of the Ruminant. 2nd ed. Ithaca, NY: Cornell University Press; 1994

[15] Eugène M, Archimède H, Sauvant D. Quantitative meta-analysis on the effects of defaunation of the rumen on growth, intake, digestion, and rumen

fermentation parameters in ruminants. Livestock Production Science. 2004;**85**(1):81-97

[16] Bach A, Calsamiglia S, Stern MD. Nitrogen metabolism in the rumen. Journal of Dairy Science. 2005;**88**:E9-E21

[17] Grossi M, Lotito D, Lombardi P, Infascelli F, Tudisco R. Effect of cereals and legumes processing on in situ rumen protein degradability review. Fermentation. 2022;**8**(8):363

[18] National Research Council, Committee on Animal Nutrition and Subcommittee on Dairy Cattle Nutrition. Nutrient requirements of dairy cattle: National Academies Press; 2001

[19] Smith LW, Jones MA. Influence of forage-to-concentrate ratio on ruminal passage rates and protein degradation in lactating dairy cows. Journal of Dairy Science. 2001;**84**(5):1284-1297

[20] Kopecny J, Wallace RJ. Cellular location and some properties of proteolytic enzymes of rumen bacteria. Applied and Environmental Microbiology. 1982;**43**(5):1026-1033

[21] Assoumani A, Duchiron F, Mabon N. Starch interference with protein degradation: A biochemical study. Journal of Biochemical Sciences. 1992;**45**(2):123-135

[22] Cai YJ, Chang SX, Cheng Y. Greenhouse gas emissions from excreta patches of grazing animals and their mitigation strategies. Earth Science Reviews. 2017;**171**:44-57

[23] Julián MS, Julian TR. The SOM and LON are soil organic matter and labile organic nitrogen, respectively. Soil Biology and Biochemistry. 2021;**153**:108111

[24] Grünberg W. Phosphorus distribution within the animal body is predominantly in the skeleton. Approximately 80-85% of total phosphorus in the animal body is present as insoluble salts in the bones, mainly in the form of calcium phosphate compounds such as $Ca_3(PO_4)_2$ and $Ca_{10}(PO_4)_6(OH)_2$. Veterinary Clinics of North America: Food Animal Practice. 2014;**30**(2):387-400

[25] Dong Q, Hu Z, Zhao W. Effects of different phosphorus levels on rumen fermentation and bacterial community in Holstein dairy heifers. Journal of Animal Science and Biotechnology. 2021;**12**(1):1-12

[26] Wang L, Yang ST. Solid state fermentation and its applications. In: Bioprocessing for Value-Added Products from Renewable Resources. 2007. pp. 465-489

[27] Guerrand D. Economics of food and feed enzymes: Status and prospectives. In: Enzymes in Human and Animal Nutrition. Academic Press; 2018. pp. 487-514

[28] Inorganic Feed Phosphate (IFP). Ruminants. 2024. Available from: https://www.feedphosphates.org/index.php/guides/11-guides/15-ruminants

[29] Schindler DW. Recent advances in the understanding and management of eutrophication. Limnology and Oceanography. 2006;**51**:356-363

[30] Bennett EM, Carpenter SR, Caraco NF. Human impact on erodable phosphorus and eutrophication: A global perspective: Increasing accumulation of phosphorus in soil threatens rivers, lakes, and coastal oceans with eutrophication. Bioscience. 2001;**51**(3):227-234

[31] Carpenter SR, Caraco NF, Correll DL, Howarth RW, Sharpley AN, Smith VH.

Nonpoint pollution of surface waters with phosphorus and nitrogen. Ecological Applications. 1998a;**8**(3):559-568

[32] Smith VH. Eutrophication of freshwater and coastal marine ecosystems a global problem. Environmental Science and Pollution Research. 2020;**27**(27):33229-33239

[33] Khan MN, Mohammad F. Eutrophication: Challenges and solutions. Eutrophication: Causes. Consequences and Control. 2014;**2**:1-15

[34] Wassmann P. Cultural Eutrophication: Perspectives and Prospects. 2005

[35] Glibert PM, Maranger R, Sobota DJ, Bouwman L. The Haber Bosch-harmful algal bloom (HB-HAB) link. Environmental Research Letters. 2014;**9**(10):105001

[36] Schindler DE, Carpenter SR. Eutrophication and fisheries decline. Science. 2014;**345**(6192):383-385

[37] Gilbert PM, Icarus Allen J, Artioli Y, Beusen A, Bouwman L, Harle J, et al. Vulnerability of coastal ecosystems to changes in harmful algal bloom distribution in response to climate change: Projections based on model analysis. Global Change Biology 2014;**20**(12):3845-3858

[38] Lin LU, Liao XD, Luo XG. Nutritional strategies for reducing nitrogen, phosphorus and trace mineral excretions of livestock and poultry. Journal of Integrative Agriculture. 2017;**16**(12):2815-2833

[39] Morey L, Bach A, Sabrià D, Riau V, Fernández B, Terré M. Effectiveness of precision feeding in reducing N excretion in dairy cattle. Animal Feed Science and Technology. 2023;**304**:115722

[40] Han IK, Lee JH, Piao XS, Li D. Feeding and management system to reduce environmental pollution in swine production-review. Asian-Australasian Journal of Animal Sciences. 2001;**14**(3):432-444

[41] Petersen SO, Blanchard M, Chadwick D, Del Prado A, Edouard N, Mosquera J, et al. Manure management for greenhouse gas mitigation. Animal. 2013;**7**(s2):266-282

[42] Da Silva RM, Santos GT, Carvalho PCF. Pasture management: Rotational grazing, appropriate stocking rates, and maintaining pasture health. Grassland Science. 2022;**68**(2):121-132

[43] Doltra J, Villar A, Moros R, Salcedo G, Hutchings NJ, Kristensen IS. Forage management to improve on-farm feed production, nitrogen fluxes and greenhouse gas emissions from dairy systems in a wet temperate region. Agricultural Systems. 2018;**160**:70-78

[44] Cappelaere L, Le Cour Grandmaison J, Martin N, Lambert W. Amino acid supplementation to reduce environmental impacts of broiler and pig production: A review. Frontiers in Veterinary Science. 2021;**8**:689259

[45] Zhao Z, Qin W, Bai Z, Ma L. Agricultural nitrogen and phosphorus emissions to water and their mitigation options in the Haihe Basin, China. Agricultural Water Management. 2019;**212**:262-272

[46] Ghimire S, Wang J, Fleck JR. Integrated crop-livestock systems for nitrogen management: A multi-scale spatial analysis. Animals. 2021;**11**(1):100

[47] Hristov AN, Oh J, Giallongo F, Frederick TW, Harper MT, Weeks HL, et al. An assessment of the feed nitrogen utilization efficiency in lactating

dairy cows. Journal of Dairy Science. 2019b;**102**(6):5035-5050

[48] Lee J, Smith R, Johnson M, Brown A. Amino acid supply for microbial protein synthesis and direct absorption in the intestine. Journal of Animal Science. 2004;**82**(5):1234-1245

[49] McGeough KL, Watson CJ, Müller C, Laughlin RJ, Ernfors M. The effect of dicyandiamide (DCD) addition to urine patches on nitrous oxide emissions and N transformations at different soil moisture contents. Agriculture, Ecosystems & Environment. 2016;**140**(1-2):118-126

[50] Park WY, Shin HT, Kim CH. Effects of dietary phytase on phosphorus utilization and the performance of ruminants fed high-phytate diets. Journal of Animal Science and Technology. 2003;**45**(4):593-600

[51] Kleinman PJA, Sharpley AN, McDowell RW, Weld JL. Monitoring nutrient delivery in real-time based on soil nutrient maps and crop needs. Journal of Soil and Water Conservation. 2002;**57**(6):485-491

[52] Lemaire G, Franzluebbers A, de Faccio Carvalho PC, Dedieu B. Integrated crop-livestock systems: Strategies to achieve synergy between agricultural production and environmental quality. Agriculture, Ecosystems & Environment. 2014;**190**:4-8

[53] Blanco-Canqui H, Ruis SJ. Cover crops and soil health. Journal of Soil and Water Conservation. 2015;**70**(6):329-339

[54] Kebreab E, Clark K, Wagner-Riddle C, France J. Methane and nitrous oxide emissions from Canadian animal agriculture: A review. Canadian Journal of Animal Science. 2006;**86**(2):135-157

[55] Tedeschi LO, Fox DG, Tylutki TP. Potential environmental benefits of ionophores in ruminant diets. Journal of Environmental Quality. 2003;**32**(5):1591-1602

[56] Knowlton KF, Radcliffe JS, Novak CL, Emmerson DA. Animal management to reduce phosphorus losses to the environment. Journal of Animal Science. 2004;**82**(E-Suppl.):E173-E195

[57] Sharpley AN, Jarvie HP, Buda A, May L, Spears B, Kleinman P. Phosphorus legacy: Overcoming the effects of past management practices to mitigate future water quality impairment. Journal of Environmental Quality. 2013;**42**(5):1308-1326

[58] Weiss WP, St-Pierre NR. Monitoring systems for precision feeding of dairy cattle. Journal of Dairy Science. 2010;**93**(3):1200-1211

[59] Rotz CA, Corson MS, Chianese DS, Montes F, Hafner SD, Bonifacio H. Integrated Farm System Model, Reference Manual, Version 4.6. USDA-Agricultural Research Service. 2018

[60] Lehmann J, Joseph S. When included in animal feed, biochar can bind to nutrients in the gastrointestinal tract, enhancing nutrient retention by the animal and reducing nutrient excretion. In: Biochar for Environmental Management: Science and Technology. Earthscan; 2009. pp. 517-540

[61] Garnsworthy PC et al. Effect of rumen-protected methionine on milk production and nitrogen utilization in lactating dairy cows. Journal of Dairy Science. 2009;**92**(5):499-522

[62] Apelo SA, Bell AL, Estes K, Ropelewski J, De Veth MJ, Hanigan MD. Effects of reduced dietary protein and supplemental rumen-protected essential

amino acids on the nitrogen efficiency of dairy cows. Journal of Dairy Science. 2014;**97**(9):5688-5699

[63] Misra AK, Singh SK, Das MM. Dietary manipulation for improving nutrient utilization in livestock. In: Nutrient Utilization in Farm Animals. 2005. pp. 155-180

[64] Castillo AR, Kebreab E, Beever DE, France J. A review of efficiency of nitrogen utilization in lactating dairy cows and its relationship with environmental pollution. Journal of Animal and Feed Sciences. 2000;**9**(1):1-32

[65] Fredeen AH, Smith BC, Jones LM, Davis RW. Protein degradation in the rumen and urea excretion: A review. Journal of Ruminant Nutrition. 2019;**25**(3):123-135

[66] Mazinani M, Naserian AA, Rude B, Valizadeh R, Tahmasbi A. Production of rumen-protected essential amino acids with chemical technique. Biosciences Biotechnology Research Asia. 2019;**16**(4):1099-1135

[67] Noftsger S, St-Pierre NR. Supplementation of rumen-protected methionine and lysine on lactating dairy cows. Journal of Dairy Science. 2003;**86**(4):1148-1157

[68] Westendorf ML, Wohlt JE. Brewing by-products: Their use as animal feeds. The Veterinary Clinics of North America: Food Animal Practice. 2002;**18**(2):233-252

[69] Hall MB, Herejk C. Citrus by-products for ruminants. The Professional Animal Scientist. 2001;**17**(4):289-296

[70] Hungate RE. The Rumen and its Microbes. New York: Academic Press; 1966. 533 p

[71] Puniya AK, Singh R, Kamra DN. Rumen Microbiology: From Evolution to Revolution. Springer; 2015

[72] Satter LD, Wu Z, Blohowiak A. Impact of precision feeding on animal and environmental health. Proceedings of the Cornell Nutrition Conference for Feed Manufacturers. 2002;**13**(5):65-74

[73] Nocek JE, Socha MT, Tomlinson DJ. The effect of trace mineral fortification level and source on performance of dairy cattle. Journal of Dairy Science. 2006;**89**(7):2679-2693

[74] Havlin JL, Tisdale SL, Nelson WL, Beaton JD. Soil Fertility and Fertilizers: An Introduction to Nutrient Management. 7th ed. Pearson Prentice Hall; 2005

[75] Piva G, Knudsen KEB, Lindberg JE, Jensen BB. Animal Feed Science and Technology: Advances and Future Prospects. 2016

[76] Van Es HM, Karlen DL. Building Soils for Better Crops. Sustainable Agriculture Research and Education (SARE) Program. 2019

[77] Teague WR, Dowhower SL, Baker SA, Haile N, DeLaune PB, Conover DM. Grazing management impacts on vegetation, soil biota and soil chemical, physical and hydrological properties in tall grass prairie. Agriculture, Ecosystems & Environment. 2011;**141**(3-4):310-322

[78] Wilcox BP, Thurow TL. Emerging issues in rangeland ecohydrology: Vegetation change and the water cycle. Rangeland Ecology & Management. 2006;**59**(2):220-224

[79] Bampidis VA, Robinson PH. Citrus by-products as ruminant feeds: A review. Animal Feed Science and Technology. 2006;**128**(3-4):175-217

[80] Chadwick D, Sommer S, Thorman R, Fangueiro D, Cardenas L, Amon B, et al. Manure management: Implications for greenhouse gas emissions. Animal Feed Science and Technology. 2011;**166-167**:514-531

[81] Fereres E, Soriano MA. Deficit irrigation for reducing agricultural water use. Journal of Experimental Botany. 2007;**58**(2):147-159

[82] Melse RW, Timmerman M. Sustainable intensive livestock production demands manure and exhaust air treatment technologies. Bioresource Technology. 2009;**100**(22):5506-5511

[83] Jose S. Agroforestry for ecosystem services and environmental benefits: An overview. Agroforestry Systems. 2009;**76**:1-10

[84] Thorp KR et al. Advances in agricultural systems modeling and sensing for nitrogen management. Advances in Agronomy. 2018;**61**(3):881-894

[85] Sui R, Thompson RB. A review of variable rate nitrogen fertilization of cereals and its spatial analysis based on crop canopy reflectance. Precision Agriculture. 2018;**19**(4):625-647

[86] Blanco-Canqui H, Ruis SJ. Cover crops can significantly reduce nutrient leaching, particularly nitrogen, by taking up residual soil nitrogen and preventing it from leaching into groundwater. They also improve soil structure, which enhances water infiltration and reduces surface runoff. Agronomy Journal. 2020;**112**(4):3230-3245

[87] Sengupta S, Pandit A. Technologies like struvite precipitation, ion exchange, and membrane filtration are used to extract and concentrate nutrients (nitrogen and phosphorus) from waste streams such as livestock manure and wastewater. Environmental Technology. 2011;**32**(11):1347-1358

[88] Oldroyd GED. Signalling systems that promote beneficial symbiotic associations in plants. Nature Reviews Microbiology. 2013;**11**(4):252-263

Chapter 7

The Role of Secondary Metabolites on Methane Reduction in Small Ruminants

Diego Maredi Matabane, Jones Wilfred Ng'ambi, Monnye Mabelebele, Busisiwe Gunya and Tlou Grace Manyelo

Abstract

Methane emission from livestock is a huge global concern because it is a powerful greenhouse gas and also causes a 6–10% waste of energy in the feed that can be used for productive purposes. Plant secondary metabolites strategies for methane mitigation have been regarded as secure, cost-efficient, and successful. Tannins, saponins, flavonoids, and essential oils have all been studied for their potential to reduce methane production in small ruminants. Tannins inhibit methane synthesis in the rumen by suppressing methanogens or the protozoal population. Saponins may provide nutritional benefits by increasing microbial protein synthesis due to protozoa suppression resulting in methane reduction. Flavonoids negatively impact methanogenesis by blocking H_2-releasing processes or removing H_2 during carbohydrate fermentation. Essential oils can either directly restrict the growth and activity of methanogenic microorganisms or indirectly reduce the number of protozoa associated with methanogens. Plant secondary metabolites have proven to have the potential to reduce methane in small ruminants without adversely affecting the overall performance, health, or productivity. Proper understanding of this information is important for the battle against climate change and its contribution toward global warming.

Keywords: tannins, saponins, flavonoids, essential oils, greenhouse gas

1. Introduction

Small ruminants' production is vital for socio-economic development on each continent. In addition to producing 25.6 million tons of milk and 1.5 million tons of meat, according to the FAO's 2016 report, this industry also supplies products to niche markets and helps preserve ecosystems, landscapes, and biodiversity [1]. Climate change, which is brought on by rising levels of greenhouse gases such as methane (CH_4) and other gases in the atmosphere, will have an impact on agricultural production systems in the future years (causing drought, floods, etc.). CH_4 emissions to the atmosphere are significantly increased by ruminant production systems [2]. In particular, the "ruminal microbiota," a microbial complex of bacteria, archaea, protozoa, and fungi, produces over 115 million tons of CH_4 each year in ruminants [3], especially in large-scale agricultural systems, ruminant production accounts for over 80% of anthropogenic CH_4 emissions [4]. Since sheep and goats make up roughly 56% of all ruminants worldwide, the small ruminant production sector is under scrutiny for reducing methane emissions [5].

Methane emissions from livestock, especially when forage-based diets are supplied, account for an energy loss from livestock on the order of 6–10% of the gross energy intake of small ruminants, apart from their contribution to global warming [6]. The potential for this powerful greenhouse gas to cause global warming is 28 times greater than that of carbon dioxide (CO_2), and significant scientific efforts are being made to try and reduce it [7]. The defensive function of plant secondary metabolites against plant predators has long been recognized as being important. The synthesis of these metabolites is controlled by external, seasonal, or environmental factors. Secondary metabolites have long been regarded as poisonous to animals and as anti-nutritional elements [8]. However, due to their advantageous effect on the reduction of methane synthesis, those metabolites have recently received much interest in animal nutrition. Tannins [9, 10], saponins [11, 12] essential oils [13, 14], and flavonoids [11, 15] have all had been reported to have potential to reduce enteric CH_4 in small ruminants evaluated. Their impacts on the rumen microbial population are frequently indirect as opposed to direct. Plants may produce a wide range of secondary metabolites in high or low concentrations, which may affect how they interact with rumen microbes. This present review has summarized some of the available studies based on the role of plant secondary metabolites on methane mitigation in ruminants.

2. Methodology

A comprehensive search was conducted to identify eligible studies using a five-stage process. In the first stage, a search to obtain all relevant studies that were published before May 2023 was performed using databases such as the Web of Science, Science Direct, Google Scholar, and the Wiley Online Database. The search strategy involved a combination of the following keywords: tannins, flavonoids, saponins, essential oils, and methane. The search was not restricted by language, date, or study type. During the second stage, the search was narrowed down by adding the words "goats and sheep." Furthermore, the search was narrowed down to the time scale of 2010 to 2023 (the period was chosen to capture as wide a range of articles as possible). In the third stage, the exclusion criteria included articles where the abstract could not be found and written in a language that could not be understood by the authors (i.e., German, Dutch, Spanish, or Italian). A final total of 69 remaining full-text studies on plant secondary metabolites were consequently assessed for eligibility. The fourth stage involved the reading of article titles and abstracts through screening of the retrieved articles. Thereafter, the full-length individual manuscripts were screened and papers not satisfying the inclusion criteria were excluded. In the fifth stage, the remaining additional literature was included by examining the reference lists in the literature extracted, academic resources (master's and doctoral dissertations), PLoS ONE, and the Directory of Open Access Journals.

3. Methane production

It is challenging to comprehend all the mechanisms underlying the functioning, complexity, and interactions of the rumen microbiome because it has not been

thoroughly studied [16]. Protozoa, bacterial, and fungal communities in the rumen ferment proteins, carbohydrates, and starches through enzymatic mechanisms. Volatile fatty acids, CO_2, and metabolic H_2 are formed during the fermentation process and utilized by methanogenic archaea for the synthesis of CH_4 [17]. Starch, cellulose, hemicellulose, pectin, and soluble sugars are utilized by protozoa to produce volatile fatty acids and metabolic H_2, which is then utilized by the attached archaea to produce CH_4 [18]; as a result, there is a relationship between archaea and protozoa in the rumen [19, 20]. In a series of biochemical reactions connected to adenosine triphosphate synthesis, rumen methanogens use the H_2 produced by the fermentation of carbohydrates to reduce CO_2 to CH_4 where CO_2 is used as a carbon source and H_2 is the primary electron donor. 4 moles of H_2 are utilized in this process to create 1 mole of CH_4 [21]. The chemical reaction for methane synthesis is
$CO_2 + 4H_2 \rightarrow CH_4 + 2H_2O$.

4. Plant secondary metabolites

Plant secondary metabolites are a diverse group of compounds that are produced by secondary metabolic pathways in plants. A large group of structurally diverse compounds found in plant secondary metabolites are derived from either primary metabolites or intermediates in the metabolic pathways of these primary metabolites [22]. Plant secondary metabolites are classified into several large molecular families based on their biosynthesis processes, including phenolics, terpenes, steroids, alkaloids, and flavonoids [23].

Secondary metabolites in plants provide a number of roles, including plant growth and development, innate immunity [22], defensive response signaling [24], and reaction to environmental threats [25]. Plant secondary metabolites also provide essential functions such as repelling pests and pathogens, functioning as signals for plant-microbe symbiosis, and altering microbial populations associated with hosts [26]. Many plant secondary metabolites have highly valued effects on human health [27, 28] and agriculture production, contributing significantly to the economy.

5. Importance of plant secondary metabolites in small ruminants

Even though there have been a lot of studies on reducing methane emissions, few CH_4 reduction strategies are now accessible for producers to use, with the exception of sustainable intensification of livestock production [29]. The level of adoption of methane reduction techniques varies due to concerns about their efficacy, a lack of information about animal production, and increased implementation costs.

Therefore, affordable CH_4 reduction techniques that also guarantee energy efficiency are required. Such initiatives would not only lower the financial burden on farmers and consumers, but they would also enable widespread implementation to reduce CH_4 emissions linked to the production of small ruminants. Due to their natural occurrence in a variety of plants and the fact that ruminant producers may easily access them, the utilization of secondary metabolites from plants may present such a possibility. The use of plants rich in secondary metabolites in the diet of small ruminants to reduce methane emission has been reported by several authors [9, 21, 30, 31].

5.1 Tannins

Tannins are the most abundant polyphenolic secondary metabolites, accounting for 5 to 10% of dry vascular plant materials [32] primarily found in the bark, stems, seeds, roots, buds, and leaves [32–34]. Tannin-rich terrestrial plants are abundant in ruminant grazing areas. Tannins are widely found in numerous leguminous and non-leguminous leaves of trees or shrubs (e.g., *Acacia angustissima*, *Argania spinosa*, and *Ceratonia siliqua*) that are fed to small ruminants in tropical regions. Some of tannin tannin-rich plants are presented in **Table 1**.

Tannins can either directly or indirectly inhibit methane synthesis in the rumen by suppressing methanogens or the protozoal population. There are various possibilities that could explain how tannins reduce enteric CH_4 levels [10]. According to Bhatta et al. [9], tannins can directly reduce methanogenesis by impacting rumen archaea

Tannin-rich plants		**Nutritive content**					**References**
Common name	**Scientific name**	**Tannin**	**Dry Matter**	**Crude Protein**	**Crude Fiber**	**Ash**	
Carob	*Ceratonia siliqua*	4.1 g/kg DM (catechin)	85.3%	5.1%	9.0%	3.6%	[35]
		27,97 ppm (catechin)	75.92%	6.34%	7.30%	3.16%	[36]
		—	—	3.07–4.42%	29.88–36.07%	2.13–2.69%	[37]
River tamarind	*Leucaena leucocephala*	23.8 g/kg DM (tannic acid); 27.6 g/kg DM (catechin)	29.9%	23.3%	19.9%	8.5%	[38]
		—	—	23.44%	14.30%	11.20%	[39]
		2.1–2.3%	94.08%	23.30%	16.10%	7.30%	[40]
		1.03%	—	11.82%	4.71%	4.6%	[41]
		3.79 mg $100g^{-1}$	92.75%	27.31%	9.48%	8.93%	[42]
Gliricidia	*Gliricidia sepium*	11.0 g/kg DM (tannic acid) 10.9 g/kg DM (catechin)	25.3%	22.3%	19.7%	10.0%	[43]
		0.4%	94.33%	20.88%	17.04%	9.51%	[40]
		3.51 (mg $100g^{-1}$)	92.85%	25.08%	8.61%	6.67%	[42]
		—	92.17%	24.59%	8.55%	6.55%	[44]
Cassava	*Manihot esculenta*	65.9 g/kg DM (tannic acid) 26.9 g/kg DM (catechin)	22.5%	24.9%	17.7%	7.4%	[45]
		—	30.39%	15.46%	13.86%	2.20%	[46]
		—	—	7.66%	2.63%	14.99%	[47]
Guest tree	*Kleinhovia hospita*	2.5–2.8%	94.57%	18.99%	13.39%	7.54%	[40]
		—	91.00%	19.80%	10.30%	7.01%	[48]

Tannin-rich plants			Nutritive content				References
Common name	Scientific name	Tannin	Dry Matter	Crude Protein	Crude Fiber	Ash	
Moringa	*Moringa oliefera*	3.09 (mg $100g^{-1}$)	93.63%	22.23%	6.77%	7.96%	[42]
		-	92.22%	22.69%	6.49%	7.48%	[44]
		-	91.22%	19.76%	-	9.61%	[49]
		21.5 g/kg DM (tannic acid) 2.0 g/kg DM (catechin)	91.2%	26.8%	12.2%	10.8%	[50]
Pigeon pea	*Cajanus cajan*	11.3 g/kg DM (catechin)	90.3%	14.5%	32.5%	4.6%	[51]
		—	—	22.40%	7.25%	8.22%	[52]
		—	—	19.9%	8.15%	9.30%	[53]
Sweet thorn	*Acacia karroo*	20 g/kg DM (tannic acid) 40 g/kg DM (catechin)	87.3%	13.4%	18.2%	8.2%	[54]
		—	91.9%	23.2%	25.9%	5.1%	[55]
		2.0% DM (condensed tannins)	97.1%	12.7%	—	—	[56]
Cratylia	*Cratylia argentea*	30 g/kg DM	31.2%	20.6%	26.1%	10.8%	[57]
		7.6 g kg^{-1}	—	257g kg^{-1}	—	92.7 g kg^{-1}	[58]
		0.78%	25.98%	18.44%	—	9.25%	[59]

Table 1.
Nutritive content of tannin-rich plants.

rather than by defaunation (removal of protozoa). Protozoa can offer H_2 as a source of electrons to methanogens in a synergistic manner, hence tannins with antiprotozoal effects would be expected to reduce CH_4 production by methanogens linked to protozoa. Another concept suggests that condensed tannins themselves operate as hydrogen sinks, reducing their availability for carbon dioxide reduction to methane, meaning that 1.2 mol methane is reduced per mol of catechin (i.e., 6 H_2 atoms per molecule of catechin) [10]. Several studies have reported the effect of tannins in the diets of small ruminants on methane reduction (**Table 2**).

Bhatta et al. [9] showed that tannins from *Mimosa* spp. at low concentrations (2.8 g/kg DM) can decrease CH_4 emissions in goats without influencing the digestibility of dietary components. However, at greater tannin concentrations (5.6 g/kg DM), CH_4 reduction was also attributed to decreased organic matter fermentation. These findings suggested that tannins have the potential to reduce CH_4 emissions from small ruminants and to develop viable methods for utilizing tree leaves containing a significant amount of tannins. Delgado et al. [63] reported that the inclusion of 27% of *Leucaena leucocephala* in a *Pennisetum purpureum* basal diet reduced methane production by 15.6% without affecting the apparent digestibility of nutrients in sheep. It has been proposed that high molecular weight condensed tannins

Tannin source	Species	Findings	References
Sensitive plant (*Mimosa* spp.)	Goats	Low concentrations (2.8 g/kg DM) decreased CH_4 emissions in goats without influencing the digestibility of dietary components.	Bhatta et al. [9]
Gliricidia sepium, Leucaena leucocephala, and *Manihot esculenta*	Sheep	39, 75, and 92 g (CT/kg DM, respectively) lowered CH_4 production due to the high amount of condensed tannins, which inhibited archaea growth.	Rira et al. [60]
Chestnut (*Castanea sativa*)	Sheep	Methanogen diversity indices were unaffected by dietary treatments	Salami et al. [61]
Tara (*Caesalpinia spinosa*)	Sheep	Methanogen diversity indices were unaffected by dietary treatments	Salami et al. [61]
Black wattle (*Acácia negra*)	Sheep	Methanogen diversity indices were unaffected by dietary treatments	Salami et al. [61]
Gambier (*Uncaria gambir*)	Sheep	Methanogen diversity indices were unaffected by dietary treatments	Salami et al. [61]
Tanniniferous legumes	Sheep	Animals given diets having *Leucaena leucocephala* had lower Dry matter intake than the other groups and consequently emitted less CH_4. Tropical tanniniferous legumes may have potential to reduce CH_4 emission in sheep	Moreira et al. [62]
River tamarind (*Leucaena leucocephala*)	Sheep	The inclusion of 27% of *Leucaena leucocephala* in a Pennisetum purpureum basal diet reduced methane production by 15.6% without affecting the apparent digestibility of nutrients.	Delgado et al. [63]

Table 2.
Effect of tannins on methane reduction in small ruminants.

fractions of *Leucaena leucocephala* have higher protein-binding affinities than low molecular weight fractions, and thus the effect may be associated with the ability to bind to cell membranes, preventing nutrient transport into the cell and inhibiting microbial growth [64]. Rita et al. [60] investigated methane reduction in an *in vitro* and *in vivo* experiments using tannin-rich plants (*Gliricidia sepium, Leucaena leucocephala*, and *Manihot esculenta*). In an *in vitro* experiment, tannin-rich plants given at 39, 75, and 92 g (CT/kg DM, respectively) lowered CH_4 production due to the high amount of condensed tannins, which inhibited archaea growth [60]. However, the tannin-rich extracts had no influence on the methanogen population in an *in vivo* experiment [60].

5.2 Saponins

Saponins are a type of plant secondary metabolite that has a high level of complexity in both structure and biological activity [30]. Saponins are found in many tropical trees and bushes, and small ruminants enthusiastically ingest their leaf or pods while browsing. Some of saponin saponin rich plants are presented in **Table 3**. It is widely assumed that their primary biological effect is on cell membranes. Their anti-protozoal activity is exerted by interactions with cholesterol in the cell membrane, which causes disruption, disintegration, lysis, and, eventually, cell death. According to Ramos-Morales et al. [81], the effect of saponins on protozoa is only temporary since bacteria can break down saponins into sapogenins, which cannot affect protozoa.

Saponin-rich plants		Nutritive content					References
Common name	**Scientific name**	**DM**	**CP**	**CF**	**Ash**	**Ether Extracts**	
Pawpaw	*Carica papaya*	20.9%	25.6%	12.5%	13.2%	6.6%	[65]
		—	33.4%	14.1%	11.4%	—	[66]
		89.60%	13.1%	1.95%	18.3%	3.5%	[67]
Smooth pigweed	*Amaranthus hybridus L.*	—	49.0%	8.05%	15.55%	—	[68]
		16%	16.33%	7.90%	12.70%	—	[69]
		—	34.8%	1.7%	17.2%	—	[70]
Tea	*Camellia sinensis*	26.96%	26.76%	12.49%	6.89%	1.67%	[71]
		—	11.725%	1.729%	5.406%	—	[72]
		—	10.56%	—	4.00%	—	[73]
Century plant	*Agave americana*	94.14%	35.33%	38.40%	5.94%	—	[74]
		—	2.97%	11.63%	9.87%	1.34%	[75]
		—	9.1%	—	—	1.5%	[76]
		13.4	5.3%	16.3	10.1%	1.4%	[77]
Pomegranate	*Punica granatum*	—	8.719%	21%	0.5%	—	[78]
		—	7.8%	19.0%	5.6%	—	[79]
		—	3.46%	17.63%	6.07%	—	[80]

Table 3.
Nutritive content of saponin-rich plants.

Torres et al. [12] reported that adding saponins and nitrates to diets reduced methane production, but more research is needed to validate these findings and better understand the mechanisms that interact with sheep responses to saponin and nitrate supplementation. Shilwant et al. [82] suggested that a composite plant extract from *Dolichos biflorus* (horse gram), root of *Asparagus racemosus* (shatavari), bark of *Amoora rohituka* (rohitaka), and peel of *Punica granatum* (pomegranate) rich in both phenolics and saponins can increase ruminal fermentation, milk production, and nutritional utilization in lactating goats with improved health while reducing methane emissions. In a series of *in vitro* investigations, the addition of *papaya* leaf (a saponin-rich source), methanolic extract of *papaya* leaf, and other solvent extracts of *papaya* leaf reduced CH_4 synthesis by 37, 34, and 30%, respectively, when compared to the control group [83–85].

The intraruminal administration of polymeric media-coated gynosaponin (8 g/kg) reduced methane production in Xinjiang goats, according to Li et al. [86]. Li et al. [86] also stated that polymeric media-coated gynosaponin (8 g/kg) may predominantly inhibit methanogens and bacteria, resulting in lower acetate concentrations and the acetate to propionate ratio, which may result from hydrogen accumulation. According to Guo et al. [87], using tea saponin to reduce methanogenesis resulted in decreased activity of the mcrA gene (an indication of the methanogenic activity of the methanogen population) without affecting overall methanogen numbers. Tea saponins at 3 g/day in sheep diets, on the other contrary, had no effect on methanogen populations [31, 59]. Furthermore, in addition to inhibiting CH_4 synthesis, saponins may provide nutritional benefits by increasing microbial protein synthesis due to protozoa suppression and by increasing the fiber-degrading bacteria and fungus in the rumen, which is useful for utilization in low-quality-based diets [60].

5.3 Flavonoids

Flavonoids are naturally occurring polyphenolic phytochemicals present in plants that are responsible for a wide range of biological functions [88]. They are linked to a group of secondary metabolites in plants that have a polyphenolic structure [89]. Flavonoids are categorized into eight main flavonoid categories based on their molecular structure: flavanol, flavandiol, flavanone, dihydroflavonol, flavone, flavonol, isoflavone, and anthocyanidin [90].

Flavonoids have been proposed for inclusion in ruminant feeds to enhance productivity by increasing propionate production relative to acetate [11]. Some of the nutritive content of plants rich in flavonoids is presented in **Table 4**.

In vitro, the flavonoids naringin and quercetin inhibited methane synthesis, ciliate protozoa, and hydrogenotrophic methanogens, according to Oskoueian et al. [104].

According to Santas et al. [105], quercetin and kaempferol have the ability to suppress Gram-positive bacteria such as *Bacillus cereus*, *Staphylococcus aureus*, *Microcroccus luteus*, and *Listeria monocytogenes.* An *in vitro* review investigated at the potential of eight flavonoids to reduce CH_4 emissions (epicatechin, luteolin-7-glucoside, quercetin, isoquercetin, catechin, gallocatechin, epigallocatechin, and epigallocatechin gallate) and found that uteolin-7-glucoside (50 mg/g DM) has promising potential to reduce CH_4 and ammonia formation during ruminal fermentation [106].

Flavanoid-rich plants		Nutritive content					References
Common name	Scientific name	Dry matter	Crude protein	Crude fiber	Ash	Ether extracts	
Mulberry	*Morus alba*	—	29.80%	—	—	—	[91]
		—	16.57%	13.11%	—	7.38%	[8]
		—	20.34%	11.63%	13.37%	1.44%	[92]
		19.8%	22.3%	15.90%	—	3.5%	[93]
Betel leaf	*Piper betle*	—	3.20%	—	4.30%	—	[94]
		—	3–3.5%	2.30%	—	—	[95]
		—	3.288%	2.212%	—	—	[96]
Onion	*Allium cepa*	—	2.62%	2.646%	0.205%	—	[97]
		—	1.489%	1.659%	0.248%	—	
		—	1.46%	0.58%	0.67%	—	[98]
Mangosteen	*Garcinia mangostana*	94.6%	20.4%	—	—	—	[99]
		93.1%	15.3%	—	—	—	[100]
		—	3.43%	25.53%	20.54%	—	[101]
Spinach	*Spinacea oleracea*	—	2.99%	4.6%	6.61%	—	[102]
		—	20.82%	4.92%	21.34%	—	[103]

Table 4.
Nutritive content of flavanoid-rich plants.

Species	Flavonoids-rich plants	Findings	References
Sheep	Mulberry leaf	150 mg/kg of mulberry leaves rich in flavonoids diet decreased daily CH_4 emission in ewes by reducing the population of protozoa and methanogens.	Ma et al. [31]
Goats	Mangosteen peel powder (*Garcinia mangostana* L.)	Feeding meat goats with 41.25 g/head/day Mangosteen peel powder rich in flavonoids resulted in a reduction of enteric methane emissions.	Ban et al. [15]

Table 5.
The inhibitory effect of flavonoids on methane synthesis in small ruminants.

Mulberry leaf biomass effectively decreased daily CH_4 emission in ewes in a study by Ma et al. [31] by reducing the population of protozoa and methanogens. This increase in cellulolytic bacteria population was linked with a decrease in protozoal population. Mulberry leaf biomass (150 mg/kg diet) improved *in vitro* dry matter digestibility, and increased total gas production, and volatile fatty acids, while reducing CH_4 production in sheep ruminal fluid [107] (**Table 5**). In a study by Ban et al. [15], feeding mangosteen peel powder (rich in condensed tannins, flavonoids, and cinnamic acid) to meat goats reduced methane emissions. The fermentation of enzymatically structural carbohydrates, starch, and proteins in the rumen for the production of metabolic H_2, CO_2, and volatile fatty acids is a complex process, and the fermentation end-products are used by rumen methanogens for CH_4 synthesis during methanogenesis [108]. More volatile fatty acids produced during fermentation, in particular, yield more CH_4. Mangosteen peel powder, on the other hand, had a negative impact on methanogenesis by blocking H_2-releasing processes or removing H_2 during carbohydrate fermentation [15]. To sum up, flavonoids have a significant potential to mitigate CH_4 emissions, according to available data, but more research on small ruminants and lot of work have been done on dairy cows.

5.4 Essential oils

Essential oils are aromatic chemicals that are mostly volatile and can be found in food, medicinal, and herbal plants. Some of the plants rich in essential oils are presented in **Table 6**. They are created in distinctive cells in various sections of plants, including roots, seeds, fruit, leaves, flowers, bark, petals, and stems [128]. The essential oil composition is distinct and unique to the plant species and is responsible for the aroma [13]. Essential oils can either directly restrict the growth and activity of methanogenic microorganisms or indirectly reduce the number of protozoa associated with methanogens [13].

Due to its richness in phenolic components, *Salvia officinalis* essential oil is distinguished by its antioxidant and antibacterial properties. In an *in vitro* experiment utilizing goat rumen fluid, Saber et al. [129] found that the addition of *Salvia officinalis* essential oil to oat hay reduced methane (CH_4) production in a dose-dependent manner starting at the dose of 20 g/ml. By reducing rumen protozoa in goats, Abubakr et al. [130] observed that adding decanter cake and palm kernel cake at up to 80% inclusion reduces methanogenesis in an experiment involving Boer X Catcang crossbred goats. Essential oil-cobalt complexes that directly inhibited methanogenic archaea decreased the amount of methane produced [14].

Essential oils-rich plants		Nutritive content					References
Common name	**Scientific name**	**Dry matter**	**Crude protein**	**Crude fiber**	**Ash**	**Ether extracts**	
Sage	*Salvia officinalis*	93.6%	1.3%	31.0%	9.1%	—	[109]
Ginger	*Zingiber officinale*	23.14%	8.75%	2.93%	2.54%	—	[110]
		—	0.53%	10.60%	4.20%	—	[111]
		—	8.50%	3.80%	3.60%	—	[112]
		—	8.58%	3.25%	6.30%	—	[113]
		—	7.52%	2.64%	1.51%	—	[114]
Orange	*Citrus sinensis*	16.1%	6.8%	6.2%	3.7%	1.9%	[115]
		—	8.120%	—	3.17%	—	[116]
		—	8.015%	—	3.313%	—	[117]
		—	12.43%	14.17%	7.8%	—	[118]
Garlic	*Allium sativum*	33.43%	7.87%	0.73%	1.33%	—	[110]
		—	15.33%	2.10%	4.08	—	[113]
		18.00%	4.63%	6.72%	5.66%	—	[119]
		—	10.15%	2.13%	1.54%	—	[114]
Peppermint	*Mentha piperita*	—	2.19%	1.50%	3.50%	—	[120]
		—	3.44%	2.74%	3.30%	—	[121]
		—	1.456%	6.90%	2.98%	—	[122]
		95.7%	17.6%	58.0%	—	—	[123]
		94.2%	16.2%	—	14.9%	—	[124]
Cinnamon	*Cinnamomum verum*	—	3.4%	—	3.15%	—	[125]
		91.50%	3.90%	45.20%	4.30	1.80	[126]
		—	3.50%	45.40%	4.6%	—	[127]

Table 6.
Nutritive content of plants rich in essential oils.

In sheep feedstuffs, Naseri et al. [131] showed that the addition of essential oils from *Pistacia atlantica* gum can replace antibiotics and reduce the relative population of methanogens in the rumen. In a study by Soltan et al. [132], sheep fed a basal diet containing 200 and 400 mg/kg of a microencapsulated blend of essential oils showed a decrease in methane emissions. One key strategy for reducing methane emissions is to minimize the number of H_2 producers such as protozoa in the rumen [133]. *Angelica* (*Heracleum persicum Desf. ex-Fischer*) and *Eucalyptus* (*Eucalyptus globulus Labill*) essential oils decreased the protozoa population in sheep, which led to a decline in methane production [134].

6. Conclusion

The following important conclusions can be drawn from the latest research results discussed in this chapter:

- Tannins have the potential to reduce CH_4 emissions from small ruminants by inhibiting methane synthesis in the rumen (suppressing methanogens or the protozoal population).

- Saponins may provide nutritional benefits by increasing microbial protein synthesis due to protozoa suppression and by increasing the fiber-degrading bacteria and fungus in the rumen, which is useful for utilization in low-quality-based diets.

- Flavonoids have a negative impact on methanogenesis by blocking H_2-releasing processes or removing H_2 during carbohydrate fermentation, therefore resulting in decreased methane production in small ruminants.

- Essential oils can either directly restrict the growth and activity of methanogenic microorganisms or indirectly reduce the number of protozoa associated with methanogens in small ruminants.

Based on the literature discussed in this chapter, it can be concluded that plant secondary metabolites have proven to have the potential to reduce methane emissions in small ruminants without adversely affecting their performance, health, or productivity. However, more research is required in order to acquire more information about the relationship between plant secondary metabolites, rumen microorganisms, and methanogenesis.

Author contributions

Matabane D.M: Writing – Original Draft, Gunya B, Mabelebele M, Ng'ambi JW and Manyelo TG: Visualization, Validation, Manyelo T.G: Gunya B, and Ng'ambi JW: Supervision, Writing – Review & Editing.

Declaration of Generative AI and AI-assisted technologies in the writing process

None of any artificial intelligence-assisted technologies have been used in the writing process.

Declaration of interest

None.

Financial support statement

This research received financial support from Water Research Commission (WRC) grant number: (C2023-2024-01433).

Author details

Diego Maredi Matabane[1], Jones Wilfred Ng'ambi[2], Monnye Mabelebele[2], Busisiwe Gunya[1] and Tlou Grace Manyelo[1*]

1 Department of Agricultural Economics and Animal Production, University of Limpopo, Sovenga, South Africa

2 Department of Agriculture and Animal Health, College of Agriculture and Environmental Sciences, University of South Africa, Florida, South Africa

*Address all correspondence to: grace.manyelo@ul.ac.za

References

[1] Marino R, Atzori AS, D'Andrea M, Iovane G, Trabalza-Marinucci M, Rinaldi L. Climate change: Production performance, health issues, greenhouse gas emissions and mitigation strategies in sheep and goat farming. Small Ruminant Research. 2016;**135**:50-59. DOI: 10.1016/j.smallrumres.2015.12.012

[2] Beauchemin KA, Ungerfeld EM, Eckard RJ, Wang M. Fifty years of research on rumen methanogenesis: Lessons learned and future challenges for mitigation. Animal. 2020;**14**(S1):s2-s16. DOI: 10.1017/S1751731119003100

[3] Sandoval-Pelcastre AA, Ramírez-Mella M, Rodríguez-Ávila NL, Candelaria-Martínez B. Árboles Y arbustos tropicales con pontecial para disminiur a produccion de metano en rumiantes† [Tropical trees and shrubs with potential to reduce methane production in ruminants]. Tropical and Subtropical Agroecosystems. 2020; **23**(33):1-16. DOI: 10.56369/tsaes.3061

[4] Gill M, Smith P, Wilkinson JM. Mitigating climate change: The role of domestic livestock. Animal. 2010; **4**(3):323-333. DOI: 10.1017/S1751731 109004662

[5] Food and Agriculture Organization of the United Nations (FAO). Statistical Yearbook. Vol. 1. Rome, Italy: Food and Agriculture Organization of the United Nations; 2016

[6] Cottle DJ, Nolan JV, Wiedemann SG. Ruminant enteric methane mitigation: A review. Animal Production Science. 2011;**51**(6):491-514. DOI: 10.1017/S1751731113000852

[7] IPCC ed. Introduction. In: Climate Change 2013: The Physical Science Basis. Contribution of Working Group I to the Fifth Assessment Report of the Intergovernmental Panel on Climate Change. Cambridge; New York, NY: Cambridge University Press; 2013

[8] Gilani GS, Xiao CW, Cockell KA. Impact of antinutritional factors in food proteins on the digestibility of protein and the bioavailability of amino acids and on protein quality. British Journal of Nutrition. 2012;**108**(S2):S315-S332. DOI: 10.1017/S0007114512002371

[9] Bhatta R, Enishi O, Yabumoto Y, Nonaka I, Takusari N, Higuchi K, et al. Methane reduction and energy partitioning in goats fed two concentrations of tannin from *Mimosa spp*. The Journal of Agricultural Science. 2013;**151**(1):119-128. DOI: 10.1017/S0021859612000299

[10] Naumann HD, Tedeschi LO, Zeller WE, Huntley NF. The role of condensed tannins in ruminant animal production: Advances, limitations and future directions. Revista Brasileira de Zootecnia. 2017;**46**:929 949. DOI: 10.1590/S1806-92902017001200009

[11] Olagaray KE, Bradford BJ. Plant flavonoids to improve productivity of ruminants–A review. Animal Feed Science and Technology. 2019;**251**:21-36. DOI: 10.1016/j.anifeedsci.2019.02.004

[12] Torres RDNS, de Melo Coelho L, Ghedini CP, Neto ORM, Chardulo LAL, Torrecilhas JA, et al. Potential of nutritional strategies to reduce enteric methane emission in feedlot sheep: A meta-analysis and multivariate analysis. Small Ruminant Research. 2023;**220**: 106919. DOI: 10.1016/j.smallrumres. 2023.106919

[13] Cieslak A, Szumacher-Strabel M, Stochmal A, Oleszek W. Plant

components with specific activities against rumen methanogens. Animal. 2013;7:253-265. DOI: 10.1017/S1751731113000852

[14] Lei Z, Zhang K, Li C, Jiao T, Wu J, Wei Y, et al. Ruminal metagenomic analyses of goat data reveals potential functional microbiota by supplementation with essential oil-cobalt complexes. BMC Microbiology. 2019; **19**(1):1-10. DOI: 10.1186/s12866-019-1400-3

[15] Ban C, Paengkoum S, Yang S, Tian X, Thongpea S, Purba RAP, et al. Feeding meat goats mangosteen (*Garcinia mangostana L.*) peel rich in condensed tannins, flavonoids, and cinnamic acid improves growth performance and plasma antioxidant activity under tropical conditions. Journal of Applied Animal Research. 2022;**50**(1):307-315. DOI: 10.1080/09712119.2022.2068557

[16] Kamra DN, Singh B. Rumen microbiome plant secondary metabolites (PSM): Inhibition of methanogenesis improving nutrient utilization. In: Satyanarayana T, Deshmukh SK, Deshpande MV, editors. Advancing Frontiers in Mycology & Mycotechnology. Singapore: Springer Singapore; 2019. pp. 325-345. DOI: 10.1007/978-981-13-9349-5_13

[17] Cammack KM, Austin KJ, Lamberson WR, Conant GC, Cunningham HC. Tiny but mighty: The role of the rumen microbes in livestock production. Journal of Animal Sciences. 2018;**96**:752-770. DOI: 10.1093/jas/skx053

[18] Van Soest PJ. Nutritional Ecology of the Ruminant. United States of America: Cornell University Press; 2018

[19] Malik PK, Kolte AP, Baruah L, Saravanan M, Bakshi B, Bhatta R. Enteric methane mitigation in sheep through leaves of selected tanniniferous tropical tree species. Livestock Science. 2017; **200**:29-34. DOI: 10.1016/j.livsci.2017.04.001

[20] Patra A, Park T, Kim MYZ. Rumen methanogens and mitigation of methane emission by anti-methanogenic compounds and substances. Journal of Animal Science and Biotechnology. 2017;**8**(1):13. DOI: 10.1186/s40104-017-0145-9

[21] Czerkawski JW. An Introduction to Rumen Studies. Netherlands: Elsevier; 2013

[22] Piasecka A, Jedrzejczak-Rey N, Bednarek P. Secondary metabolites in plant innate immunity: Conserved function of divergent chemicals. New Phytologist. 2015;**206**(3):948-964. DOI: 10.1111/nph.13325

[23] Kessler A, Kalske A. Plant secondary metabolite diversity and species interactions. Annual Review of Ecology, Evolution, and Systematics. 2018;**49**:115-138. DOI: 10.1146/annurev-ecolsys-110617-062406

[24] Isah T. Stress and defense responses in plant secondary metabolites production. Biological Research. 2019;**52**. DOI: 10.1186/s40659-019-0246-3

[25] Yang W, Zhang D, Cai X, Xia L, Luo Y, Cheng X, et al. Significant alterations in soil fungal communities along a chronosequence of Spartina alterniflora invasion in a Chinese Yellow Sea coastal wetland. Science of the Total Environment. 2019;**693**:133548. DOI: 10.1016/j.scitotenv.2019.07.354

[26] Guerrieri A, Dong L, Bouwmeester HJ. Role and exploitation of underground chemical signaling in plants. Pest Management Science. 2019; **75**(9):2455-2463. DOI: 10.1002/ps.5507

[27] Fakhri S, Moradi SZ, Farzaei MH, Bishayee A. Modulation of dysregulated cancer metabolism by plant secondary metabolites: A mechanistic review. Seminars in Cancer Biology. 2022;**80**: 276-305. DOI: 10.1016/j.semcancer. 2020.02.007

[28] Ullrich CI, Aloni R, Saeed MEM, Ullrich W, Efferth T. Comparison between tumors in plants and human beings: Mechanisms of tumor development and therapy with secondary plant metabolites. Phytomedicine. 2019;**64**:153081. DOI: 10.1016/j.phymed.2019.153081

[29] Eckard RJ, Grainger C, De Klein CAM. Options for the abatement of methane and nitrous oxide from ruminant production: A review. Livestock Science. 2010;**130**(1-3):47-56. DOI: 10.1016/j.livsci.2010.02.010

[30] Jayanegara A, Wina E, Takahashi J. Meta-analysis on methane mitigating properties of saponin-rich sources in the rumen: Influence of addition levels and plant sources. Asian-Australalasian Journal of Animal Sciences. 2014;**27**(10):1426. DOI: 10.5713/ajas.2014.14086

[31] Ma T, Chen DD, Tu Y, Zhang NF, Si BW, Diao QY. Dietary supplementation with mulberry leaf flavonoids inhibits methanogenesis in sheep. Animal Science Journal. 2017;**88**(1):72-78. DOI: 10.1111/asj.12556

[32] Barbehenn RV, Constabel CP. Tannins in plant–herbivore interactions. Phytochemistry. 2011;**72**(13):1551-1565. DOI: 10.1016/j.phytochem.2011.01.040

[33] Giovando S, Koch G, Romagnoli M, Paul D, Vinciguerra V, Tamantini S, et al. Spectro-topochemical investigation of the location of polyphenolic extractives (tannins) in chestnut wood structure and ultrastructure. Industrial Crops and Products. 2019;**141**:111767. DOI: 10.1016/j.indcrop.2019.111767

[34] Tomak ED, Gonultas O. The wood preservative potentials of valonia, chestnut, tara and sulphited oak tannins. Journal of Wood Chemistry and Technology. 2018;**38**(3):183-197. DOI: 10.1080/02773813.2017.1418379

[35] Heuzé V, Tran G, Sauvant D, Lessire M, Lebas F. Carob (*Ceratonia siliqua*). In: Feedipedia, a Programme by INRAE, CIRAD, AFZ and FAO. France; 2016. Available from: https://feedipedia.org/node/320 [Accessed: 22 May 2023]

[36] Youssef MKE, El-Manfaloty MM, Ali HM. Assessment of proximate chemical composition, nutritional status, fatty acid composition and phenolic compounds of carob (*Ceratonia siliqua L.*). Food and Public Health. 2013;**3**(6): 304-308. Available from: https://www.researchgate.net/publication/287648598

[37] Sigge GO, Iipumbu L, Britz TJ. Proximate composition of carob cultivars growing in South Africa. South African Journal of Plant and Soil. 2011; **28**(1):17-22. DOI: 10520/EJC88004

[38] Heuzé V, Tran G. Papaya (Carica papaya) fruits, leaves and by-products. In: Feedipedia, a Programme by INRAE, CIRAD, AFZ and FAO. France; 2015a. Available from: https://www.feedipedia.org/node/522 [Accessed: 25 June 2023]

[39] Zanu HK, Mustapha M, Addo Nartey M. Response of broiler chickens to diets containing varying levels of Leucaena (*Leucaena leucocephala*) leaf meal. Online Journal of Animal and Feed Research. 2012;**2**(2):108-112. Available from: https://www.researchgate.net/publication/304499236

[40] Ahmed MA, Jusoh S, Alimon AR, Ebrahimi M, Samsudin AA. Nutritive

and anti-nutritive evaluation of *Kleinhovia hospita, Leucaena leucocephala* and *Gliricidia sepium* with respect to their effects on *in vitro* rumen fermentation and gas production. Tropical Animal Science Journal. 2018;**41**(2):128-136. DOI: 10.5398/tasj.2018.41.2.128

[41] Agbo AN, Balogun JK, Oniye SJ, Auta J. Effect of different processing methods on nutritional composition of *Leucaena leucocephala* (Lam De Wit) leaves as inclusion in fish feed. Journal of Applied Sciences and Environmental Management. 2017;**21**(4):719-725. DOI: 10.4314/jasem.v21i4.12

[42] Aye PA, Adegun MK. Chemical composition and some functional properties of Moringa, Leucaena and Gliricidia leaf meals. Agriculture and Biology Journal of North America. 2013; **4**(1):71-77. DOI: 10.5251/abjna.2013.4.1.71.77

[43] Heuzé V, Tran G. Leucaena (*Leucaena leucocephala*). In: Feedipedia, a Programme by INRAE, CIRAD, AFZ and FAO. France; 2015. Available from: https://feedipedia.org/node/282 [Accessed: 22 May 2023]

[44] Kikelomo AM. Voluntary feed intake and nutrient utilization of West African Dwarf sheep fed supplements of *Moringa oleifera* and *Gliricidia sepium* fodders. American Journal of Agriculture and Forestry. 2014;**2**(3):94-99. DOI: 10.11648/j.ajaf.20140203.16

[45] Heuzé V, Tran G. Cassava leaves and foliage. In: Feedipedia, a Programme by INRAE, CIRAD, AFZ and FAO. France; 2016. Available from: https://www.feedipedia.org/node/528 [Accessed: 22 May 2023]

[46] Anaeto M, Sawyerr AF, Alli TR, Tayo GO, Adeyeye JA, Olarinmoye AO. Cassava leaf silage and cassava peel as dry season feed for west African dwarf sheep. Global Journal of Science Frontier Research Agriculture and Veterinary Sciences. 2013;**13**(2):1-4. Available from: https://www.researchgate.net/publication/258049934

[47] Bichi A, Ahmad M. Growth performance and nutrient utilization of African catfish (*Clarias gariepinus*) fed varying dietary levels of processed cassava leaves. Bayero Journal of Pure and Applied Sciences. 2010;**3**(1):118-122. DOI: 10.4314/bajopas.v3i1.58739

[48] Ahmed MA, Adeyemi KD, Jahromi MF, Jusoh S, Alimon AR, Samsudin AA. Effects of dietary *Kleinhovia hospita* and *Leucaena leucocephala* leaves on rumen fermentation and microbial population in goats fed treated rice straw. Tropical Animal Health and Production. 2017;**49**: 1749-1756. DOI: 10.1007/s11250-017-1388-3

[49] Hammouda Y, El-Nadi A, AboZaid H. Evaluation of feeding raw moringa (Moringa oleifera Lam.) leaves meal in Nile tilapia fingerlings (*Oreochromis niloticus*) diets. Global Veterinaria. 2014; **13**(1):105-111. Available from: https://www.researchgate.net/publication/331744723

[50] Heuzé V, Tran G, Boudon A, Lebas F. Sweet thorn (*Acacia karroo*). In: Feedipedia, a Programme by INRAE, CIRAD, AFZ and FAO. France; 2019. Available from: https://www.feedipedia.org/node/349 [Accessed: 30 August 2023]

[51] Heuzé V, Thiollet H, Tran G, Delagarde R, Bastianelli D, Lebas F. Pigeon pea *(Cajanus cajan)* forage. In: Feedipedia, a Programme by INRAE, CIRAD, AFZ and FAO. France; 2017. Available from: https://www.feedipedia.org/node/22444 [Accessed: 30 August 2023]

[52] Oke DG. Proximate and phytochemical analysis of *Cajanus cajan* (*Pigeon pea*) leaves. Chemical Science Transactions. 2014;**3**(3):1172-1178. Available from: http://ir.bowen.edu.ng:8080/jspui/handle/123456789/1002

[53] Kolhe PH, Patil RP. Phytochemical and proximate determination from leaf of *Cajanus cajan* (L.) Millsp. Think India Journal. 2019;**22**(31):11-17. Available from: https://thinkindiaquarterly.org/index.php/think-india/article/download/17528/12544

[54] Heuzé V, Tran G, Hassoun P, Bastianelli D, Lebas F. *Moringa (Moringa oleifera)*. In: Feedipedia, a Programme by INRAE, CIRAD, AFZ and FAO. France; 2019b. Available from: https://www.feedipedia.org/node/124 [Accessed: 30 August 2023]

[55] Marume U, Chimonyo M, Dzama K. Influence of dietary supplementation with Acacia karroo on experimental haemonchosis in indigenous Xhosa lop-eared goats of South Africa. Livestock Science. 2012;**144**(1-2):132-139. DOI: 10.1016/j.livsci.2011.11.007

[56] Brown D, Ng'ambi JW. Effects of dietary *Vachelia karroo* leaf meal inclusion on meat quality and histological parameters in Pedi bucks fed a *Setaria verticillata* hay-based diet. Applied Ecology and Environmental Research. 2019;**17**(2):2893-2909. DOI: 10.15666/aeer/1702_28932909

[57] Heuzé V, Thiollet H, Tran G, Boval M, Lebas F. Cratylia (*Cratylia argentea*). In: Feedipedia, a Programme by INRAE, CIRAD, AFZ and FAO. France; 2018. Available from: https://www.feedipedia.org/node/17365 [Accessed: 31 August 2023]

[58] Heinritz SN, Hoedtke S, Martens SD, Peters M, Zeyner A. Evaluation of ten tropical legume forages for their potential as pig feed supplement. Livestock Research for Rural Development. 2012;**24**(1). Available from: http://www.lrrd.org/lrrd24/1/hein24007.htm

[59] Zhou H, Li M, Zi X, Xu T, Hou G. Nutritive value of several tropical legume shrubs in Hainan province of China. Journal of Animal and Veterinary Advances. 2011;**10**(13):1640-1648. DOI: 10.3923/javaa.2011.1640.1648

[60] Rira M, Morgavi DP, Archimède H, Marie-Magdeleine C, Popova M, Bousseboua H, et al. Potential of tannin-rich plants for modulating ruminal microbes and ruminal fermentation in sheep. Journal of Animal Science. 2015;**93**(1):334-347. DOI: 10.2527/jas.2014-7961

[61] Salami SA, Valenti B, Bella M, O'Grady MN, Luciano G, Kerry JP, et al. Characterisation of the ruminal fermentation and microbiome in lambs supplemented with hydrolysable and condensed tannins. FEMS Microbiology Ecology. 2018;**94**(5):fiy061. DOI: 10.1093/femsec/fiy061

[62] Moreira GD, Lima PDMT, Borges BO, Primavesi O, Longo C, McManus C, et al. Tropical tanniniferous legumes used as an option to mitigate sheep enteric methane emission. Tropical Animal Health and Production. 2013;**45**:879-882. DOI: 10.1007/s11250-012-0284-0

[63] Delgado DC, Galindo J, Cairo J, Orta I, Dorta N. Supplementation with foliage of *L. leucocephala*. Its effect on the apparent digestibility of nutrients and methane production in sheep. Cuban Journal of Agricultural Science. 2013;**47**(3):257-265

[64] Saminathan M, Tan HY, Sieo CC, Abdullah N, Wong CMVL, Abdulmalek E, et al. Polymerization degrees, molecular weights and protein-binding affinities of condensed tannin fractions from a *Leucaena leucocephala* hybrid. Molecules. 2014;**19**(6):7990-8010. DOI: 10.3390/molecules19067990

[65] Heuzé V, Tran G. Gliricidia (*Gliricidia sepium*). In: Feedipedia, a Programme by INRAE, CIRAD, AFZ and FAO. France; 2015c. Available from: https://feedipedia.org/node/552 [Accessed: 22 May 2023]

[66] Maisarah AM, Asmah R, Fauziah O. Proximate analysis, antioxidant and anti proliferative activities of different parts of *Carica papaya*. Journal of Tissue Science & Engineering. 2014;**5**(1):1. DOI: 10.4172/2157-7552.1000133

[67] Nath R, Dutta M. Phytochemical and proximate analysis of papaya (*Carica papaya*) leaves. Scholars Journal of Agriculture and Veterinary Sciences. 2016;**3**(2):85-87. Available from: https://citeseerx.ist.psu.edu/document?repid=rep1&type=pdf&doi=9c66d0757a55bd767eecf6818818fef5f2a1f577

[68] Asaolu SS, Adefemi OS, Oyakilome IG, Ajibulu KE, Asaolu MF. Proximate and mineral composition of Nigerian leafy vegetables. Journal of Food Research. 2012;**1**(3):214. DOI: 10.5539/jfr.v1n3p214

[69] Oyelola O, Banjoko I, Ajioshin I. Nutritional content of common *Amaranthus hybridus* vegetable (Efo Tete) in Nigeria. The FASEB Journal. 2014;**28**(1):828. Available from: https://www.academia.edu/26086495

[70] Adeyeye EI, Omolayo FO. Chemical composition and functional properties of leaf protein concentrates of *Amaranthus hybridus* and *Telfairia occidentalis*. Agriculture and Biology Journal of North America. 2011;**3**:499-511. DOI: 10.5251/abjna.2011.2.3.499.511

[71] Bhowmik DP. Proximate Analysis of Green Tea *(Camellia sinensis)* Leaf Powder. Khulshi, Chattagram, Bangladesh: Chattogram Veterinary and Animal Sciences University; 2022. Available from: http://dspace.cvasu.ac.bd/jspui/handle/123456789/932

[72] Uba JO, Onyeike EN, Ogunka-Nnoka CU, Ikewuchi CC. Bioactive and nutrient composition of *Camellia sinensis* (Tea plant) leaves. Journal of Medicinal Plants Studies. 2022;**10**(6):06-14. DOI: 10.22271/plants.2022.v10.i6a.1481

[73] Ndomou SCH, Djikeng FT, Teboukeu GB, Doungue HT, Foffe HAK, Tiwo CT, et al. Nutritional value, phytochemical content, and antioxidant activity of three phytobiotic plants from West Cameroon. Journal of Agriculture and Food Research. 2021;**3**:100105. DOI: 10.1016/j.jafr.2021.100105

[74] Bouaziz MA, Rassaoui R, Besbes S. Chemical composition, functional properties, and effect of inulin from Tunisian *Agave americana L.* leaves on textural qualities of pectin gel. Journal of Chemistry. 2014;**2014**. DOI: 10.1155/2014/758697

[75] King BR, Hoon JH. The Influence of Moisture Content on the Dry Matter Intake of American aloe (*Agave americana*). Middelburg: Grootfontein Agricultural Development Institute; 2011. Available from: http://gadi.agric.za/articles/King_BR/moisture.php

[76] Santra A, Karim SA. Nutritional evaluation of some Indian tree leaves and herbs as fodder and defaunating agent in sheep. Indian Journal of Animal Sciences. 2019;**89**(10):1128-1134. DOI: 10.56093/ijans.v89i10.95018

[77] Heuzé V, Tran G, Hassoun P, Lebas F. Century plant (Agave Americana). In: Feedipedia, a Programme by INRAE, CIRAD, AFZ and FAO. France; 2020. Available from: https://www.feedipedia.org/node/192 [Accessed: 30 September 2023]

[78] Ullah N, Ali J, Khan FA, Khurram M, Hussain A, Rahman IU, et al. Proximate composition, minerals content, antibacterial and antifungal activity evaluation of pomegranate (*Punica granatum L.)* peels powder. Middle-East Journal of Scientific Research. 2012;**11** (3):396-401. Available from: https://www.researchgate.net/publication/265052028

[79] Sharma K, Akansha CE. Comparative studies of proximate, mineral and phytochemical compositions of pomegranate (*Punica granatum*) in peel, seed and whole fruit powder. Methods. 2018;**17**:18. Available from: https://www.researchgate.net/publication/372240679

[80] Romelle FD, Rani A, Manohar RS. Chemical composition of some selected fruit peels. European Journal of Food Science and Technology. 2016;**4**(4):12-21. Available from: https://www.researchgate.net/profile/Feumba-Dr/publication/326579276

[81] Ramos-Morales E, Arco-Pérez A, Martín-García AI, Yáñez-Ruiz DR, Frutos P, Hervás G. Use of stomach tubing as an alternative to rumen cannulation to study ruminal fermentation and microbiota in sheep and goats. Animal Feed Science and Technology. 2014;**198**:57-66. DOI: 10.1016/j.anifeedsci.2014.09.016

[82] Shilwant S, Hundal JS, Singla M, Patra AK. Ruminal fermentation and methane production *in vitro*, milk production, nutrient utilization, blood profile, and immune responses of lactating goats fed polyphenolic and saponin-rich plant extracts. Environmental Science and Pollution Research. 2023;**30**(4):10901-10913. DOI: 10.1007/s11356-022-22931-y

[83] Jafari S, Goh YM, Rajion MA, Jahromi MF, Ebrahimi M. Ruminal methanogenesis and biohydrogenation reduction potential of *papaya (Carica papaya)* leaf: An *in vitro* study. Journal of Animal Science. 2016a;**15**: 157-165. DOI: 10.1080/1828051X.2016.1141031

[84] Jafari S, Meng GY, Rajion MA, Jahromi MF, Ebrahimi M. Manipulation of rumen microbial fermentation by polyphenol rich solvent fractions from *papaya* leaf to reduce green-house gas methane and biohydrogenation of C18 PUFA. Journal of Agricultural and Food Chemistry. 2016b;**64**(22):4522-4530. Available from: https://pubs.acs.org/doi/abs/10.1021/acs.jafc.6b00846

[85] Jafari S, Goh YM, Rajion MA, Jahromi MF, Ahmad YH, Ebrahimi M. Papaya (*Carica papaya*) leaf methanolic extract modulates *in vitro* rumen methanogenesis and rumen biohydrogenation. Animal Science Journal. 2016c;**88**(2):267-276. DOI: 10.1111/asj.12634

[86] Li P, Mehmood IM, Chen W. Effects of polymeric media-coated Gynosaponin on microbial abundance, rumen fermentation properties and methanogenesis in Xinjiang goats. Animals. 2022;**12**(16):2035. DOI: 10.3390/ani12162035

[87] Guo YQ, Liu JX, Lu Y, Zhu WY, Denman SE, McSweeney CS. Effect of tea saponin on methanogenesis, microbial community structure and expression of mcrA gene, in cultures of

rumen micro-organisms. Letters in Applied Microbiology. 2008;**47**(5):421-426. DOI: 10.1111/j.1472-765X.2008.02459.x

[88] Samanta A, Das G, Das SK. Roles of flavonoids in plants. Carbon. 2011;**100** (6):12-35. Available from: https://www.researchgate.net/publication/279499208

[89] Feng W, Hao Z, Li M. Isolation and structure identification of flavonoids [Internet]. In: Flavonoids – From Biosynthesis to Human Health. United Kingdom: Intech Open; 2017. pp. 17-43. DOI: 10.5772/67810

[90] Halbwirth H. The creation and physiological relevance of divergent hydroxylation patterns in the flavonoid pathway. International Journal of Molecular Sciences. 2010;**11**(2):595-621. DOI: 10.3390/ijms11020595

[91] Al-Kirshi RA, Alimon A, Zulkifli I, Atefeh S, Zahari MW, Ivan M. Nutrient digestibility of mulberry leaves (*Morus alba*). Italian Journal of Animal Science. 2013;**12**(2):e36. DOI: 10.4081/ijas.2013.e36

[92] Olteanu M, Panaite T, Ciurescu G, Diana Criste R. Effect of dietary mulberry leaves on performance parameters and nutrient digestibility of laying hens. Indian Journal of Animal Sciences. 2012;**82**(8):914. Available from: https://www.researchgate.net/profile/Rodica-Diana-Criste/publication/280633216

[93] Vu CC, Verstegen MWA, Hendriks WH, Pham KC. The nutritive value of mulberry leaves (*Morus alba*) and partial replacement of cotton seed in rations on the performance of growing Vietnamese cattle. Asian-Australasian Journal of Animal Sciences. 2011;**24**(9):1233-1242. DOI: 10.5713/ajas.2011.90328

[94] Sarma C, Rasane P, Kaur S, Singh J, Singh J, Gat Y, et al. Antioxidant and antimicrobial potential of selected varieties of *Piper betle L.* (Betel leaf). Anais da Academia Brasileira de Ciências. 2018;**90**:3871-3878. DOI: 10.1590/0001-3765201820180285

[95] Shah SK, Garg G, Jhade D, Patel N. *Piper betle*: Phytochemical, pharmacological and nutritional value in health management. International Journal of Pharmaceutical Sciences Review and Research. 2016;**38**(2):181-189. Available from: https://www.researchgate.net/publication/305425617

[96] Mazumder A. Measurement of antioxidant capacity and chemical constituents of betel leaf (*Piper Betle L.*) and producing antioxidant riched dahi [Doctoral dissertation]. Chattogram Veterinary & Animal Sciences University; 2022. Available from: http://dspace.cvasu.ac.bd/jspui/handle/123456789/893

[97] Bhattacharjee S, Sultana A, Sazzad MH, Islam MA, Ahtashom M, Asaduzzaman M. Analysis of the proximate composition and energy values of two varieties of onion (*Allium cepa* L.) bulbs of different origin: A comparative study. International Journal of Nutrition and Food Sciences. 2013;**2** (5):246-253. DOI: 10.11648/j.ijnfs.20130205.16

[98] Dalhat MH, Adefolake FA, Musa M. Nutritional composition and phytochemical analysis of aqueous extract of *Allium cepa* (onion) and *Allium sativum* (garlic). Asian Food Science Journal. 2018;**3**(4):1-9. DOI: 10.9734/AFSJ/2018/43165

[99] Wanapat M, Chanthakhoun V, Phesatcha K, Kang S. Influence of mangosteen peel powder as a source of plant secondary compounds on rumen

microorganisms, volatile fatty acids, methane and microbial protein synthesis in swamp buffaloes. Livestock Science. 2014;**162**:126-133. DOI: 10.1016/j.livsci.2014.01.025

[100] Foiklang S, Wanapat M, Norrapoke T. Effect of grape pomace powder, mangosteen peel powder and monensin on nutrient digestibility, rumen fermentation, nitrogen balance and microbial protein synthesis in dairy steers. Asian-Australasian Journal of Animal Sciences. 2016;**29**(10):1416. DOI: 10.5713/ajas.15.0689

[101] Tjahjani S. Antimalarial activity of *Garcinia mangostana L* rind and its synergistic effect with artemisinin in vitro. BMC Complementary and Alternative Medicine. 2017;**17**:1-5. DOI: 10.1186/s12906-017-1649-8

[102] Agarwal A, Raj N, Chaturvedi N. A comparative study on proximate and antioxidant activity of Brassica oleracea (kale) and Spinacea oleracea (spinach) leaves. International Journal of Advanced Research in Biological Sciences. 2017;**4**(4):22-29. DOI: 10.22192/ijarbs.2017.04.04.004

[103] Hussain J, Rehman NU, Khan AL, Hamayun M, Hussain SM, Shinwari ZK. Proximate and essential nutrients evaluation of selected vegetables species from Kohat region, Pakistan. Pakistan Journal of Botany. 2010;**42**(4):2847-2855. Available from: https://www.researchgate.net/publication/230845261

[104] Oskoueian E, Abdullah N, Oskoueian A. Effects of flavonoids on rumen fermentation activity, methane production, and microbial population. BioMed Research International. 2013; **2013**:349129. DOI: 10.1155/2013/349129

[105] Santas J, Almajano MP, Carbó R. Antimicrobial and antioxidant activity of crude onion (*Allium cepa, L.*) extracts. International Journal of Food Science & Technology. 2010;**45**(2):403-409. DOI: 10.1111/j.1365-2621.2009.02169.x

[106] Sinz S, Kunz C, Liesegang A, Braun U, Marquardt S, Soliva CR, et al. In vitro bioactivity of various pure flavonoids in ruminal fermentation, with special reference to methane formation. Czech Journal of Animal Science. 2018; **63**:293-304. DOI: 10.17221/118/2017-CJAS

[107] Al-Bayati M, Hassan A. Effects of *in vitro* supplementation of mulberry leaf flavonoids on microbial flora, methanogenesis and fermentative products in rumen fluid of sheep. Journal of Research in Ecology. 2018;**6**:2067-2077. Available from: https://ecologyresearch.info/documents/EC0610.pdf

[108] Ku-Vera JC, Jiménez-Ocampo R, Valencia-Salazar SS, Montoya-Flores MD, Molina-Botero IC, Arango J, et al. Role of secondary plant metabolites on enteric methane mitigation in ruminants. Frontiers in Veterinary Science. 2020;**7**:584

[109] Khalil E, Esoh R, Rababah T, Almajwal AM, Alu MH. Minerals, proximate composition and their correlations of medicinal plants from Jordan. Journal of Medicinal Plants Research. 2012;**6**(47):5757-5762. Available from: https://academicjournals.org/article/article1380715654_Khalil%20et%20al.pdf

[110] Odebunmi EO, Oluwaniyi OO, Bashiru MO. Comparative proximate analysis of some food condiments. Journal of Applied Sciences Research. 2010;**6**(3):272-274. Available from: https://www.researchgate.net/profile/Omolara-Oluwaniyi/publication/287786326

[111] Osabor VN, Bassey FI, Umoh UU. Phytochemical screening and quantitative evaluation of nutritional values of *Zingiber officinale* (Ginger). American Chemical Science Journal. 2015;**8**(4):1-6. DOI: 10.9734/ACSJ/2015/16915

[112] Oforma CC, Udourioh GA, Ojinnaka CM. Characterization of essential oils and fatty acids composition of stored ginger (*Zingiber officinale roscoe*). Journal of Applied Sciences and Environmental Management. 2019;**23**(12):2231-2238. DOI: 10.4314/jasem.v23i12.22

[113] Otunola GA, Oloyede OB, Oladiji AT, Afolayan AJ. Comparative analysis of the chemical composition of three spices–*Allium sativum L. Zingiber officinale Rosc.* and *Capsicum frutescens L.* commonly consumed in Nigeria. African Journal of Biotechnology. 2010;**9**(41):6927-6931. DOI: 10.5897/AJB10.183

[114] Lawal AR, Olayinka BU, Murtadha RA, Ayinla A, Etejere EO. Comparative analysis of phytochemical and proximate composition of *Allium sativum L.* and *Zingiber officinale Rosc*. Nigerian Journal of Basic and Applied Sciences. 2018;**26**(2):82-87. DOI: 10.5455/NJBAS.265778

[115] Heuzé V, Tran G, Hassoun P, Lebas F. Citrus pulp, fresh. In: Feedipedia, a Programme by INRAE, CIRAD, AFZ and FAO. France; 2017. Available from: https://www.feedipedia.org/node/679 [Accessed: 14 September 2023]

[116] Mhiri N, Ioannou I, Ghoul M, Boudhrioua NM, Mezghenni H, Hamrouni L, et al. Proximate chemical composition of orange peel and variation of phenols and antioxidant activity during convective air drying. Journal of New Sciences. 2015;**9**:881-990. Available from: https://www.researchgate.net/publication/326271874

[117] Kammoun Bejar A, Ghanem N, Mihoubi D, Kechaou N, Boudhrioua Mihoubi N. Effect of infrared drying on drying kinetics, color, total phenols and water and oil holding capacities of orange (Citrus sinensis) peel and leaves. International Journal of Food Engineering. 2011;**7**(5). DOI: 10.2202/1556-3758.2222

[118] Gotmare S, Gade J. Orange peel: A potential source of phytochemical compounds. International Journal of ChemTech Research. 2018;**11**:240-243. DOI: 10.20902/IJCTR.2018.110229

[119] Ayoola AA, Yusuf AO, Oki DG. Phytochemical screening and proximate analysis of *newbouldia laevis* and *allium sativum*. Nigerian Journal of Animal Science. 2016;**18**(1):242-256. Available from: https://www.researchgate.net/publication/309560547

[120] Mainasara MM, Bakar MFA, Waziri AH, Musa AR. Comparison of phytochemical, proximate and mineral composition of fresh and dried peppermint (*Mentha piperita*) leaves. Journal of Science and Technology. 2018;**10**(2). DOI: 10.30880/jst.2018.10.02.014

[121] Uribe E, Marín D, Vega-Gálvez A, Quispe-Fuentes I, Rodríguez A. Assessment of vacuum-dried peppermint (*Mentha piperita L.*) as a source of natural antioxidants. Food Chemistry. 2016;**190**:559-565. DOI: 10.1016/j.foodchem.2015.05.108

[122] Javaid A, Imran A, Arshad MU, Afzaal M, Asif Shah M. Formulation and characterization of micro-emulsions of peppermint and coriander oils extracted by using a supercritical fluid system. International Journal of Food Properties. 2023;**26**(1):2379-2387. DOI: 10.1080/10942912.2023.2246684

[123] Mehri M, Sabaghi V, Bagherzadeh-Kasmani F. *Mentha piperita* (peppermint) in growing Japanese quails diet: Performance, carcass attributes, morphology and microbial populations of intestine. Animal Feed Science and Technology. 2015;**207**:104-111. DOI: 10.1016/j.anifeedsci.2015.05.022

[124] Abdel-Wareth AAA, Lohakare JD. Effect of dietary supplementation of peppermint on performance, egg quality, and serum metabolic profile of Hy-Line Brown hens during the late laying period. Animal Feed Science and Technology. 2014;**197**:114-120. DOI: 10.1016/j.anifeedsci.2014.07.007

[125] Sontakke MD, Syed HM, Sawate AR. Studies on extraction of essential oils from spices (cardamom and cinnamon). International Journal of Chemical Studies. 2018;**6**(2):2787-2789. Available from: https://www.academia.edu/download/85030847/6-2-296-678.pdf

[126] Gaikwad DS, Fulpagare YG, Deokar DK, Bhoite UY, Nimablkar CD. Effect of dietary feed supplementation of cinnamon and ginger on proximate composition of broilers meat. Plant Archive. 2018;**18**(2):1947-1950. Available from: http://www.plantarchives.org/18-02/1947-1950%20(4470).pdf

[127] Al Dhaheri AS, Alkhatib DH, Jaleel A, Tariq MNM, Feehan J, Apostolopoulos V, et al. Proximate composition and mineral content of spices increasingly employed in the Mediterranean diet. Journal of Nutritional Science. 2023;**12**:e79. DOI: 10.1017/jns.2023.52

[128] Ugbogu EA, Elghandour MM, Ikpeazu VO, Buendía GR, Molina OM, Arunsi UO, et al. The potential impacts of dietary plant natural products on the sustainable mitigation of methane emission from livestock farming. Journal of Cleaner Production. 2019;**213**:915-925. DOI: 10.1016/j.jclepro.2018.12.233

[129] Saber J, Houcine S, Foued A, Ameni D, Houcem S, Chaabane A, et al. Antioxidant and antibacterial properties of Salvia officinalis essential oils and their effects on In vitro feed fermentation with goat rumen liquor. Animal Nutrition and Feed Technology. 2022;**22**(2):297-310. DOI: 10.5958/0974-181X.2022.00024.5

[130] Abubakr AR, Alimon AR, Yaakub H, Abdullah N, Ivan M. Digestibility, rumen protozoa, and ruminal fermentation in goats receiving dietary palm oil by-products. Journal of the Saudi Society of Agricultural Sciences. 2013;**12**(2):147-154. DOI: 10.1016/j.jssas.2012.11.002

[131] Naseri V, Kafilzadeh F, Jahani-Azizabadi H. Effects of Pistacia atlantica gum essential oil on ruminal methanogen, protozoa, selected bacteria species and fermentation characteristics in sheep. Small Ruminant Research. 2022;**209**:106650. DOI: 10.1016/j.smallrumres.2022.106650

[132] Soltan YA, Natel AS, Araujo RC, Morsy AS, Abdalla AL. Progressive adaptation of sheep to a microencapsulated blend of essential oils: Ruminal fermentation, methane emission, nutrient digestibility, and microbial protein synthesis. Animal Feed Science and Technology. 2018;**237**:8-18. DOI: 10.1016/j.anifeedsci.2018.01.004

[133] Morgavi D, Forano E, Martin C, Newbold CJ. Microbial ecosystem and methanogenesis in ruminants. Animal. 2010;**4**:1024-1036. DOI: 10.1017/S1751731110000546

[134] Nooriyan SM, Rouzbehan Y. Effect of essential oils of eucalyptus (*Eucalyptus globulus labill*) and angelica (*Heracleum persicum desf*. Ex fischer) on *in vitro* ruminal fermentation, protozoal population and methane emission using afshari sheep inoculum. Journal of Agricultural Sciences and Technology. 2017;**19**:553-567. Available from: https://www.sid.ir/en/VEWSSID/J_pdf/84820170305.pdf

Chapter 8

Enhancing Production, Nutritional Qualities and Utilization of Fibrous Crop Residues in Smallholder Crop-Livestock Systems: Potential Intervention Options and Progress toward Sustainable Livestock Production

Mesfin Dejene, Aemiro Kehaliew, Fekede Feyissa, Gezahegn Kebede, Getu Kitaw, Geberemariyam Terefe, Mulugeta Walelegne, Bethlehem Mekonnen, Kasa Biratu and Diriba Geleti

Abstract

Large quantities of cereals and grain legume crop residues (CRs) such as straw, stover and haulms are produced every year. They are used as a major and cheap source of livestock feed in developing countries especially during the dry season. However, the overall contribution of CRs as feed for ruminants is much less than the potential estimates because of several factors. In crop-livestock systems, most estimate of cereal CRs production and quality traits available in literature are based on the whole residue and do not represent farmer's practices/context related to the various uses of residue fractions. In addition, there has been a strong focus on post-harvest interventions, but little adoption has been observed, with less emphasis on pre-harvest interventions and residue handling, storage and utilization. This book chapter aims to review the determinant factors and the reasons for low adoption and explores potential intervention options for improving whole-farm productivity and sustainability as a 'win-win' solution. Overall, understanding the local/on-farm socio-economic factors and practices/methods is crucial to estimate the production and quality of CRs/CR fractions actually available as feed for ruminants, and to select and promote the possible intervention options that are more practical for wide adoption by the smallholder farmers.

Keywords: dual-purpose, feedstuffs, food-feed, haulms, ruminants, smallholder, Stover, straw

1. Introduction

Due to the growing population and the associated changes in urbanization, income increase and change in dietary preferences by the growing middle class, the total demand for meat, milk and eggs is projected to almost double worldwide by 2050, particularly in the developing world [1, 2]. These necessitate an increase in feed production and efficient utilization for improving livestock productivity to meet the ever-increasing demands for animal-source food (ASF) consumption. However, the competition for food and feed on a fixed land base present significant challenges towards sustainable feed and livestock production system [1, 3, 4]. Poor or inadequate livestock feed, seasonal variability of feed gaps and imbalanced feeding to livestock have been identified as the major constraint to animal production in most developing countries [2, 5]. Recent estimates indicated that 61% of all herds faced a metabolizable energy (ME) feed gap, and 55% a crude protein (CP) gap between actually supplied feed and calculated requirements at attainable milk production levels in East African smallholder farms [2]. Shortages of arable land and water in the smallholder system constrained options for improving the feed resource base through increasing the cultivated area under improved forages or intensive pastures management [6]. Moreover, concentrate ingredients or compound feeds are generally either not accessible or in short supply and most often expensive for wider use as supplement in low-quality forage-based diet of ruminants. Feed losses are most often high (up to 30–50%) in cut-and-carry systems [2]. Feed can contribute up to 70% of total production costs of ruminants [5, 7]. This triggers efficient utilization of available feed resources for ruminant feeding particularly those not competing with human food like crop residues (CRs) including reduction in wastage and widening the feed resource base through exploring non-conventional potential feed resources [5, 6, 8]. Globally, CRs production has increased from 3.8 billion metric tons in 2004–2005 [9] to about 5.3 billion metric tons in 2020–2021 [10], with both cereals and legumes contributing 82% while the rest are contributed by sugar crops 10%, tubers 5%, and oil crops 3% [9]. Crop residues contribute about 70% of feed resources in India on DM basis [11]. With increasing land allocation for crop production and decreasing grazing lands, dependence on fibrous CRs mainly from cereal and legume crops such as straw, stover and haulms for livestock feeding is expected to increase including crop thinning during crop growing period [12–15]. Case studies in Ethiopia also revealed this scenario [16, 17]. Crop residues may be the only source of feed in late dry seasons or drought periods particularly in semi-arid areas with low and erratic rainfall [18]. The large quantities of CRs are contributed by cereals which usually accounting over 50% of the crop biomass dry matter (DM) [18, 19]. Generally, the potential of CRs as ruminant feed has not been fully exploited in smallholder crop-livestock systems, particularly given the ever-increasing land allocation to crop cultivation at the expense of grazing lands. This is partly due to the fact that: i) CRs particularly from cereals are bulky and generally have low nutritive value that limits voluntary intake (VI) [20–22], ii) Improper management of the bulky and fibrous CRs contributing to DM and nutrient losses and low productivity of ruminant livestock in the tropical regions [5], iii) the bulky nature of CRs that requires significant investment and labor for collecting, storing, handling, transporting, and processing also limits the use of CRs [10, 22, 23], and iv) competing demands for CRs in smallholder systems, most importantly for soil fertility, and for household energy and construction, and other uses [14, 15, 24–26].

All of these factors led to inadequate supply CRs for ruminants particularly during the dry season in sub-Saharan Africa (SSA). This necessitates improved CR production in the same unit of land and efficient utilization of CRs for livestock feeding [5, 15, 27–32] in smallholder farming systems. First, improving the production of CRs in the same unit of land does not require additional water or land or other farm inputs to produce [15, 29]. Second, ruminant livestock have a huge potential to utilize low-quality fibrous CRs and convert them into high-quality human food [3]. A new analysis of the feed/food debate also revealed that to produce the equivalent amount of ASF (meat, milk, or eggs) much less human-edible feed is needed in ruminant systems than in monogastric systems (6 vs. 16 kg of human-edible feed dry matter (DM) per kilogram of protein products) [33]. However, less information is available on feed interventions related to CRs (less than one in ten articles dealt with CRs) compared to cultivated forages and fodder trees, despite the huge contribution and potential of CRs as a ruminant feedstuff in small-scale ruminant systems across tropical regions [34]. There have been few studies focused on either pre-harvest [12, 15, 31, 35] or post-harvest [5, 32, 36, 37] intervention options for enhancing the production, nutritive value and utilization of CRs as feed for ruminants. Many attempts have been made to upgrade post-harvest CRs using physical, chemical and biological treatments but little adoption has been reported. This stimulated targeted improvement of CRs pre-harvest through breeding and selection at source [15, 28–30, 38].

The increasing global demand for biomass as food, feed, industrial raw material and a source of energy results in an increasing challenge on sustainable agriculture particularly in SSA [39]. Crop residues are a key element of the interaction between crops (soil mulching) and livestock in many smallholder crop-livestock systems in developing countries, and residue management is a major issue affecting the sustainability of crop-livestock systems. On the other hand, the most estimate of CRs production and quality traits available in literature either is based on the whole residue especially from tick-stemmed cereal crops and do not represent farmer's practices/context related to the various uses of residue fractions. This calls for revisiting this traditional methodological problems and optimizing allocation of crop residues for improving whole-farm productivity. Hence, in addition to increasing CRs production and nutritive value, and reducing losses during harvest and post-harvest management of CRs, balancing the use of residues for other competing uses such as for soil amendment and forage has also been suggested [26, 40, 41] as an important strategy for improving whole-farm productivity and agricultural sustainability in smallholder crop-livestock systems [3] including the likely adoption of the technology. Through this book chapter, the authors sought to bridge the gap between the conventional research approach/methodology and practical application, providing a comprehensive assessment of fibrous CRs in system wide perspective, recommend possible approach while estimating the amount and quality of CRs that is actually available for feeding livestock and other uses according to farmer's practices/context and also contribute to the global effort toward more sustainable use of CRs as a 'win-win' solution for improving whole-farm productivity.

This chapter contributes to the existing literature on CRs by i) synthesizing the quality attributes and feeding values of cereal and legume CRs for ruminants, ii) summarizing determinant factors for the availability, nutritive value and utilization of CRs as feed for ruminants, iii) describing methodological problems and recommending possible solutions for characterizing the quality attributes of residue fractions and/or whole residue, thereby estimating the amount of CRs that is actually available for feeding livestock and optimizing allocation of crop residues for improving whole-farm productivity and iv) exploring potential intervention options for improving the production, quality and utilization of CRs as feedstuff for ruminants in smallholder crop-livestock system as a 'win-win' solution for improving whole-farm productivity and sustainability. As a pre-harvest intervention, we focused on cultivar/varietal choice and those crop agronomy aspects that affect the yield and quality of CRs and could likely be easily modified in smallholder crop-livestock, mainly on cereals and grain legumes or pulses CRs since they are commonly used as livestock feedstuffs in smallholder systems.

Therefore, the aim of this chapter is to present the potential intervention options suitable for smallholder farmers that could likely be easily applied and adopted in smallholder crop-livestock systems

- to improve the production and quality of CRs as ruminant feed
- that reduce feed wastage during harvest, storage and feeding, and improve the feed utilization efficiency by ruminants

A further goal is to provide the scientific community on key gaps and recommend possible approach while estimating the amount and quality of CRs that is actually available for feeding livestock and other uses according to farmer's practices/context and also to contribute to the global effort toward more sustainable use of CRs as a 'win-win' solution for improving whole-farm productivity.

2. Quality attributes and feeding values of cereal and legume crop residues for ruminants

Generally, senescent cereal CRs are characterized by a high fiber and low N (<1.12% DM) contents and low digestibility [13, 21, 42–45], an unbalanced mineral composition [45, 46] and low VI [20, 22, 47]. For instance, the voluntary DM intakes of ruminants fed on cereal CRs alone ranged from 1.4–2.0% of live weight (LW)/day for maize stover, < 2.0% of LW for rice straw, 1.6–2.3% of LW for tef [*Eragrostis tef* (Zucc.) Trotter] straw and 1.1–2.1% of LW for wheat straw [13, 43–45, 48, 49]. As a result, the feeding value of low-quality forages like cereal CRs is also generally far below the maintenance requirements of adult ruminants; when fed exclusively CRs diets ruminants most often lose weight with low VI [43, 45, 50]. For instance, sheep-fed maize stover alone for about 63 days [45] and 92 days [13] in Ethiopia resulted in the live weight and carcass weight loss by about 42 and 26 g/head/day, respectively, and this was likely because of the negative nitrogen balance as observed in [13]. Similarly, feeding tef straw alone did not support the maintenance requirements of cross-bred calves in Ethiopia. There was a LW loss of about 75.8 g/head/day during the feeding period of 111 days [43]. In contrast, haulms of grain legumes such as cowpea, groundnut, haricot bean and faba bean can have better nutritive value compared to cereal CRs and supported daily LW gain in sheep [51–54] and Arsi bulls (47 g/head/day) [55] when fed as sole diet.

Nonetheless, cereal CRs have the potential to be used as a coping strategy for a certain period of time during critical feed shortage/drought with an acceptable body weight losses but without or with minimum losses of live animal through death. For instance, Singh et al. [51] reported that feeding exclusively chopped coarse-stemmed cereal CRs diets such as millet, sorghum and maize as expected resulted in the weight loss of the Yankassa rams by 45.4, 59.7 and 65.9 g/head/day, respectively, during 70 days of the dry season in Nigeria, but there was no single mortality or sickness observed. This shows that low-quality forages like cereal CRs can be used to keep the animals alive for some time during critical periods.

3. Determinants of crop residues availability, quality and utilization as feed for ruminants

3.1 Harvest and post-harvest management and utilization practices

Crop residues which are the major roughage source during the dry season are either stored opportunistically or grazed in situ in smallholder crop-livestock systems in SSA [35]. In areas where there are relatively high demands for CRs as feed for ruminants, the harvest and post-harvest management and utilization practice of CRs in smallholder are often associated with considerable levels of dry matter (DM) and nutrient losses due to delayed harvesting of the residue after grain maturity [20, 56, 57], during post-harvest residue management practices such as condition/method and duration of CRs storage [32, 56, 58, 59] and feeding practices such as during stubble grazing or during harvesting, transporting, processing and stall feeding practices like with or without feeding troughs [32, 60–62]. Several authors reported the substantial losses of forage DM and nutrients during harvest, storage and feeding in smallholder system mainly due to lack of appropriate feed harvesting, processing and conserving technologies and exacerbated feed shortage in SSA [36, 58, 59, 63, 64].

Crop residue utilization practices through direct stubble grazing result in wastage through trampling and spoilage, but allow animals to select the most nutritious plant parts and the return of nutrients to the soil [60, 62]. Different studies in Eastern and Southern Africa [58, 61, 63, 65–67] have shown that collection and storage of CRs is a common practice to mitigate dry season feed shortage. But the extent of practicing collection of CRs and storage for later use varied among farmers depending up on several factors such as the relative importance of the residue as feed, the bulkiness and difficulties for transportation, and other competing uses [63, 66], and agro-ecology, production system, labor availability, intensification and market access [20]. In smallholder systems traditionally CRs are stored throughout the dry season mostly in loose form without cover. Moreover, baling of CRs and use of feeding troughs and storage sheds were uncommon in most reports [58, 61, 68]. Crop residues stored in open without having any cover that exposed in rain and temperature extremes accelerate a sharp decline in their DM and feeding value probably due to rotting, exposure to rainfall or destruction by termites [68]. The extent of such losses limits the amount of CRs that is actually available for feeding livestock. However, studies in East Africa [32, 69] indicated that using storage shades and feeding troughs has a huge potential to reduce feed loss during storage and utilization.

3.2 Competing demands for crop residues

In smallholder mixed crop-livestock system, CRs (straws and stovers) are increasingly important as feed for ruminants in developing countries [18] and have many uses other than as ruminant feed [18, 20, 24, 25] such as to enhance soil fertility through soil mulching, to provide material for construction, to provide household energy and other uses [14]. Among the competing demands for CRs, the demand for CRs for soil mulching is one of the interventions under conservation agriculture (CA), and sustainable intensification practices has been increasing and exacerbated the situation in most crop–livestock systems. Retaining part of the CRs produced in crop fields is being advocated as one of the bases of CA to sustain agricultural intensification [14, 18, 24, 70, 71]. However, the relative contribution of CRs as feed for ruminants showed substantial variation depending on the combined population and livestock density gradients in South Asia and SSA. For instance, the contribution of CRs in livestock feeds in 2011 increased from low-density to high-density areas and can range from 50 to 78% in South Asia and from 10–60% in SSA [18]. Most farmers in Burkina Faso and Western Kenya retain around 80% or more cereal residues on their fields [18, 25]. As a result, many studies reported crop residue trade-offs in smallholder crop–livestock systems [18, 24, 25, 72]. On top of these uses of CRs, CRs markets are emerging in SSA and India [22, 73–75] triggered by feed shortage. On the other hand, burning of CRs is also common practice in many regions in Africa and Asia [5, 23, 76] mainly associated with high cost, labor shortages, lack of suitable technology for efficient utilization of CRs without delay of the subsequent cropping season and lack of technical knowledge and market access of the CRs [23], which also has an adverse effect on the soil, environmental and human health [5, 76]. As a result of the recent government regulations against open field burning of rice straw and the increasing use of straw for various purposes such as fodder for ruminants, for mushroom production, for fuel (heating and biogas) source, for board or paper production and also for organic fertilizer production, mechanized collection of CRs such as rice straw in baled form is becoming popular in Asia [77]. The extent of such competing uses and burning of CRs limits the amount of CRs that is actually available for feeding livestock.

In summary, though large quantities of CRs are potentially available for feeding to ruminants, but the overall contribution of CRs as feed for ruminants is much less than the potential estimates indicated above, because of: a) the other competing uses, b) the losses associated with the harvest and post-harvest CRs management practices through direct stubble grazing and/or in harvesting, processing, condition and duration of storage and feeding practices and c) the burning of CRs. All these factors need to be considered in national and regional assessments of crop residue inventory and feed balance and promoting increased use of this resource as ruminant feed. Promoting suitable technology that may have a strong likelihood of adoption and improving farmers' technical knowledge for efficient residue management and utilization, balancing the use of residue fractions for various uses for improving whole-farm productivity and linking farmers to CRs markets are potential intervention areas. Furthermore, the traditional methods need to be revisited and discussed below.

4. Revisiting the traditional methodological problems

As discussed above, CRs have various competing uses in smallholder farmers and unlikely that whole residue exclusively used as feed for ruminants. For instance, cutting height at harvest of whole plant cereal species varies within smallholder crop-livestock systems. Farmers either cut high or low at ground level depending up on method of harvest, the livestock density, labor availability, access to fodder market, and the type of crop species. For instance, many combine-harvested crops such as wheat and barley are cut high. However, crops on small-scale farms where there is no combine harvester and straw are scarce and may be cut at ground level manually using sickle [78]. Among thin-stemmed cereals in Ethiopia, wheat is harvested at higher cutting height (about 20–30 cm or more from the ground) than tef which is harvested close to the ground so as to maximize the volume of straw harvested. Similarly thick-stemmed cereals like maize and sorghum, stover are usually harvested either to ground level or at high stubble height; the upper part of the stover usually removed from the field or stored in situ for later use as feed during the dry season while the lower part of the stover most often left in the field as mulch, or for stubble grazing, or other uses [14, 26]. In addition, the maize ears are also removed from the stalk right in the field leaving the rest for in situ grazing in North-western Ethiopia (**Figure 1**).

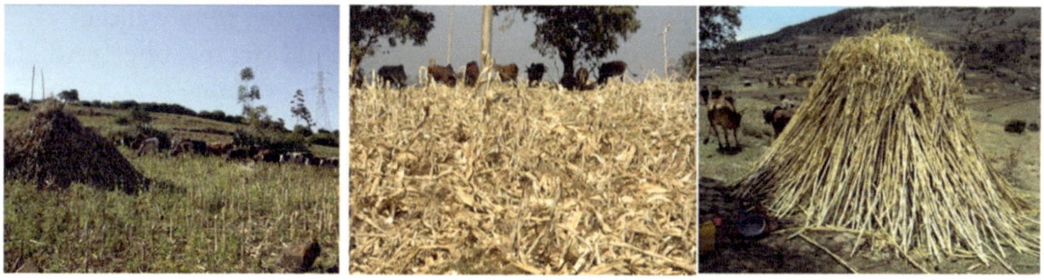

Figure 1.
Maize cut at high stubble height; the lower stover left in the field for stubble grazing, while the upper part of the stover is stored in situ for later use during the dry season in North-western Ethiopia (left) (Source and Photo credit: 136), maize ear removed from the stalk in the field leaving the rest for in situ grazing in Western Ethiopia (middle) (Source and Photo credit: 67), and sorghum grain removed from the stalk in the field and the stover cut at ground level and conserved for dry season feeding in Chiro district, Eastern Ethiopia (right).

Generally, the extent of CRs removal from fields usually increased with increased labor availability, livestock density and market access [14, 79]. For instance, [25] reported that much straw or stover is used as mulch in an agro-pastoral system of Burkina Faso, because of low quality as feed for ruminants, absence of livestock or shortage of labor. This has implications for how CRs are allocated to various purposes, conserved and fed and the measurement of the nutritive value of those parts of the stover actually used as a ruminant feedstuff. However, in contrast to this practice, in most reports found in literature regarding estimates of the cereal CRs production and nutritive value available as feed for ruminants refer to the whole residue harvested at ground level especially from tick-stemmed cereal crops and do not represent farmer's practices/context related to the various uses of residue fractions. Such measurements and literature values may be poor indicators of nutritive value and the contributions of the stover used for ruminant feeding and mislead feed budgeting and prediction of animal performances. Hence, the traditional methods need to be revisited and should represent farmer's practices/context related to the various uses of residue fractions while estimating the production and the proportion of the residue fractions allocated for various uses and characterizing the quality of CRs fractions actually available as feed for ruminants.

5. Optimizing allocation of crop residues for improving whole-farm productivity

In addition to increasing CRs production and nutritive value and reducing losses during harvest and post-harvest management of CRs, balancing the use of residues from thick-stemmed cereals such as maize stover for other competing uses particularly for soil amendment and forage has been reported as an important strategy for enhancing both crop and livestock productivity and sustainability [26, 41]. Optimal allocation of CRs like maize/sorghum stover for feed and soil mulching can be attained through manipulating the cutting height at harvest according to the circumstances and demands for CRs. Increasing the cutting height of whole plant cereal species can increase the quality of CRs removed from crop fields as feed for ruminants while leaving some amount of the lower part of the CRs in the field either to be grazed or used as soil mulching and for other uses [26, 41, 80, 81]. In line with this, manipulating cutting height at two internodes below the lowest ear of maize stover at grain maturity provided nearly about two-third of the stover as upper part for feed (6.38 t/ha) and the rest one-third of the stover as lower part (3.82 t/ha) could be left in the field available for mulch, stubble grazing or other purposes [26]. Similarly, available literature in China suggested that the upper fraction of the maize stover could be removed from the field for feed while the lower stover fraction is of comparable value for soil amendment and found as a feasible option to enhance both crop and livestock productivity through best use of maize stover fractions [41, 81]. This simple harvest management strategy of the residues from thick-stemmed cereals coupled with choice and use of suitable dual-purpose food-feed varieties provides the most appropriate proportions of upper and lower stover fractions according to circumstances and need for optimal allocation and improves whole-farm productivity.

6. Enhancing the production, nutritive value and utilization of crop residues for ruminants: potential intervention options

Improving voluntary intake and digestibility of low-quality CRs through upgrading and/or supplementation has been the major emphasis [13, 45, 82]. However, little adoption of upgrading post-harvest CRs technologies has been reported [83]. Much less effort has been put into pre-harvest intervention strategies mainly crop management factors, multidimensional crop improvement and post-harvest residue management, utilization and feeding practices [83, 84]. The importance of focusing more on pre-harvest strategies also highlighted [34] for improving crop residue yields and quality in the same unit of land without affecting the primary product which may have a strong likelihood of adoption.

6.1 Pre-harvest intervention options

6.1.1 Enhancing whole plant value: progress towards developing dual-purpose crops through multidimensional crop improvement approaches

Plant breeding and selection criteria using multi-trait and whole-plant (i.e. food and fodder) model against the single (grain)-trait model has been the focus of research in public and private crop-improvement programs towards whole-plant improvement/optimization [11, 15, 85]. Using dual-purpose/food–feed crops improve both grain/pod yield and biomass yield and residue quality without requiring additional land and water [86] and enhance animal productivity [52, 53, 87]. The following subsections discuss the two separate approaches towards developing dual-purpose crops through multidimensional crop improvement [15].

6.1.1.1 Exploiting cultivar-dependent variation for improving ruminant productivity

This approach is through exploiting the variations among the existing cereal and grain legume cultivars in both grain/pod and residue yields and residue quality traits such as nutrient composition, digestibility, voluntary intake and animal productivity, which is relatively quick and requires lower investment than the second approach, that is, targeted genetic enhancement [88]. Substantial variation in CRs quality among genotypes within cereal crop species without sacrificing grain yield has been reported. Chemical composition and in vitro digestibility of CRs vary among genotypes within species of maize [30, 89, 90], sorghum and pearl millet [15, 29, 86, 87, 91], wheat [92–94], barley [50, 95] and rice [11, 96]. For instance, the stover CP content and in-vitro organic matter digestibility (IVOMD) of sorghum cultivars varied by about 5.5 and 10 percentage units, respectively [91] while rice cultivars varied in straw IVOMD by about 5 to 10% units [88]. This has a great potential to improve ruminant productivity. For instance, calculations from feeding standards [97, 98] indicate that an increase of 5 percentage units in dry matter digestibility (DMD) would be expected to increase ME intake of ruminants by about 20% and could, for example, increase growth rate of a 300 kg animal from 0.15 to 0.30 kg/day. In addition, an increase in forage NDF digestibility by a one percentage unit could increase the dry matter intake (DMI) and milk production by about 0.17 and 0.25 kg/day, respectively [99].

In an experiment using a sorghum stover of the lower and higher quality varieties (IVOMD 47 and 52%, respectively) resulted in milk improvement from (10 to 15 kg/day) in dairy buffalo fed in densified total mixed ration having about 50% of sorghum stover inclusion rate, due to higher IVOMD and hence higher feed intake [15]. Large variation ($P < 0.05$) was observed among barley genotypes in daily live weight (LW) gain of sheep ranged from −143–18 g/head/day as a result of the higher straw digestible organic matter intake (DOMI) (as g/kg $LW^{0.75}$/day) for the superior barley cultivar than for the inferior one when fed as sole diets [100].

There also appears to be large potential for selecting dual-purpose genotypes of the CRs of grain legumes such as cowpea and groundnut [52, 73, 101–103], faba bean [54, 104], chickpea [105, 106], lentil [107, 108] and common bean [109] without sacrificing pod/seed yield. In addition, the variation in leaf loss observed among common beans genotypes while approaching seed maturity [110] suggesting the need to include this trait as a selection criteria [101]. For instance, sheep fed exclusively groundnut haulms diet from 10 different cultivars in India, nitrogen retention was positive and 70% higher (from 6.7 to 11.4 g/head/day) while weight gains in sheep were more than two-fold (from 65 to 137 g/day) for the superior groundnut genotype than for the poor-quality genotype [52].

Generally, the variation observed among cultivars in most crops in terms of grain and residue yield and residue quality traits [15, 28, 30, 90] was found to be promising for simultaneous selection of superior cultivars both for grain and straw traits. However, the recent advances in dual purpose rice and wheat research [88] suggest that this approach is not promising for all crops. For instance, it looks promising for rice but not for wheat that may need targeted genetic enhancement for simultaneous selection of superior wheat cultivars both for grain and straw traits [88]. Furthermore, the differences observed in residue quality traits among cultivars in most studies were relatively smaller than the differences in the grain yield and residue yield. However, the overall increased in nutrient yields (e.g., both digestible dry matter and ME productivity of the residue) per hectare through use of dual-purpose cultivars has a great potential to improve ruminant productivity/ha/year.

6.1.1.2 Targeting genetic improvement towards specific traits: recent advances toward developing dual-purpose crop cultivars

The second approach towards developing food-feed (dual-purpose) crop cultivars is through targeted genetic enhancement, using conventional [42, 111, 112] and molecular breeding approaches [113, 114], and has greater potential for impact. The recent results [115] demonstrated the feasibility of incorporating genomic prediction as a tool to improve maize stover quality traits such as IVOMD and ME through genome-wide association study. This will allow maize breeders to select for stover quality traits more quickly and cost-effectively while avoiding the need for field or lab-based phenotyping and significantly reducing the need for additional testing resources and to develop new dual purpose maize varieties without sacrificing grain yield. However, these approaches require more investment and time compared to simply exploitation of already existing variations [15].

6.1.2 Crop management options

Exploring the potential crop management options that can contribute to the improvement of yield and quality of CR has been reviewed by [12]. As simple crop management options to improve the production and quality of CRs as ruminant feed that could likely be easily applied and adopted in smallholder crop–livestock systems such as i) manipulation of plant density, ii) improved crop protection practices and use of disease-tolerant food-feed crops and iii) fertilization are discussed below.

6.1.2.1 Modification of planting density

In most maize growing areas of Africa, farmers use lower plant densities at harvest than the recommended rates (e.g., in Nigeria 5.3 plants/m^2 irrespective of varietal difference, environment or management practice, and in Ethiopia it varied from 4.4 plants/m2 to 5.3 plants/m2, depending on cultivar maturity), imply that maize yield gap could potentially be due to lower plant density [116–118]. On the other hand, maize plant densities up to 8.5 plants/m^2 are recommended under intensive production in North America [119], because the newer maize hybrids were more tolerant to high plant population than the older hybrids [118]. As a simple management option, increasing maize plant density of medium maturing genotypes from the recommended 5 to 7 plants/m^2 in Ethiopia increased dry matter yields of both grains, by 9% (from 6.5 to 7.1 t/ha) and of stover by about 21% (from 11.7 to 14.1 t/ha), while the stover digestible dry matter yield/ha was increased by about 20% (all $P < 0.05$) [120]. This is in accord with the previous findings in North America [121] who reported that increasing maize grain and whole plant yield through increasing plant density from 4 to 10 plants/m^2. This might be attributed to the higher crowding stress tolerance of modern hybrids [122] and has higher optimum plant densities for grain yield than older hybrids even under sub-optimal nutrient conditions [123] and suggests the potential of improving maize residue yield through higher plant density with modern hybrids without compromising grain yield and residue quality. However, several factors could influence the optimum maize plant population density; most importantly moisture availability, soil fertility, hybrid maturity group and row spacing [124] need to be considered.

Recent study using sorghum varieties released for grain in Ethiopia [125] indicated that increasing the plant density of sorghum from the recommended 12.5 to 100 kg/ha resulted in similar total biomass yield but increased the stover IVOMD and decreased concentrations of fiber fractions and stalk thickness. This will have a great potential for improving animal production associated with higher intake as a result of higher quality and thin-stemmed stover. In another study, the possibility of increasing sorghum grain and stover yield through increasing the plant density from the recommended 26,600 plants/ha to 53,300 plants/ha has been demonstrated in Mali, albeit it varied depending on plant density, N fertilization, and variety [126]. Generally, the potential constraints to the adoption of technologies are the more nutrients and water needed with higher plant densities.

6.1.2.2 Improved crop protection practices and use of disease-tolerant food-feed crops

There are also substantial amounts of forage dry matter and nutrient losses due to poor management crop diseases, pests and weed. There also appears to be a huge potential for enhancing the productivity and feeding value of cereal and legume CRs and thereby improving animal productivity and profitability in smallholder crop–livestock systems in SSA through improved management of crop diseases, pests and weeds [35, 127]. Moreover, high adoption rate has also been reported through development and promotion of disease-tolerant, food–feed crops such as groundnut and sorghum in India [35]. This is due to the substantial benefits obtained by farmers in terms of not only in improved fodder availability by >50% and > 60% in groundnut and sorghum, respectively, but also in improved fodder nutritive value (dry matter digestibility and dry matter intake by 10–15% and by 10–32%, respectively). As a result, milk yield and net returns to farmers increased by about 0.44 kg/day and 25–29%, respectively. Similarly, Lukuyu et al. and Lenné and Thomas [31] and [35] also reported that improved fodder availability (green maize fodder through thinning's and dry residue/stover after grain maturity) by about 40–166% and 118–409 kg/season, respectively, through the use of improved management practices such as resistant/tolerant dual-purpose maize varieties for streak virus disease and/or stem-borer along with the higher planting population density than the recommended and the push-pull strategy for stem-borer and weed management.

6.1.2.3 Fertilization

Improving total plant biomass both crop residue and grain yields including crop residue quality particularly the N concentration of the crop residue through application of fertilizers (particularly N and P) at sowing and/or days after crop emergence has been well documented [12, 56, 71, 128, 129]. Improving yields of pearl millet grain and stover, the yields of both digestible dry matter and ME of the stover and stover N content have been reported in India through increasing N fertilizer rate [128]. This could potentially have large effects on the amount and feedstuff quality of the CRs available for livestock, thereby reducing the feed deficit gaps [129]. According to [129] increasing fertilizer level over farmers practice in the semiarid region of Karnataka, southern India resulted more increase in residue yield than residue quality attributes, but the overall increase in residue nutrient yields/ha (e.g., ME productivity/ha) potentially has large effects in ruminant productivity (up to 40% higher milk productivity/ha/year). The appropriate use of fertilizer to enhance CRs availability for both CA and fodder for ruminants in smallholder systems in Africa has also been discussed [71]. However, cost of fertilizer, poor market access and the recurrent drought are some of the constraints for adoption in smallholder farmers [70, 84, 130].

6.1.3 Timely harvesting and rapid removal of the CRs soon after grain maturity

Farmers usually harvest grain crops either soon after grain maturity or sometime after grain maturity. In SSA, cereal CRs are often harvested when they are fully matured, dried, and senesced on the field [37]. In the latter case, farmers intentionally left to dry in the field for about 1 to 4 weeks after grain maturity of most cereal crops depending up on labor availability, season (main vs. short rainy season), and cropping system (double/relay cropping) [19, 20, 37, 57]. However, the reduction in nutritive value of CRs as a result of delayed harvesting after grain physiological maturity associated to the greater loss of the most digestible plant parts such as of leaves due to sun-drying and lignifications [20, 37, 57, 128]. For instance [57] reported that maize harvested at a grain DM content ranging from about 70 to 80% gave higher leaf-to-stem ratio, higher CP and lower NDF contents in stover without significant change in grain and stover yield than harvested at grain DM content about 88–90%. Similarly, delayed harvest of finger millet straws for about 10 days after grain maturity of the crop in India resulted in decrease ($P < 0.05$) in IVOMD and in vitro cell wall digestibility by about 4 (from 61–57%) and 5 (from 48–43%) percentage units, respectively [56]. Leaf loss and losses through senescence could be greatly minimized through removal of the CRs from the field soon after grain maturity [20, 57, 128]. These highlight the need for training farmers and awareness creation toward the benefits of timely harvesting and rapid removal of the CRs soon after grain maturity.

6.2 Post-harvest intervention options

Straw/stover is underutilized in some African countries mainly due to lack of appropriate feed harvesting/collection, transportation, processing, conserving/storage and feeding technologies for efficient utilization [32, 36, 58, 59, 63, 64, 69, 131, 132]. Labor shortage during harvest, lack of transportation, cost effectiveness and lack of awareness are also other factors contributing for the inefficient utilization of CRs by smallholder farmers [61]. Previous studies [32, 69] showed that proper handling of bulky CRs during harvesting and transportation and use of appropriate storage and feeding facilities that minimizes losses may improve feed availability and utilization that would help in coping with dry season feed shortages. In this regard recently [37] reviewed straw and stover collection, preservation and storage practices and technologies to improve crop residue quality using physical (chopping, pelleting and densification), chemical with acids and alkalis and biological treatments with selected micro-organisms or their products in SSA. However, the following sections focus on the potential intervention options suitable for smallholder farmers that reduce feed wastage during storage and feeding including recent technology like spin-off technologies from second-generation biofuel to improve the quality of CRs suitable for small and medium business enterprises. In addition, options for improved utilization of low-quality CRs on farms such as through supplementation, residue management while feeding and including animal management options also discussed.

6.2.1 Box baling of crop residues

Box baling technology, used to make bales made by trampling CRs into wooden frames placed on the ground and manually tied with locally available rope inserted in the frames, before the CRs, is simple and cheaper method for conserving roughages that do not require mechanization [36]. The potential and limitations of this technology summarized (see [68]). Box baling of CRs reduces transport cost, suitable for storage, and helps in feed budgeting, but it requires initial capital and labor. However, box baling or baling of CRs has not been promoted widely in East Africa and was uncommon in most reports in smallholder crop–livestock systems most importantly due to less awareness by smallholder farmers [36]. Farmers commonly store CRs in loose form resulted in dry matter and nutrients losses. However, there are few exceptions. For instance, 71% of the surveyed respondents in Kebbi state, Nigeria, employed baling of the CRs, and 22% of them store and preserve the CRs in silos, while few (7%) of the respondents use metallic drum to store and preserve the CRs [133].

6.2.2 Using storage sheds and feeding troughs for reducing losses

Poor conservation/storage of straws and stover has been reported in smallholder crop-livestock systems in SSA [58, 59, 64, 131, 134] and southeast Asia [44]. About 90% of farmers in East Shoa, Ethiopia, store CRs in the open uncovered [65]. However, there are few exceptions. For instance, in South Gondar zone, Ethiopia where cereal CRs stacked after threshing under a roof shade made of grass and wood, around homesteads and covered with plastic sheets, and inside their house and on trees [135], and in peri-urban dairy producers in Ethiopia where CRs most often stored under roof in loose form [136]. In southeast Asia, livestock farmers collect and stock-pile rice straw in a simple shed usually made from locally available materials or stored in piles outdoors [44]. Improper storage and feeding methods can lead to substantial amounts of forage waste. Maize and sorghum stover are collected and stacked mostly in the field uncovered for later use [131, 134]. These practices reduce the quality and efficiency of utilization compared to the crop residue conserved around homesteads and under shade conditions. For instance, dry matter loss of cereal CRs can reach up to 20–25% in Alamata district, northern Ethiopia [131] and about 10% in Southern Ethiopia [132], and that of pulse residues up to 7%. Part of this loss is attributed to the traditional uncovered storage practices of CRs that is exposed to temperature fluctuations, termites and untimely precipitation [131]. As rain leaches through uncovered stacks, it also washes away soluble carbohydrates and reduces the quality of the residue and animal performance.

Storage conditions and duration are also the major factors that influence the DM and nutrient losses mainly during bad weather condition [35, 137]. In line with this [58] reported that the CP concentrations and IVOMD of both tef and wheat straws showed consistently decreasing trends with the increased storage durations from 0 to 6 months in central highlands of Ethiopia but the nutrient losses were higher in straws stored in open air than those stored under shelter. The results of another study in Ghana using grain legume residues such as cowpea, groundnut and soybean haulms stored under various conditions over a duration of 120 day [59] also showed that DM quantity reduced by 14% and 35% when haulms stored in the best (using polythene bags and under roof/rooms) and worst (on rooftops or tree-forks) conditions, respectively. Storing CRs in an open field uncovered is also associated with the formation of mycotoxins. Storage of CRs under cover not only reduces the DM and nutrient losses but also reduces the absorption of moisture especially during bad weather conditions and hence reduces the formation of mycotoxins compared with the storage of CRs without cover [137]. These losses can be further minimized using improved feeding practices such as using improved wooden feed troughs along with feed storage sheds. For instance, it has been reported that using feed storage sheds and wooden feed troughs reduced feed wastage during storage and feeding by ~30–50% in Ethiopia [32] while in Tanzania 20–30% feed wastage reduced through the use of feed troughs during feeding [69]. The technologies have been successfully demonstrated in Ethiopia and received acceptance by farmers in intensifying systems since they can also save labor time by about 10–20% and economically feasible [32].

6.2.3 Pre-treatments of low-quality CRs for improving fiber utilization

Technologies to overcome the poor digestibility, low animal intake, and very low protein content of CRs have been developed for pretreatment of CRs before feeding to animals. Pretreatments of low-quality fibrous CRs by chemical, physical and biological treatments with fungi or their combinations to improve their nutritive value (digestibility and VI) and fiber utilization are well documented [37, 120, 138–140]. Chemical treatments of low-quality fibrous forages with acid or alkali break down fiber and improve their digestibility and VI [141]. Urea treatment may also increase the nitrogen content of the forage, which is the critical nutrient in low-quality fibrous CRs for ruminants, but its efficacy depends on sufficient urease and moisture [140]. The most practical chemical treatment is urea treatment since urea is widely available and easy to handle compared with NaOH, H2O2, acids or KOH. However, with the exception of some Asian countries like India and China, urea-ammonia treatment of CRs, has limited adoption and impact in smallholder farmers in SSA [83], due to its limitations for large-scale application, seasonality, costs involve and hazard issues, such as toxicity and environmental pollution, variable efficacy that depend on the presence of urease and quality of the residue to be treated and the type of residue like fine vs. course-stemmed cereal residues, are among others. Treatment of straw with lime solution [CaO/Ca(OH)2] improves fiber degradability and provides complementary effects in combination with urea in increasing degradability and incrementing both the calcium and nitrogen contents of the treated straw, but it has longer solubility in water compared to NaOH or urea [44].

Physical treatments are applied to reduce the particle size of CRs and improve VI as a result of the reduced ruminal fermentation time [83, 139], thus providing easy entries or access of the rumen microorganisms for degradation. These physical treatments include soaking, chaffing, chopping, shredding, pulverizing, pelleting, steaming pressure and gamma irradiation. Among which, soaking straw/stover overnight in water which brings softness between the lignin and cellulose component of the residue to enhance intake and digestibility is a common and economical treatment of CRs [44]. Chopping also has relevance for field application and most often practiced by smallholder farmers, but the lack of low cost and suitable chopper has been the main determinant for its adoption. Grinding, chopping or pelleting had beneficial effects in breaking down the cell wall contents of cereal residues [44]. Crop residue densification through compacting, briquetting or pelletizing may also enhance the use of bulky forage like CRs as livestock feeds [5, 77, 142] through enhancing handling, storage and transportation and reducing the associated costs [77, 143], and also allow formulating total mixed diet or mixing with other feed additives. This needs initial investment to purchase pelletizing or compacting machine which has been beyond the reach of smallholder farmers, and the benefits derived may be not attractive, but it could be suitable for cooperatives/unions and private sector to commercialize crop residue based densified products. Reduced particle size or processing strategies such as pelleting increase the rumen outflow rate and enhance VI [144], with possible negative effects on feed utilization [145]. This causes less time for rumination and less exposure to microbial degradation, and consequently reducing degradation and digestibility of the straw. Hence, the balance between the particle size and the retention time/passage rate of the ingested treated straw should be properly considered while using these techniques [44]. Recently spin-off technologies from second-generation biofuel such as ammonia fiber expansion that uses steam-pressure-thermal treatment has been reported [146] and found to be promising to degrade lignocellulose and improve digestibility, intake, productivity and profitability. For instance, steam explosion improved VI by 4% of live weight in male sheep and total live weight gain of 3.92 kg. But this does not use any chemicals, does not take much treatment time and is generally simple. A treatment cost-benefit ratio is of at least 1:2 [15], but it appears not feasible on smallholder condition and should target small and medium business enterprises [146].

Most studies on biological treatment techniques have inconsistent results. The major drawback is the strain of the fungi to be used and its capacity to degrade lignocelluloses [44]. Among the biological technologies, white-rot fungi are well known for their potential for degradation of lignocelluloses, but several strains degrade easily digestible carbohydrates and often resulted in dry matter and nutrient losses [140]. Although efforts have been made to reduce DM loss while treating straw using solid state fermentation with ligninolytic fungi [83], generally many biologically treated CRs are not economical, and the process has not yet optimized under field conditions [147]. Incubation period is another limitation for its practical application in treating CRs [44]. Recently, [148] also reported that potential adoption of biological treatments of CRs has limited due to suitable strains used to avoid or minimize carbohydrate degradation (loss), the inconsistencies in animal response, and the high technical skills needed. In addition, the limitations on availability of resources to produce and handle large quantities of fungi or their enzymes for practical and field application, and the concerns and problems to be addressed and overcome (e.g., some fungi produce toxins so proper care should be considered) while using biological treatment of straw [44]. It has been recommended that more research is needed to improve the aforementioned constraints for enhancing crop residue quality and improving fiber utilization through biological treatments [37, 140]. Enzyme treatment of CRs to increase degradability and animal performance is not common under smallholder production systems because of the additional input costs involved as well as the limitation of skills for using enzyme products [44].

Generally, treated low-quality fibrous CRs usually support modest level of animal productivity and require additional supplements to provide sufficient nutrients for high-producing animals.

6.2.4 Supplementation of cereal crop residue forage diets for improved utilization and animal performance

Low-quality fibrous CRs, particularly those from cereals, are usually high fiber content, poor digestibility, very low VI and deficient in nitrogen, sulphur, phosphorous and other micro and macro minerals as feed for ruminants. The critical ones are nitrogen followed by sulphur as they are the main determinants primarily to inhibit fermentation process for fiber digestion in the rumen and thus reduce VI [138]. Forage legumes and legume straw (haulm) generally have high nutritive value (digestible energy and CP), which can decrease the use of purchased concentrate ingredient or compound feed supplements and of associated costs [102, 149, 150]. For instance, supplementation with locally available feed resources like legume straw (haulm) may provide N for N-deficient cereal straw/stover to stimulate fiber digestion in the rumen and thus increase ME intake of cereal CRs [13, 102, 149]. Utilization of low-quality fibrous CRs would be improved, and modest level of animal productivity could be obtained through supplementation 0. For instance, supplementation of small amounts of legume haulms ranging from 150 to 450 g DM/head/d improved dry matter and nutrient intake, N balance and enhanced animal performance (carcass weight and body weight gain) in sheep in East and West Africa [13, 45, 102]. Moreover, supplementation of non-protein nitrogen (NPN) (e.g. urea) is also another option for improved utilization of low-quality forages [138]. However, this needs simple and practical management options to provide NPN supplements with low risk in smallholder systems. Among the categories of various safe ways of supplementing urea as NPN supplements like in the form of urea–molasses multi-nutrient block

(UMB), slow-release forms of urea, and using a sticky urea–molasses solution that are common in Australia, Europe and North America [120], providing the urea in UMB supplements has been widely promoted in SSA and Asia, so ruminants can only consume small amounts through the day [83]. In addition to NPN supplementation, including some sulphur in the form of ammonium sulphate or elemental sulphur is also needed as substrates of rumen microorganisms to optimize the rumen microbial fermentation and fiber utilization [120]. These improve feed efficiency and potentially would reduce the intensity of enteric methane emission per animal product produced [144, 151].

6.2.5 Residue management: increasing the amount on offer

One simple physical method to increase voluntary intake and productivity is increasing the amount on offer without changing the diet composition for improved intake and animal productivity [144]. Depending up on the nature of the feed, the optimum level of excess feed on offer ranges from 15 to over 40%, so that ruminants have a chance to preferentially select and consume the more nutritious parts of the residue such as leaves than the thick stems, maximizing intake and thereby improving productivity [139, 152–155]. On the other hand, increasing the feed intake of ruminants decreases the retention time of feed in the rumen due to higher passage rates, decreases the proportion of ingested and absorbed nutrients and energy associated with animal maintenance, leading to a decline in CH4 losses per unit of DMI [144]. In contrast to stubble grazing approach, in the hand-feeding CRs approach obviously there are more refusals available that should be integrated with improved refusal management so that refusals can be effectively returned to cropland as organic matter or used for other purpose as a 'win-win' intervention so as to improve whole-farm productivity with little additional labor associated with handling, that is, for example, see [40]. Moreover, the latter approach should also have the greatest potential in the areas where supply exceeds the demands for CRs as feed for ruminants [120].

6.3 Animal management options: improved utilization efficiency of low-quality fibrous CRs

The two approaches that have been suggested to enhance the efficient utilization of low-quality fibrous feedstuffs under animal management option are 1) selectively breeding for better suited animals for improved feed efficiency [156, 157] and smaller metabolic body weight [158], and 2) the application of rumen biotechnology such as altering the rumen microbial composition or using genetically engineered rumen microbes [159–162], or a combination of both approaches [144]. However, genotyping an animal for feed efficiency is costly, particularly high capital requirement and multiplication of superior animals have been cited as the major determinant factors for improved adoption of ruminants selected for efficient utilization of low-quality fibrous forages [20, 144]. According to the recent report [144], genetic selection for feed efficiency is not yet a breeding objective in most ruminant systems due to the lack of genomic tools designed to predict feed efficiency. On the other hand, several technical difficulties must be solved before the latter approach will be possible [161]. Some of the constraints of genetic manipulation as listed by [162] are categorized mainly related with the incompatibility of modified microbes in the rumen environment and the existing regulatory concerns of the public.

7. Conclusions

From the scientific findings discussed in this chapter, the following important conclusions can be drawn:

1. Given the diverse characteristics of smallholder farmers, understanding the local/on-farm socio-economic factors and practices/methods on CRs management and use is crucial to select and promote the possible intervention options that are more practical for wide adoption by the stallholder farmers.

2. As a pre-harvest intervention options that may have a strong likelihood of adoption for enhancing CRs yields and quality in the same unit of land without affecting the primary product:

    a. Development and use of suitable dual-purpose crop genotypes and crop management practices would increase the availability (digestible dry matter and ME yields of CRs) fodder for ruminants.

    b. Timely harvesting and rapid removal of the CRs soon after grain maturity would also reduce the loss of the most palatable and digestible plant parts such as leaves and leaf sheaths and lignified.

3. Promoting post-harvest intervention options such as

    a. Simple, low cost and practical forage conservation technologies (e.g., box baling) along with proper storage practices (e.g., storing under shed/cover), and the use of feed troughs while feeding would help in reducing feed losses and coping with dry season feed shortages.

    b. Applying suitable crop residue treatment options (e.g., chopping) and locally available low-input supplementation for livestock and residue management while feeding (increasing the amount on offer) would increase the residue quality, intake and ruminant productivity.

    c. Optimal allocation of CRs of residue fractions mainly from thick-stemmed cereals as feedstuff and mulch including the use of feed refusals/leftovers and animal manure as fertilizer enhance both livestock and crop production and sustainability that also needs the close integration of animal nutritionists and plant/soil scientists.

4. Furthermore,

    a. The traditional methods need to be revisited and should represent farmer's context related to the various uses of residue fractions while estimating the production and quality of CRs/CR fractions actually available as feed for ruminants and other uses.

    b. Linking farmers to CRs markets and improving farmers' knowledge through continuous promotion and training on the improved technologies/practices are also crucial for improved availability and adoption.

Author contributions

All authors have made significant contribution.

Conflict of interest

The authors declare no conflict of interest.

Author details

Mesfin Dejene[1*], Aemiro Kehaliew[1], Fekede Feyissa[2], Gezahegn Kebede[1], Getu Kitaw[1], Geberemariyam Terefe[1], Mulugeta Walelegne[1], Bethlehem Mekonnen[1], Kasa Biratu[3] and Diriba Geleti[2]

1 Ethiopian Institute of Agricultural Research (EIAR), Holetta Research Center, Addis Ababa, Ethiopia

2 EIAR, Addis Ababa, Ethiopia

3 EIAR, Jimma Research Center, Jimma, Ethiopia

*Address all correspondence to: mesfindegene@yahoo.co.uk; mesfindejene47@gmail.com

References

[1] Henchion M, Moloney AP, Hyland J, Zimmermann J, McCarthy S. Review: Trends for meat, milk and egg consumption for the next decades and the role played by livestock systems in the global production of proteins. Animal. 2021;**15**:100287. DOI: 10.1016/j.animal.2021.100287

[2] Paul BK, Birnholz C, Nzogela B, Notenbaert A, Herrero M, Bwire J, et al. Livestock Feeding Systems and Feed Gaps in East African Smallholder Farms. Nairobi, Kenya: The Alliance of Bioversity International and the International Center for Tropical Agriculture (CIAT); 2021

[3] Ayantunde AA, Duncan AJ, van Wijk MT, Thorne P. Review: Role of herbivores in sustainable agriculture in sub-Saharan Africa. Animal. 2018;**12**(S2):s199-s209. DOI: 10.1017/S175173111800174X

[4] Marshall K, Gibson JP, Mwai O, Mwacharo JM, Haile A, Getachew T, et al. Livestock genomics for developing countries – African examples in practice. Frontiers in Genetics. 2019;**10**:297. DOI: 10.3389/fgene.2019.00297

[5] FAO. Crop residue based densified total mixed ration – A user-friendly approach to utilise food crop by-products for ruminant production, by Walli TK, Garg MR, Makkar HPS. In: Animal Production and Health Paper No. 172. Rome, Italy: FAO; 2012

[6] Makkar HPS. Review: Feed demand landscape and implications of food-not *feed* strategy for food security and climate change. Animal. 2018;**12**(8):1744-1754. DOI: 10.1017/S175173111700324X

[7] Yang K, Qing Y, Yu Q, Tang X, Chen G, Fang R, et al. By-product feeds: Current understanding and future perspectives. Agriculture. 2021;**11**:207. DOI: 10.3390/agriculture11030207

[8] Wadhwa M, Bakshi MPS, Makkar HPS. Utilization of Fruit and Vegetable Wastes as Livestock Feed and as Substrates for Generation of Other Value-Added Products. Bangkok, Thailand: FAO; 2013

[9] Lal R. World crop residues production and implications of its use as a biofuel. Enviroment International. 2005;**31**(4):575-584

[10] Shinde R, Shahi DK, Mahapatra P, Singh CS, Naik SK, Thombare N, et al. Management of crop residues with special reference to the on-farm utilization methods: A review. Industrial Crops and Products. 2022;**181**:114772. DOI: 10.1016/j.indcrop.2022.114772

[11] Samireddypalle A, Prasad KVSV, Ravi D, Khan AA, Reddy R, Angadi UB, et al. Embracing whole plant optimization of rice and wheat to meet the growing demand for food and feed. Field Crops Research. 2019;**244**:107634. DOI: 10.1016/j.fcr.2019.107634

[12] Reddy B, Reddy PS, Bidinger F, Blümmel M. Crop management factors influencing yield and quality of crop residues. Field Crops Research. 2003;**84**:57-77

[13] Koralagama K, Mould F, Fernandez-Rivera S, Hanson J. The effect of supplementing maize Stover with cowpea (*Vigna unguiculata*) haulms on the intake and growth performance of Ethiopian sheep. Animal. 2008;**2**:954-691

[14] Duncan AJ, Bachewe F, Mekonnen K, Valbuena D, Rachier G, Lule D, et al.

Crop residue allocation to livestock feed, soil improvement and other uses along a productivity gradient in eastern Africa. Agriculture, Ecosystems and Environment. 2016;**228**:101-110. DOI: 10.1016/j.agee.2016.1005.1011

[15] Blümmel M, Samireddypalle A, Zaidi PH, Vadez V, Reddy R, Janila P. Multidimensional crop improvement by ILRI and partners: Drivers, approaches, achievements and impact. In: McIntire J, Grace D, editors. The Impact of the International Livestock Research Institute. Nairobi, Kenya: ILRI, and Wallingford, UK: CABI; 2020b. pp. 481-505

[16] Mekasha A, Gerard B, Tesfaye K, Nigatu L, Duncan AJ. Inter-connection between land use/land cover change and herders'/farmers' livestock feed resource management strategies: A case study from three Ethiopian eco-environments. Agriculture, Ecosystems and Environment. 2014;**188**:150-162

[17] Mekuria W, Mekonnen K, Thorne P, Bezabih M, Tamene L, Abera W. Competition for land resources: Driving forces and consequences in crop-livestock production systems of the Ethiopian highlands. Ecological Processes. 2018;**7**:30. DOI: 10.1186/s13717-018-0143-7

[18] Valbuena D, Erenstein O, Tui SHK, Abdoulaye T, Claessens L, Duncan AJ, et al. Conservation agriculture in mixed crop–livestock systems: Scoping crop residue trade-offs in sub-Saharan Africa and South Asia. Field Crops Research. 2012;**132**:175-184

[19] Dejene M. Options for Improving the Yield and Nutritive Value of Maize and Grain Legume Residues for Ruminants in East African Farming Systems [Doctoral dissertation]. Brisben: The University of Queensland; 2018. DOI: 10.14264/uql.2018.138

[20] Williams TO, Fernández-Rivera S, Kelley TG. The influence of socioeconomic factors on the availability and utilization of crop residues as animal feeds. In: Renard C, editor. Crop Residues in Sustainable Mixed Crop/Livestock Farming Systems. Wallingford, UK: CAB International; 1997. pp. 25-39

[21] Ertiro BT, Twumasi-Afriyie S, Blümmel M, Friesen D, Negera D, Worku M, et al. Genetic variability of maize Stover quality and the potential for genetic improvement of fodder value. Field Crops Research. 2013a;**153**:79-85

[22] Amole T, Augustine A, Balehegn M, Adesogoan AT. Livestock feed resources in the west African Sahel. Agronomy Journal. 2022;**114**:26-45. DOI: 10.1002/agj2.20955

[23] Lin M, Begho T. Crop residue burning in South Asia: A review of the scale, effect, and solutions with a focus on reducing reactive nitrogen losses. Journal of Environmental Management. 2022;**314**(15):115104. DOI: 10.1016/j.jenvman.2022.115104

[24] Jaleta M, Kassie M, Shiferaw B. Tradeoffs in crop residue utilization in mixed crop–livestock systems and implications for conservation agriculture. Agricultural Systems. 2013;**121**:96-105

[25] Andrieu N, Vayssières J, Corbeels M, Blanchard M, Vall E, Tittonell P. From farm scale *synergies* to village scale trade-offs: Cereal crop residues use in an agro-pastoral system of the Sudanian zone of Burkina Faso. Agricultural Systems. 2015;**134**:84-96. DOI: 10.1016/j.agsy.2014.08.012

[26] Dejene M, Dixon RM, Walsh KB, McNeill D, Seyoum S, Duncan AJ. High-cut harvesting of maize Stover and genotype choice can provide improved feed for ruminants and stubble for

conservation agriculture. Agronomy Journal. 2022;**114**:187-200. DOI: 10.1002/agj2.20874

[27] Renard C. Crop Residues in Sustainable Mixed Crop/Livestock Farming Systems. Wallingford, UK: CAB International; 1997

[28] Lenné J, Fernandez-Rivera S, Blümmel M. Approaches to improve the utilization of food–feed crops—Synthesis. Field Crops Research. 2003;**84**:213-222

[29] Sharma K, Pattanaik AK, Anandan S, Blümmel M. Food–feed crop research: A synthesis. Animal Nutrition and Feed Technology. 2010;**10S**:1-10

[30] Blümmel M, Grings EE, Erenstein O. Potential for dual-purpose maize varieties to meet changing maize demands: Synthesis. Field Crops Research. 2013a;**153**:107-112. DOI: 10.1016/j.fcr.2013.10.006

[31] Lukuyu BA, Murdoch A, Romney D, Mwangi D, Njuguna J, McLeod A, et al. Integrated maize management options to improve forage yield and quality on smallholder farms in Kenya. Field Crops Research. 2013;**153**:70-78

[32] Bezabih M, Mekonnen K, Adie A, Thorne P, Duncan AJ, Ebrahim M, et al. Postharvest Handling and Utilization of Crop Residues in the Highlands of Ethiopia [Poster Presentation]. Addis Ababa, Ethiopia: Africa RISING Ethiopia Review and Planning Meeting; 2016

[33] Mottet A, Haan C, Falcucci A, Tempio G, Opio C, Gerber P. Livestock: On our plates oreating at our table? A new analysis of the feed/food debate. Global Food Security. 2017;**14**:1-8

[34] Baltenweck I, Cherney D, Duncan A, Eldermire E, Lwoga ET, Labarta R, et al. A scoping review of feed interventions and livelihoods of small-scale livestock keepers. Nature Plants. 2020;**6**(10):1242-1249. DOI: 10.1038/s41477-020-00786-w

[35] Lenné J, Thomas D. Integrating crop—Livestock Research and Development in sub-Saharan Africa: Option, imperative or impossible? Outlook on Agriculture. 2006;**35**:167-175

[36] Makini FW, Mose LO, Kamawu GK, Mulinge WW, Salasya B, Makelo MN. Innovation Opportunities in Dairy Livestock in Kenya. Guide Book. Accra, Ghana: Forum for Agricultural Research in Africa; 2019

[37] Balehegn M, Ayantunde A, Amole T, Njarui D, Nkosi BD, Müller FL, et al. Forage conservation in sub-Saharan Africa: Review of experiences, challenges, and opportunities. Agronomy Journal. 2022;**114**:75-99. DOI: 10.1002/agj2.20954

[38] Reed JD, Capper B, PJH N, editors. Plant breeding and the nutritive value of crop residues. In: Proceedings of a Workshop, 7-10 December 1987, Addis Ababa. Ethiopia: ILCA; 1988

[39] Callo-Concha D, Jaenicke H, Schmitt CB, Denich. Food and non-food biomass production, processing and use in sub-Saharan Africa: Towards a regional bioeconomy. Sustainability. 2020;**12**:1-9. DOI: 10.3390/su12052013

[40] Larbi A, Smith JW, Adekunle IO, Agyare WA, Gbaraneh LD, Tanko RJ, et al. Crop residues for mulch and feed in crop–livestock systems: Impact on maize grain yield and soil properties in the west african humid forest and savanna zones. Experimental Agriculture. 2002;**38**(3):253-264. DOI: 10.1017/S0014479702003010

[41] Tian SZ, Liu Z, Wang BW, Wang Y, Li ZJ, Lal R, et al. Balancing

the use of maize residues for soil amendment and forage. Plant, Soil and Environment. 2016;**62**(11):490-496. DOI: 10.17221/470/2016-PSE

[42] Ertiro BT, Zeleke H, Friesen D, Blümmel M, Twumasi-Afriyie S. Relationship between the performance of parental inbred lines and hybrids for food-feed traits in maize (*Zea mays* L.) in Ethiopia. Field Crops Research. 2013b;**153**:86-93. DOI: 10.1016/j.fcr.2013.02.008

[43] Ebro A, Nsahlai I, Yami A, Umunna N. Effect of supplementing graded levels of forage legumes on performance of crossbred calves fed tef (*Eragrostis tef*) straw. Journal of Applied Animal Research. 2004;**26**:107-112

[44] Aquino D, Barrio AD, Trach NX, Hai NT, Khang DN, Toan NT, et al. Rice straw-based fodder for ruminants. In: Gummert M, Hung N, Chivenge P, Douthwaite B, editors. Sustainable Rice Straw Management. Cham: Springer; 2020. DOI: 10.1007/978-3-030-32373-8_7

[45] Tolera A, Sundstøl F. Supplementation of graded levels of Desmodium intortum hay to sheep feeding on maize Stover harvested at three stages of maturity: 1. Feed intake, digestibility and body weight change. Animal Feed Science and Technology. 2000;**85**:239-257

[46] Gulilat L, Chekol Y. Mineral in crop residues and interaction with soil minerals contents in Ethiopia: Review. MOJ Food Processing and Technology. 2020;**8**(2):40-44. DOI: 10.15406/mojfpt.2020.08.00240

[47] Wilson J, Kennedy P. Plant and animal constraints to voluntary feed intake associated with fibre characteristics and particle breakdown and passage in ruminants. Australian Journal of Agricultural Research. 1996;**47**:199-225

[48] Devendra C. Crop residues for feeding animals in Asia: Technology development and adoption in crop/livestock systems. In: In: Renard C, eiditor., editor. Crop Residuals in Sustainable Mixed Crop/Livestock Farming System. Wallingford: CAB International; 1997. pp. 241-267

[49] Aredo TA, Musimba N. Study on the chemical composition, intake and digestibility of maize Stover, tef straw and haricot bean haulms in Adami Tulu District, Ethiopia. Kasetsart Journal. 2003;**37**:401-407

[50] Herbert F, Thomson E, Capper B. Effect of genotype on the morphological characteristics, chemical composition and feeding value of nine barley straws, and responses to soya-bean meal supplementation. Animal Science. 1994;**58**:117-126

[51] Singh BB, Musa A, Ajeigbe HA, Tarawali SA. Effect of feeding crop residues of different cereals and legumes on weight gain of Yankassa rams. International Journal of Livestock Production. 2011;**2**(2):017-023

[52] Prasad K, Khan A, Vellaikumar S, Devulapalli R, Ramakrishna Reddy C, Nigam S, et al. Observations on livestock productivity in sheep fed exclusively on haulms from ten different genotypes of groundnut. Animal Nutrition and Feed Technology. 2010;**10S**:121-126

[53] Etela I, Dung D. Utilization of Stover from six improved dual-purpose groundnut (*Arachis hypogaea* L.) cultivars by west African dwarf sheep. African Journal of Food, Agriculture, Nutrition and Development. 2011;**11**:4538-4545

[54] Wegi T. Effects of Feeding Different Varieties of Faba Bean (*Vicia faba* L.) Straws with Concentrate on Feed Intake, Digestibility, Body Weight Gain

and Carcass Characteristics of Arsi-Bale Sheep [MSc Thesis]. Dire Dawa: Haramaya University, Ethiopia; 2016

[55] Ebro A, Tadesse T, Abebe T. The supplementation of haricot bean residue with lablab (*Lablab purpureus*) hay in the diet of Arsi bulls and heifers (*Bos indicus*). Tropical Science. 2005;**45**:114-117

[56] Subba Rao A, Prabhu UH, Seetharam A, Gowda BTS, Oosting SJ, Sampath KT, et al. Finger millet. In: Singh K, Schiere JB, editors. Handbook for Straw Feeding Systems. New Delhi, India: ICAR; 1995. pp. 353-366

[57] Tolera A, Sundstùl F, Said AN. The effect of stage of maturity on yield and quality of maize grain and Stover. Animal Feed Science and Technology. 1998;**75**:157-168

[58] Feyissa F, Kebede G, Assefa G. Dynamics in nutritional qualities of tef and wheat straws as affected by storage method and storage duration in the central highlands of Ethiopia. African Journal of Agricultural Research. 2015;**10**(38):3718-3725. DOI: 10.5897/AJAR2015.9903

[59] Akakpo DB, de Boer IJM, Adjei-Nsiah S, Duncan AJ, Giller KE, Oosting SJ. Evaluating the effects of storage conditions on dry matter loss and nutritional quality of grain legume fodders in West Africa. Animal Feed Science and Technology. 2020;**262**:114419. DOI: 10.1016/j.anifeedsci.2020.114419

[60] Klopfenstein T, Erickson G, Berger L. Maize is a critically important source of food, feed, energy and forage in the USA. Field Crops Research. 2013;**153**:5-11. DOI: 10.1016/j.fcr.2012.1011.1006

[61] Gizaw S, Ebro A, Tesfaye Y, Mekuriaw Z, Mekasha Y, Hoekstra D, et al. Feed resources in the highlands of Ethiopia: A value chain assessment and intervention options. In: LIVES Working Paper 27. Nairobi, Kenya: International Livestock Research Institute (ILRI); 2017

[62] Petzel EA, Smart AJ, St-Pierre B, Selman SL, Bailey EA, Beck EE, et al. Estimates of diet selection in cattle grazing cornstalk residues by measurement of chemical composition and near infrared reflectance spectroscopy of diet samples collected by ruminal evacuation. Journal of Animal Science. 2018;**96**(5):1914-1928. DOI: 10.1093/jas/sky1089

[63] Ndathi AJN, Nyangito MM, Musimba NKR, Mitaru BN. Smallholder farmers' feed material conservation strategies in the tropical dry-lands of South-Eastern Kenya. Livestock Research for Rural Development. 2012;**2012**(24):96. Available from: http://www.lrrd.org/lrrd24/6/ndat24096.htm

[64] Seglah PA, Wang Y, Wang H, Bi Y. Estimation and efficient utilization of straw resources in Ghana. Sustainability. 2019;**11**:4172. DOI: 10.3390/su11154172

[65] Tesfaye A, Chairatanayuth P. Management and feeding systems of crop residues: The experience of east Shoa zone, Ethiopia. Livestock Research for Rural Development. 2007;**19**:31. Available from: http://www.lrrd.org/lrrd19/3/tesf19031.htm

[66] Gurmessa G, Tolemariam T, Tolera A, Beyene F. Production and utilization of crop residues in Horro and Guduru districts, Western Ethiopia. Food Science and Quality Management. 2016;**48**:77-84

[67] Duguma B, Janssens GPJ. Assessment of livestock feed resources and coping strategies with dry season feed scarcity in mixed crop–livestock farming systems around the Gilgel gibe catchment, Southwest Ethiopia. Sustainability.

2021;**13**(19):10713. DOI: 10.3390/su131910713

[68] Lukuyu BA, Kitalyi A, Franzel S, Duncan A, Baltenweck I. Constraints and options to enhancing production of high quality feeds in dairy production in Kenya. In: Uganda and Rwanda ICRAF Working Paper no. 95. Nairobi, Kenya: World Agroforestry Centre; 2009

[69] Lukuyu BA, Ravichandran T, Maass B, Laswai G, Bwire J, Duncan AJ. Enhancing livestock productivity through feed and feeding interventions in India and Tanzania. In: ILRI Project Report. Nairobi, Kenya: International Livestock Research Institute (ILRI); 2015

[70] Twomlow SJ, Urolov JC, Jenrich M, Oldrieve B. Lessons from the field Zimbabwe's conservation agriculture task force. Journal of SAT Agricultural Research. 2008;**6**:1-11

[71] Vanlauwe B, Wendt J, Giller KE, Corbeels M, Gérard B, Nolte C. A fourth principle is required to define conservation agriculture in sub-Saharan Africa: The appropriate use of fertilizer to enhance crop productivity. Field Crops Research. 2014;**155**:10-13

[72] Tittonell P, Gérard B, Erenstein O. Tradeoffs around crop residue biomass in smallholder crop-livestock systems–What's next? Agricultural Systems. 2015;**134**:119-128

[73] Samireddypalle A, Boukar O, Grings E, Fatokun CA, Kodukula P, Devulapalli R, et al. Cowpea and groundnut haulms fodder trading and its lessons for multidimensional cowpea improvement for mixed crop livestock Systems in West Africa. Frontier in Plant Science. 2017;**8**:30. DOI: 10.3389/fpls.2017.00030

[74] Konlan SP, Ayantunde AA, Addah W, Dei HK, Karbo N. Emerging feed markets for ruminant production in urban and peri-urban areas of northern Ghana. Tropical Animal Health Production. 2018;**50**(1):169-176. DOI: 10.1007/s11250-017-1418-1

[75] Duncan A, Samaddar A, Blümmel M. Rice and wheat straw fodder trading in India: Possible lessons for rice and wheat improvement. Field Crops Research. 2020;**2020**(246):107680. DOI: 10.1016/j.fcr.2019.107680

[76] Cassou E. Field Burning. Agricultural Pollution. World Bank. Washington, DC: World Bank; 2018

[77] Balingbing C, Hung NV, Nghi NT, Hieu NV, Roxas AP, Tado CJ, et al. Mechanized collection and densification of Rice straw. In: Gummert M, Hung N, Chivenge P, Douthwaite B, editors. Sustainable Rice Straw Management. Cham: Springer; 2020. DOI: 10.1007/978-3-030-32373-8_2

[78] Suttie JM. Hay and straw conservation: For small-scale farming and pastoral conditions. In: FAO Plant Production and Protection Series No. 29. Rome, Italy: Food and Agriculture Organisation of the United Nations; 2000

[79] Rusinamhodzi L, van Wijk MT, Corbeels M, Rufino MC, Giller KE. Maize crop residue uses and trade-offs on smallholder crop livestock farms in Zimbabwe: Economic implications of intensification. Agriculture, Ecosystems and Environment. 2015;**214**:31-45

[80] Dong CF, Shen YX, Ding CL, Xu NX, Cheng YH, Gu HR. The feeding quality of rice (*Oryza sativa* L.) straw at different cutting heights and the related stem morphological traits. Field Crops Research. 2013;**141**:1-8

[81] Liang M, Wang G, Liang W, Shi P, Dang J, Sui P, et al. Yield and quality of maize Stover: Variation among

cultivars and effects of N fertilization. Journal of Integrative Agriculture. 2015;**14**(8):1581-1587

[82] Singh K, Schiere JB, editors. Feeding of ruminants on fibrous crop residues: Aspects of treatment, feeding, nutrient evaluation, research and extension. In: Proceedings of a Workshop; 4-8 February 1991; National Dairy Research Institute (NDRI)-Karnal. New Delhi, India: Indian Council of Agricultural Research (ICAR); 1993

[83] Owen E, Smith T, Makkar HPS. Successes and failures with animal nutrition practices and technologies in developing countries: A synthesis of an FAO e-conference. Animal Feed Science and Technology. 2012;**174**:211-226

[84] Balehegn M, Duncan A, Tolera A, Ayantunde AA, Issa S, Karimou M, et al. Improving adoption of technologies and interventions for increasing supply of quality livestock feed in low-and middle-income countries. Global Food Security. 2020;**26**:100372. DOI: 10.1016/j.gfs.2020.100372

[85] Schiere J, Joshi A, Seetharam A, Oosting S, Goodchild A, Deinum B, et al. Grain and straw for whole plant value: Implications for crop management and genetic improvement strategies. Experimental Agriculture. 2004;**40**:277-294

[86] Somegowda VK, Vemula A, Naravula J, Prasad G, Rayaprolu L, Rathore A, et al. Evaluation of fodder yield and fodder quality in sorghum and its interaction with grain yield under different water availability regimes. Current Plant Biology. 2021;**25**:100191. DOI: 10.1016/j.cpb.2020.100191

[87] Umutoni C, Bado V, Whitbread A, Ayantunde A, Gangashetty P. Evaluation of chemical composition and in vitro digestibility of stovers of different pearl millet varieties and their effect on the performance of sheep in the west African Sahel. Acta Agriculturae Scandinavica, Section A — Animal Science. 2021;**70**(2):91-99

[88] Blümmel M, Duncan AJ, Lenné JM. Recent advances in dual purpose Rice and wheat research: A synthesis. Field Crops Research. 2020a;**253**:107823. DOI: 10.1016/j.fcr.2020.107823

[89] Tolera A, Berg T, Sundstøl F. The effect of variety on maize grain and crop residue yield and nutritive value of the Stover. Animal Feed Science and Technology. 1999;**79**:165-177

[90] Erenstein O, Blummel M, Grings E. Potential for dual-purpose maize varieties to meet changing maize demands: Overview. Field Crops Research. 2013;**153**:1-4

[91] Blümmel M, Zerbini E, Reddy B, Hash C, Bidinger F, Khan A. Improving the production and utilization of sorghum and pearl millet as livestock feed: Progress towards dual-purpose genotypes. Field Crops Research. 2003;**84**:143-158

[92] Habib G, Shah S, Inayat K. Genetic variation in morphological characteristics, chemical composition and in vitro digestibility of straw from different wheat cultivars. Animal Feed Science and Technology. 1995;**55**:263-274

[93] Bezabih M, Adie A, Ravi D, Prasad KVSV, Jones C, Abeyo B, et al. Variations in food-fodder traits of bread wheat cultivars released for the Ethiopian highlands. Field Crops Research. 2018;**229**:1-7. DOI: 10.1016/j.fcr.2018.09.006

[94] Joshi AK, Kumar U, Mishra VK, Chand R, Chatrath R, Naik R, et al.

Variations in straw fodder quality and grain–straw relationships in a mapping population of 287 diverse spring wheat lines. Field Crops Research. 2019;**243**:107627. DOI: 10.1016/j.fcr.2019.107627

[95] Erickson D, Meyer D, Foster A. The effect of genotypes on the feed value of barley straws. Journal of Animal Science. 1982;**55**:1015-1026

[96] Flachowsky G, Tiroke K, Schein G. Botanical fractions of straw of 51 cereal varieties and in *sac o* degradability of various fractions. Animal Feed Science and Technology. 1991;**34**:279-289

[97] CSIRO. Nutrient Requirements of Domesticated Ruminants. Collingwood, Victoria, Australia: CSIRO publishing; 2007

[98] Dixon RM, Mayer R. Estimating the voluntary intake by sheep of tropical grasses from digestibility, regrowth-age and leaf content: A meta-analysis. Animal Production Science. 2020;**60**(14):1694-1703. DOI: 10.1071/AN19531

[99] Oba M, Allen MS. Evaluation of the importance of the digestibility of neutral detergent fiber from forage: Effects on dry matter intake and milk yield of dairy cows. Journal of Dairy Science. 1999;**82**:589-596. DOI: 10.3168/jds.S0022-0302(99)75271-9

[100] Capper B, Thomson E, Rihawi S. Voluntary intake and digestibility of barley straw as influenced by variety and supplementation with either barley grain or cottonseed cake. Animal Feed Science and Technology. 1989;**26**:105-118

[101] Larbi A, Dung D, Olorunju P, Smith J, Tanko R, Muhammad I, et al. Groundnut (*Arachis hypogaea*) for food and fodder in crop-livestock systems: Forage and seed yields, chemical composition and rumen degradation of leaf and stem fractions of 38 cultivars. Animal Feed Science and Technology. 1999;**77**:33-47

[102] Singh B, Ajeigbe H, Tarawali SA, Fernandez-Rivera S, Abubakar M. Improving the production and utilization of cowpea as food and fodder. Field Crops Research. 2003;**84**:169-177

[103] Nigam S, Blummel M. Cultivar-dependent variation in food-feed-traits in groundnut (*Arachis hypogaea* L.). Animal Nutrition and Feed Technology. 2010;**10S**:39-48

[104] Gebremeskel Y, Estifano A, Melau S. Effect of selected faba bean (*Vicia faba* L.) varietal difference on straw DM yield, chemical composition and nutritional quality. Journal of the Dry Lands. 2011;**4**:333-340

[105] Kafilzadeh F, Maleki E. Chemical composition, in vitro digestibility and gas production of straws from different varieties and accessions of chickpea. Journal of Animal Physiology and Animal Nutrition. 2012;**96**:111-118

[106] Wamatu J, Alemu T, Tolera A, Beyan M, Alkhtib A, Eshete M, et al. Selecting for food-feed traits in desi and kabuli genotypes of chickpea (*Cicer arietinum*). Journal of Experimental Biology and Agricultural Sciences. 2017a;**5**(6):852-860

[107] Erskine W, Rihawi S, Capper B. Variation in lentil straw quality. Animal Feed Science and Technology. 1990;**28**:61-69

[108] Wamatu J, Mersha A, Tolera A, Beyan M, Alkhtib A, Eshete M, et al. Selecting for food-feed traits in early and late maturing lentil genotypes (*Lens culinaris*). Journal of Experimental Biology and Agricultural Sciences. 2017b;**5**(5):697-705

[109] Dejene M, Dixon RM, Duncan AJ, Wolde-meskel E, Walsh KB, McNeill D. Variations in seed and post-harvest residue yields and residues quality of common bean (*Phaseolus vulgaris* L.) as a ruminant feedstuff. Animal Feed Science and Technology. 2018;**244**:42-55. DOI: 10.1016/j.anifeedsci.2018.07.017

[110] Dejene M, Dixon RM, Duncan AJ, Walsh KB, McNeill D, Wolde-meskel E. Yields and the nutritive value of early harvested common bean (*Phaseolus vulgaris* L.) crop residues for ruminants. Livestock Research for Rural Development. 2021;**33**(113):1-8. Available from: http://www.lrrd.org/lrrd33/9/33113mesfi.html

[111] Bidinger FR, Blümmel M, Hash CT, Choudhary S. Genetic enhancement for superior food-feed traits in a pearl millet [*Pennisetum glaucum* (L.) R. Br.] variety by recurrent selection. Animal Nutrition and Feed Technology. 2010;**10S**:61-68

[112] Zaidi PH, Vinayan MT, Blümmel M. Genetic variability of tropical maize Stover quality and the potential for genetic improvement of food feed value in India. Field Crops Research. 2013;**153**:94-101. DOI: 10.1016/j.fcr.2012.11.020

[113] Nepolean T, Blümmel M, Bhasker Raj AG, Senthilvel S, Hash CT. QTLs controlling Stover yield and quality traits in pearl millet. International Sorghum and Millets Newsletter. 2006;**47**:149-152

[114] Vinayan MT, Raman B, Jyothsna T, Zaidi PH, Blümmel M. A note on potential candidate genomic regions with implications for maize Stover fodder quality. Field Crops Research. 2013;**153**:102-106. DOI: 10.1016/j.fcr.2013.03.018

[115] Vinayan MT, Seetharam K, Babu R, Zaidi PH, Blummel M, Nair SK. Genome wide association study and genomic prediction for Stover quality traits in tropical maize (*Zea mays* L.). Scientific Reports. 2021;**11**:686. DOI: 10.1038/s41598-020-80118-2

[116] Sani BM, Oluwasemire KO, Mohammed HI. Effect of irrigation and plant density on the growth, yield and water use efficiency of early maize in the Nigerian Savanna. Journal of Agricultural and Biological Science (JABS). 2008;**3**:8

[117] Balemi T, Kebede M, Abera T, Hailu G, Gurmu G, Getaneh F. Some maize agronomic practices in Ethiopia: A review of research experiences and lessons from agronomic panel survey in Oromia and Amhara regions. African Journal of Agricultural Research. 2019;**14**(33):1749-1763. Available from: http://www.academicjournals.org/AJAR

[118] Adnan AA, Diels J, Jibrin JM, Kamara AY, Craufurd P, Shaibu AS, et al. Optimum stand density of tropical maize varieties: An on-farm evaluation of grain yield responses in the Nigerian Savanna. Frontiers in Agronomy. 2022;**4**:773012. DOI: 10.3389/fagro.2022.773012

[119] Li J, Xie RZ, Wang KR, Ming B, Guo YQ, Zhang GQ, et al. Variations in maize dry matter, harvest index, and grain yield with plant density. Agronomy Journal. 2015;**107**:829-834. DOI: 10.2134/agronj14.0522

[120] Dejene M, Dixon R. Options to improve availability, nutritive value and utilisation of crop residue feedstuffs for ruminants. In: Wilkus E, Mekuria M, Rodriguez D, Dixon J, editors. The Sustainable Intensification of Maize–Legume Systems for Food Security in Eastern and Southern Africa (SIMLESA): Lessons and Way Forward, ACIAR Monograph No. 211. Canberra: Australian Centre for International Agricultural Research; 2021. pp. 151-174

[121] Cox WJ. Whole-plant physiological and yield responses of maize to plant density. Agronomy Journal. 1996;**88**:489-496

[122] Tokatlidis I, Koutroubas S. A review of maize hybrids' dependence on high plant populations and its implications for crop yield stability. Field Crops Research. 2004;**88**:103-114

[123] Di Matteo JA, Ferreyra JM, Cerrudo AA, Echarte L, Andrade FH. Yield potential and yield stability of argentine maize hybrids over 45 years of breeding. Field Crops Research. 2016;**197**:107-116. DOI: 10.1016/j.fcr.2016.07.023

[124] Sangoi L. Understanding plant density effects on maize growth and development: An important issue to maximize grain yield. Ciência Rural. 2001;**31**:159-168

[125] Mekasha A, Min D, Bascom N, Vipham J. Seeding rate effects on forage productivity and nutritive value of sorghum (*Sorghum bicolor* L.). Agronomy Journal. 2022;**114**:201-215. DOI: 10.1002/agj2.20856

[126] Dembele JSB, Gano B, Kouressy M, Dembele LL, Doumbia M, Ganyo KK, et al. Plant density and nitrogen fertilization optimization on sorghum grain yield in Mali. Agronomy Journal. 2021;**113**:4705-4720. DOI: 10.1002/agj2.20850

[127] Murdoch AJ, Njuguna JM, Dorward PT, Romney D, Lukuyu BA, Mwangi DM, et al. Lessons learned in developing IPM options to improve maize forage yield and quality for small-scale dairy farmers in Central Kenya. In: Harris D, Richards JI, Silverside P, Ward AF, Witcombe JR, editors. Pathways out of Poverty, Aspects of Applied Biology. Vol. 75. Homerton College: Cambridge; 2005. pp. 53-60

[128] Bidinger FR, Blümmel M. Determinants of ruminant nutritional quality of pearl millet [*Pennisetum glaucum* (L.) R. Br.] Stover: I. Effects of management alternatives on Stover quality and productivity. Fields Crops Research. 2007;**103**:119-128. DOI: 10.1016/j.fcr.2007.05.006

[129] Haileslassie A, Blümmel M, Wani S, Sahrawat KL, Pardhasaradhi G, Samireddypalle A. Extractable soil nutrient effects on feed quality traits of crop residues in the semiarid rainfed mixed crop–livestock farming systems of southern India. Environment, Development and Sustainability. 2013;**15**:723-741. DOI: 10.1007/s10668-012-9403-3

[130] Chilowa W. The impact of agricultural liberalization on food security in Malawi. Food Policy. 1998;**23**:553-569

[131] Tesfay Y. Feed Resource Availability in Tigray Region, Northern Ethiopia, for Production of Export Quality Meat and Livestock. Addis Ababa, Ethiopia: USAID; 2010. 84p

[132] Tolera A, Said AN. Assessment of feed resources in Welayta Sodo. Ethiopian Journal of Agricultural Science. 1994;**14**:69-87

[133] Illo AI, Kamba AA, Umar S, Abubakar A. Analysis of crop residues availability for animal feed in Kebbi state, Nigeria. International Journal of Agricultural Extension. 2018;**06**(02):89-97

[134] Tegegne F, Assefa G. Feed Resource Assessment in the Amhara Regional Staste. Addis Ababa, Ethiopia: USAID; 2010. 104p

[135] Debela T. Assessment of available livestock feed resources in South Gondar

zone, Amhara National Regional State, Ethiopia. American Journal of Agriculture and Forestry. 2021;**9**(4):269-275. DOI: 10.11648/j.ajaf.20210904.24

[136] Tolera A, Feyissa F, Geleti D, Duressa D, Kebede D, Gurmessa S, et al. Assessment of Livestock Feed Production and Utilization Systems and Analysis of Feed Value Chain in Diga District. Ethiopia: ILRI; 2014. 26p

[137] Ncube S, Mubaiwa E, Mpofu D. The Feeding Value of Stover Stored in Two Different Ways. Harare: Annual Report, Division of Livestock and Pastures, department of research and specialist services; 1993. 94p

[138] Minson D. Forage in Ruminant Nutrition. San Diego: Academic Press; 1990. 483p

[139] Osafo ELK, Owen E, Said AN, Gill M, Sherington J. Effects of amount offered and chopping on intake and selection of sorghum Stover by Ethiopian sheep and cattle. Animal Science. 1997;**65**:55-62

[140] Adesogan AT, Arriola KG, Jiang Y, Oyebade A, Paula EM, Pech-Cervantes AA, et al. Symposium review: Technologies for improving fiber utilization. Journal of Dairy Science. 2019;**02**:5726-5755. DOI: 10.3168/jds.2018-15334

[141] Schiere J, Nell A. Feeding of urea treated straw in the tropics. I. A review of its technical principles and economics. Animal Feed Science and Technology. 1993;**43**:135-147

[142] Mani S, Tabil LG, Sokhansanj S. Effects of compressive force, particle size and moisture content on mechanical properties of biomass pellets from grasses. Biomass and Bioenergy. 2006;**30**:648-654. DOI: 10.1016/j.biombioe.2005.01.004

[143] Bonfante E, Palmonari A, Mammi L, Canestrari G, Fustini M, Formigoni A. Effects of a completely pelleted diet on growth performance in Holstein heifers. Journal of Dairy Science. 2016;**99**:9724-9731. DOI: 10.3168/jds.2016-11033

[144] FAO. Methane Emissions in Livestock and Rice Systems – Sources, Quantification, Mitigation and Metrics. Rome: FAO; 2023. DOI: 10.4060/cc7607en

[145] Makkar HPS, Beever D. Optimization of feed use efficiency in ruminant production systems. In: Proceedings of the FAO Symposium; 27 November 2012; Bangkok, Thailand: FAO Animal Production and Health No. 16. Rome: FAO and Asian-Australasian Association of Animal Production Societies; 2013

[146] Blümmel M, Teymouric F, Moorec J, Nielsonc C, Videtoc J, Kodukulaa P, et al. Ammonia Fiber expansion (AFEX) as spin off technology from 2nd generation biofuel for upgrading cereal straws and stovers for livestock feed. Animal Feed Science and Technology. 2018;**236**:178-186. DOI: 10.1016/j.anifeedsci.2017.12.016

[147] Mahesh MS, Mohini M. Biological treatment of crop residues for ruminant feeding: A review. African Journal of Biotechnology. 2013;**12**(27):4221-4231. DOI: 10.5897/AJB2012.2940

[148] Asmare B. Biological treatment of crop residues as an option for feed improvement in the tropics: A review. Animal Husbandry, Dairy and Veterinary Science. 2020;**4**:1-6. DOI: 10.15761/AHDVS.1000176

[149] McMeniman N, Elliott R, Ash A. Supplementation of rice straw with crop by-products. I. Legume straw supplementation. Animal Feed Science and Technology. 1988;**19**:43-53

[150] Schultze-Kraft R, Rao IM, Peters M, Clements RJ, Bai C, Liu G. Tropical forage *legumes* for environmental benefits: An overview. Tropical Grasslands-Forrajes Tropicales. 2018;**6**(1):1-14. DOI: 10.17138/tgft(6)1-14

[151] Garg MR, Sherasia P, Phondba BT, Hossain SA. Effect of feeding a balanced ration on milk production, microbial nitrogen supply and methane emissions in field animals. Animal Production Science. 2014;**54**:1657-1661. DOI: 10.1071/AN14163

[152] Fernandez-Rivera S, Midou A, Marichatou H. Effect of food allowance on diet selectivity and intake of pearl millet (*Pennisetum glaucum*) Stover leaves by sheep. Animal Production. 1994;**58**:249-256

[153] Subba Rao A, Prabhu UH, Sampath SR, Schiere JB. The effect of level of allowance on the intake and digestibility of finger millet (*Eleusine corsicana*) straw in crossbred heifers. Animal Feed Science and Technology. 1994;**49**:37-41

[154] Savadogo M, Zemmelink G, Nianogo AJ. Effect of selective consumption on voluntary intake and digestibility of sorghum (*Sorghum bicolor* L. Moench) Stover, cowpea (*Vigna unguiculata* L. Walp.) and groundnut (*Arachis hypogaea* L.) haulms by sheep. Animal Feed Science and Technology. 2000;**84**:265-277

[155] Methu JN, Owen E, Abate AL, Tanner JC. Botanical and nutritional composition of maize Stover, intakes and feed selection by dairy cattle. Livestock Production Science. 2001;**71**:87-96

[156] Løvendahl P, Difford GF, Li B, Chagunda MGG, Huhtanen P, Lidauer MH, et al. Review: Selecting for improved feed efficiency and reduced methane emissions in dairy cattle. Animal. 2018;**12**:s336-s349. DOI: 10.1017/S1751731118002276

[157] Beauchemin KA, Ungerfeld EM, Eckard RJ, Wang M. Review: Fifty years of research on rumen methanogenesis: Lessons learned and future challenges for mitigation. Animal. 2020;**14**(S1):s2-s16. DOI: 10.1017/S1751731119003100

[158] VandeHaar MJ, Armentano LE, Weigel K, Spurlock DM, Tempelman RJ, Veerkamp R. Harnessing the genetics of the modern dairy cow to continue improvements in feed efficiency. Journal of Dairy Science. 2016;**99**(6):4941-4954

[159] Ørskov ER, Flint HJ. Manipulation of rumen microbes or feed resources as methods of improving feed utilization. In: Proceedings of Biotechnology in Livestock in Developing Countries; 4-8 September 1989; Edinburgh. Scotland: Centre for Tropical Veterinary Medicine; 1991. pp. 123-138

[160] Wallace RJ. Rumen microbiology, biotechnology and ruminant nutrition: Progress and problems. Journal of Animal Science. 1994;**72**(11):2992-3003. DOI: 10.2527/1994.72112992x

[161] McSweeney CS, Dalrymple BP, Gobius KS, Kennedy PM, Krause DO, Mackie RI, et al. The application of rumen biotechnology to improve the nutritive value of fibrous feedstuffs: Pre- and post-ingestion. Livestock Production Science. 1999;**59**(2-3):265-283

[162] Kulkarni NA, Chethan HS, Shashank CG. Rumen manipulation: An important strategy to improve livestock productivity. Epashupalan. 2021;**4**(2):279-288. Available from: https://wp.me/pbYZMt-2BH

Chapter 9

Effects of Concentrate Supplementation on Skin Quality Attributes in Crossbred Sheep

Ayele Abebe, Gebeyehu Goshu, Asfaw Bisrat, Tesfaye Zewdie, Tsegaab Bekele and Tesfaye Getachew

Abstract

This study examined the effects of concentrate supplementation levels on skin quality in crossbred sheep (Awassi X Bonga; AB, Awassi X Washera; AW, and Dorper X Menz; DM). The lambs (44 in total) were randomly assigned to different breed and supplementation groups. They grazed on natural pasture and received 300, 600, or 900 grams of concentrate feed with 21% crude protein and 14 MJ/kg metabolizable energy. After 90 days, the animals were culled, and their skins were assessed. Higher concentrate supplementation (900 g) significantly improved skin weight, size, thickness, and tear load ($p < 0.05$). Moisture content, fat content, and hide substance percentage were not significantly affected by the supplementation level ($p > 0.05$). DM breed showed higher thickness, tear load, and moisture content for raw skin compared to AB and AW ($p < 0.05$). Skins from DM with 900 g supplementation exhibited superior quality. The study concluded that skins from different breeds with concentrate supplementation (300 to 900 g) showed improved leather production within acceptable standards. Further research is recommended for indigenous sheep breeds in different regions, considering crossbreeding levels.

Keywords: Awassi, Bonga, crossbreeding, Dorper, leather, skin quality, Washera

1. Introduction

Ethiopia is home to a diverse population of livestock, including a substantial sheep population, making it the second-largest in Africa with approximately 30.7 million heads [1]. In the study conducted by Galal [2], the sheep breeds in the country were classified into four primary groups based on their tail type. These groups consist of short fat-tailed, long fat-tailed, thin-tailed, and fat-rumped sheep.

Another researcher [3] expanded on this classification and identified fourteen sheep breeds in Ethiopia. Among them, Washera, Bonga, and Menz sheep are specifically adapted to the Western, Southwestern, and Northern regions of the country, respectively.

Small ruminants, such as sheep and goats, possess unique characteristics, including efficient reproduction cycles, faster growth rates, and adaptability to diverse environments, making them an important source of protein and income for farmers in the tropics and subtropics [4]. However, the productivity of Ethiopian sheep breeds remains low, with most sheep breeds yielding less than 10 kg of carcass weight at 1 year of age [5]. Factors contributing to this low productivity include limited availability of quality feed throughout the year, inadequate management practices, limited veterinary services, and slow growth rates in indigenous sheep breeds.

The main emphasis in Ethiopia has been on enhancing the meat production of indigenous sheep breeds, with efforts directed towards improving productivity. Crossbreeding programs, involving the introduction of improved exotic sheep breeds, have been implemented to enhance the growth traits of indigenous sheep breeds [6, 7]. However, the impact of crossbreeding on the quality of sheep skins, particularly for leather production, remains a concern. Skins obtained from crossbred sheep in Ethiopia have often received lower acceptance and lower market prices, or have been rejected entirely [6, 7].

The international trade of raw and manufactured hides, skins, and leather has experienced significant growth, reaching around US$53.8 billion with an annual average increase of 12% over the past 30 years [8]. As trade patterns have evolved, the evaluation and classification of skins have become essential [9]. Therefore, it is crucial to understand the quality attributes of skins from crossbred sheep, particularly those subjected to different levels of concentrate supplementation, to optimize the benefits of crossbreeding programs in Ethiopia.

The aim of this study was to investigate the quality attributes of skins from F_1 crossbred sheep with varying levels of concentrate supplementation, in addition to grazing, to inform the design of crossbreeding programs and enhance leather production in the country.

2. The materials and methods used in this study are as follows

2.1 Study site description

The study was conducted at the Debre Berhan Agricultural Research Center, situated in the central highlands of Ethiopia. The center is positioned approximately 120 km northeast of Addis Ababa, at an elevation of 2780 m above sea level. Its geographical coordinates are 39° E longitude and 10° N latitude. The grazing area within the research site is characterized by natural vegetation, primarily dominated by Andropogon longipes grass. Additionally, the area contains varying proportions of Pennisetum and Festuca species, along with the legume Trifolium species. The climate of the study area exhibits distinct seasonal patterns. It experiences a long rainy season from June to September, accounting for 75% of the total annual rainfall. There is also a short rainy season from February/March to April/May, followed by a dry season from October to January. The average annual rainfall recorded at the research center is approximately 920 mm. The monthly minimum air temperatures, measured at a height of 0.5 m above the ground, range from 2°C in November to 8°C in August. Correspondingly, the monthly maximum temperatures range from 18°C in September to 23°C in June.

2.2 Management of experimental animals

A total of 44 half-bred lambs, comprising male lambs of AW, AB, and DM crossbreeds, were included in the study. The Dorper sheep breed was sourced from

South Africa, while the Awassi breed was imported from Israel, respectively, with the aim of improving the productivity of indigenous sheep breeds. These lambs were a subset of animals from a larger experiment focused on evaluating the early finishing ability of crossbreed ram lambs for commercial production.

The experimental sheep were randomly assigned to three treatment groups and three genotypes, taking age and initial live weight into consideration during the stratification process. The treatment groups consisted of grazing supplemented with 300, 600, and 900 g/d of concentrate feed, corresponding to three feeding levels. At the start of the experiment, the average age of the sheep was 7.26 months, and they weighed 23.92 kg. The lambs were slaughtered at approximately 10 months of age. The concentrate feed used in the experiment was purchased from the Kality feed processing plant in Addis Ababa. On a dry matter basis, it contained 49.5% wheat bran, 49.0% Noug cake (*Guizotia abyssinica*), 1% limestone, and 0.5% salt. This composition provided 21% crude protein and 14 MJ/kg metabolizable energy. The concentration of the commercial concentrate is as follows: Wheat bran - 830.3 g/kg, Noug seed cake - 139.7 g/kg, common salt - 10 g/kg, and limestone - 20 g/kg.

The experiment took place from May to July. The animals were grazed together during the day, and group batches of concentrate feed were provided twice daily at 12:00 am and at night. Fresh skins from the 44 male lambs were obtained which had an average age of 7.26 months and an initial weight of 23.99 kg at the beginning of the experiment, were used to assess the skin/leather quality attributes. The study consisted of a 15-day acclimatization period, followed by a 90-day experimental period. During the experimental period, the animals had unrestricted access to grazing, and watering took place twice daily. Prior to the commencement of the experiment, the animals underwent internal parasite drenching and external parasite deworming, following the established protocol of the research center.

3. Preparation of natural pasture HAH and commercial concentrate

Feed samples were subjected to drying in an air-forced oven at 60°C for 48 hours and then ground to pass through a 1 mm sieve mill. The ground samples were stored in a sealed plastic bag at room temperature until analysis. Analysis of dry matter (DM), ash, crude protein (CP), neutral detergent fiber (NDF), and acid detergent fiber (ADF) followed the methods outlined by AOAC [10] and Van Soest et al. [11]. The nitrogen (N) content was measured using the Kjeldahl method [10], and the crude protein (CP) was calculated as N multiplied by 6.25.

3.1 Skin grading and physical tests

Fresh skins were gathered for analysis and promptly dispatched to the Leather Industry Development Institute (LIDI) on the day of animal slaughter. The weight of the fresh skins was recorded immediately after slaughter. At the Leather Industry Development Institute Testing and Research Laboratory in Ethiopia (LIDI), the measurement of size and the grading of quality for the fresh skins were performed.

Trained technicians at LIDI measured the size of the skins in square inches and classified them into three categories: medium, large, and extra-large.

The wet salting process adhered to the guidelines prescribed by the Ethiopian Standards Authority. Prior to salt application, the skins were cleaned in accordance with the ESA code B.J6.003 (1990). The quantity of salt utilized was equivalent to 50% of the weight of the fresh skin. It is worth mentioning that skins from all breeds underwent identical wet salting conditions. Following the wet salting process, the skins from all breeds underwent curing under identical conditions (wet salted) and were subsequently tanned using the same method (chrome tanned). This ensured that any observed differences in the leather quality among the different groups could be attributed to variations in breed, diet, and properties of the raw materials. Chemical and physico-mechanical characteristics were evaluated to assess the leather quality of the ram lambs. Tensile strength (N/mm^2) and percent elongation (%) were measured using the methodology described in ISO 3376-1 [12].

The skin processing involved multiple stages, including soaking, liming, washing, fleshing, trimming, deliming, pickling, tanning, basification, slamming, neutralization, re-tanning, drying, and smoothing. Following the tanning process, the leather was conditioned according to ISO 2419 [13], and samples were taken for testing based on the procedure outlined in ISO 2418 [14]. The physical tests were conducted under controlled environmental conditions, with a temperature of 20 ± 2°C and a relative humidity of 65 ± 5%. Samples were collected from both parallel and perpendicular orientations to the backbone of the leather. These physical tests assessed the strength of the leather and its resistance to stretching before the upper grain layers cracked, potentially causing surface damage. Although the specific physical tests conducted at LIDI were not explicitly mentioned, they were performed as part of the evaluation process.

3.2 Tensile strength

Tensile strength quantifies the force necessary to fracture a dumbbell-shaped leather specimen. The sample is firmly secured between two clamps, which gradually separate at a consistent speed of around 100 mm per minute. During this separation, the force required to stretch the leather is automatically recorded. Eventually, the leather sample will rupture. The force at which the sample breaks is known as the tensile strength and is expressed in Newtons (N).

"To determine the tensile strength, samples were taken from both along and across the length of the skin. The samples were cut into a specific size, taking into account the thickness (mm) and width (mm) of the leather. The tensile strength was then calculated by dividing the measured breaking load (N) by the cross-sectional area of the sample, which is the product of the thickness and width of the leather. The result is expressed in units of N/mm^2. The measurement and calculation of tensile strength were performed following the ISO 3376-1 [12] procedure.

$$\text{Measured breaking load}\left(N^2\right)=\frac{\text{Tensile strength}\left(N/mm\right)}{\left(\text{Thickness}\left(mm\right)\times\text{Width}\left(mm\right)\right)} \quad (1)$$

3.3 Elongation at break

During the tensile strength test described earlier, the elongation at break is also measured. As the leather sample stretches under the applied force, it eventually reaches a point where it breaks. At this point, the percentage of stretch the sample underwent before breaking is referred to as the elongation at break.

The elongation at break is calculated by comparing the change in length of the leather sample at the point of breakage to its original length. The difference is expressed as a percentage of the original length, representing the amount of stretch the leather underwent before it broke. This measurement provides valuable information about the ductility and flexibility of the leather. It indicates the extent to which the leather can be stretched before reaching its breaking point.

$$\text{Elongation } at \text{ break}(\%) = \left(\frac{\text{Length } at \text{ break}(\text{mm}) - \text{Initial length}(\text{mm})}{\text{Initial length}(\text{mm})}\right) \times 100 \quad (2)$$

3.4 The tear load

The slit tear strength test involves a well-defined procedure using a rectangular leather sample with a small cut or slit. One clamp is fastened to the bottom of the sample, while another clamp is inserted through the slit. The clamps then apply tension to the sample until the slit initiates tearing. The point at which the tear commences is considered the slit tear strength. To facilitate standardized comparison across various leather samples, the slit tear strength is expressed relative to the average thickness of the leather.

To determine the average tear load or arithmetic mean, multiple samples are tested, and the tear load values are averaged. This provides a representative measure of the tear strength of the leather. Tear resistance is another parameter that is determined using the test method specified by the International Organization for Standardization. ISO 3377-2 [15] defines the test method for determining tear resistance, while ISO 3376-1 [12] outlines the test method for slit tear strength.

Samples used for the tests were conditioned according to ISO 2419 [13], which specifies the conditioning procedure for leather samples. The sampling method followed ISO 2418 [14], and the sampling location adhered to ISO 2418 [14]. Additionally, the thickness of the samples was measured in accordance with ISO 2589 [16], which provides guidelines for measuring the thickness of leather. By following these standardized procedures and test methods, the slit tear strength, average tear load, and tear resistance of the leather samples can be accurately determined and compared.

$$\text{Tear resistance}(\text{N/mm}) = \left(\frac{\text{Force } at \text{ tear}(\text{N})}{\text{Skin thickness}(\text{mm})}\right) \quad (3)$$

3.5 Double edge tear force (N)

The Double Edge Tear Force is the maximum load at which tearing occurs, as determined by following the ISO 3377-2 [15] procedure.

3.6 Chemical quality test of skin/leather

3.6.1 The fat content

Fat content is determined using the dichloromethane extraction method, which involves the following formula for the determination of fat and other soluble substances:

$$Fat\ \text{content}\,(\%) = \left[\frac{(\text{Weight of extracted } fat)}{(\text{Weight of the moisture-free sample})}\right] \times 100 \qquad (4)$$

To calculate the fat content, the weight of the extracted fat is divided by the weight of the moisture-free sample and then multiplied by 100 to express the result as a percentage.

The process for determining the fat content involves the following steps:

The moisture-free samples are subjected to Soxhlet extraction using dichloromethane as the solvent. The extraction process continues for a minimum of 5 hours to ensure complete extraction of the fat.

After the extraction, the solvent is distilled from the flask, leaving behind the extracted materials.

The extracted materials are then dried at a temperature of 102 ± 2°C until a constant weight is achieved. This drying process helps remove any residual solvent and moisture.

If there is a reduction in weight of more than 0.1% compared to the original weight of the sample, the samples are re-dried to ensure accurate measurements.

The total drying time should not exceed 8 hours to prevent over-drying of the sample.

Using the formula and following the specified procedure, the fat content of the moisture-free samples can be accurately determined. This information provides insights into the lipid composition of the leather material.

$$\text{The extractable substance in}\,(\%) = \left(\frac{\text{gram extract}}{\text{gram weight of the sample}}\right) \times 100 \qquad (5)$$

3.6.2 Moisture content

The moisture content of the skin samples was assessed as a percentage of mass using the ES 1195 test method [17].

3.6.3 Percent hide substance

The 'hide substance' H, is expressed as a percentage by mass, is given by the formula: H = N x 5.62. Where Nitrogen (N) is expressed as a percentage by mass, is given by the formula;

The hide substance (H), which is expressed as a percentage by mass, was calculated using the formula: H = N x 5.62. Here, Nitrogen (N) was also expressed as a percentage by mass and can be calculated using the formula:

$$N = (V/m) \times 0.7 \qquad (6)$$

Where:

V represents the volume, measured in milliliters, of the standard volumetric sulfuric or hydrochloric acid solution (5.5) utilized for the titration. It is adjusted for the blank test (**Table 1**).

Variable (n)	Age (months)	Initial Weight (kg)	Raw skin weight (kg)	Skin Size, Raw (Sq ft)
Overall (44)	7.26 ± 0.36	23.99 ± 1.39	3.62 ± 0.19	7.75 ± 0.30
Breed and blood level	ns	ns	***	**
Awassi x Bonga 50% (10)	7.1 ± 0.45	26.24 ± 1.70	4.23 ± 0.23[b]	8.54 ± 0.36[b]
Awassi x Washera 50% (13)	7.6 ± 0.36	24.05 ± 1.39	3.74 ± 0.19[b]	8.11 ± 0.30[b]
Dorper x Menz 50% (21)	7.2 + 0.29	22.64 ± 1.10	3.14 ± 0.15[a]	7.05 ± 0.23[a]
Treatment	ns	ns	***	*
Grazing +300 g concentrate (12)	7.6 ± 0.42	23.85 ± 1.60	3.11 ± 0.21[a]	7.43 ± 0.34[a]
Grazing +600 g concentrate (16)	7.0 ± 0.33	24.27 ± 1.26	3.57 ± 0.17[a]	7.74 ± 0.27[a]
Grazing +900 g concentrate (16)	7.3 ± 0.33	24.81 ± 1.26	4.43 ± 0.17[b]	8.54 ± 0.27[b]
CV (%)	18.03	20.91	18.53	13.71

*Means with different superscripts for a class within a column differ significantly, ***P < 0.001; **P < 0.01; *P < 0.05, ns - non-significant.*
"a" was denoted for lower values and "b" is for the next higher values etc.

Table 1.
Least squares means (LSM) ± standard error (SE) of initial age (months), initial weight (kg), and raw skin weight (kg) for crossbred lambs under different supplementation levels.

3.7 Data recorded and analysis

Each experimental animal's initial live weight, as well as their weight and body condition scores every fortnight, were meticulously recorded. Body weight measurements were taken at the beginning of the experiment, every 15 days throughout the 90 days, and finally at the end. To analyze the live weights and body condition scores, a general linear model from SAS (2004) was employed. The model included the concentrate level as the main factor, while initial age and weight were used as covariates. The inclusion of a covariate in the model was determined only if it yielded statistically significant results. Tukey-Kramer tests were employed to assess the variation among the groups being compared.

4. Results and discussion

4.1 The initial weight and age of the experimental sheep

The initial age and body weight of the ram lambs used in this specific experiment were found to be similar (P > 0.05), with an average age of 7.26 ± 0.19 months and an average body weight of 23.92 ± 1.39 kg. **Table 2** provides the specific values for the initial age in months and body weight in kg.

	DM%	OM%	CP%	NDF%	ADF%	ME MJ/Kg DM
Natural pasture hay	89.2	80.8	6.5	75.1	35.4	7.88
Commercial concentrate	93.6	89.4	18.8	46.3	19.1	11.8

Table 2.
Type of feed used and methods of preparation.

4.2 Raw skin weight and size

4.2.1 The weight and dimensions of the raw skin

4.2.1.1 Evaluation and classification of the skin based on its mass and dimensions

The average weight and size of the raw skins were determined to be 3.62 ± 0.19 kg and 7.75 ± 0.30 square feet, respectively. Notably, the skins from the DM crossbreeds exhibited significantly lower weight and size ($p < 0.05$) compared to those from the AW and AB crossbreeds. This difference can be attributed to the larger size of the lambs born from Awassi rams, as opposed to the smaller size of the Dorper meat breed. As per the Ethiopian Specification for lambskin (code ES B.J6.003), all three crossbreeds' skins evaluated in this study were classified as extra-heavy (1.50–1.80 kg, standard) and extra-large based on their weight and size. Interestingly, our findings contradict those of Salehi et al. [18], who reported no significant weight differences between Kashmir and Hairy goat types. Given that the market value of fresh skins is determined by their weight and size, our observations indicate that the skins from crossbred sheep hold a high value. Furthermore, the level of concentrate feeding also played a role in determining the weight and size of the raw skins in this experiment. Lambs fed a higher concentrate level (900 g/h/d) demonstrated a 42% increase in skin weight and a 15% increase in size compared to their counterparts receiving 300 g of concentrate supplementation. These findings indicate that implementing enhanced feeding practices can have a favorable impact on the dimensions and mass of crossbreed sheepskin.

4.3 The physical characteristics of leather derived from the skin of crossbreed lambs

4.3.1 The thickness of the skin

In this specific study involving crossbreed lambs, the skin thickness showed a significant improvement, measuring 1.35 mm, which was notably higher than the standard thickness of 0.6 mm.

Specifically, Dorper X Menz (DM) lambs produced a skin thickness of 1.43 mm, while AB and AW crossbreed lambs yielded a thickness of 1.23 mm. These results indicate that sheepskin derived from crossbreed lambs, supplemented with 300–900 g of concentrate in addition to grazing, is highly suitable for producing high-quality upper leather.

It is worth noting that our findings surpass those of Getachew et al. [6, 7] concerning indigenous Washera sheep (0.99 mm) and indigenous Menz sheep (1.18 mm), although they align with the Awassi X Menz 50% sheep (1.23 mm). This suggests that the supplementation of crossbreed lambs has a substantial impact on skin thickness, leading to superior results. In our study, ram lambs supplemented with 900 g/h/d exhibited a skin thickness of 1.49 mm, whereas lambs supplemented with 300 g/h/d yielded a thickness of 1.17 mm. This signifies a thickness advantage of 27% for the higher supplementation level. Getachew et al. [6, 7] conducted a comparable study that likewise showed a 19% increase in thickness due to improved supplementation levels in crossbreed and indigenous sheep breeds such as Washera and Menz sheep.

4.3.2 The tensile strength

Table 2 displays the range of tensile strength values obtained in this study, which varied from 9.33 to 12.22 N/mm^2. Our findings indicate that the tensile strength is lower compared to the results reported by Teklebrhan et al. [19], which ranged from 18.1 to 24.6 N/mm^2, and by Getachew et al. [6, 7], which ranged from 16.11 to 18.94 N/mm^2. In our study, breed and diet did not have a significant effect on tensile strength ($p > 0.05$).

It is important to note that the tensile strength values obtained in this study fall below the standard requirement of 20 N/mm^2 for skins to be utilized in upper leather production. It is noteworthy to mention that all the lamb breeds examined in our study yielded leather that complied with the quality standards outlined by the leather industry, as stated by BASF [20]. According to BASF [20], lamb garments are required to have a minimum tensile strength of 12 N/mm^2.

4.3.3 The elongation at break

The average percentage of elongation at break in this study was determined to be 49.73%, with a range of 46–51%. Statistical analysis indicated no significant impact ($p > 0.05$) of the treatment groups and genotypes on the elongation at break percentage. Specifically, the AB, AW, and DM sheep breeds exhibited elongation at break values of 47, 50, and 51%, respectively. The average elongation at break percentages obtained for these three genotypes (ranging from 47 to 51%) aligns with the findings of Jacinto et al. [21], who reported a value of 53% for crossbreed sheep such as Texel × Native and Santa Inês × Native. A notable trend of improvement can be observed among the different levels of supplementation (46–51%) for the groups receiving 300, 600, and 900 g of concentrate supplementation. This suggests that higher levels of supplementation may enhance the physical properties of the leather compared to lower supplementation levels.

In contrast to our study, Getachew et al. [6, 7] reported higher elongation at break values of 66 and 65%, indicating greater flexibility compared to our findings. Additionally, a study conducted by Teklebrhan et al. [19] on different sheep breeds, including Blackhead Ogaden, Hararghe Highland, Dorper X Blackhead Ogaden, and Dorper X Hararghe Highland, revealed percentage elongation values of 48%, 56%, 52%, and 44%, respectively, which align closely with the results obtained in our study. The elongation at break percentages observed in this particular study falls within the acceptable range of 40–80% and meets the recommended value for sheepskin, signifying that the leather products are well-suited for use by the leather industry in terms of their flexibility and stretchability.

4.3.4 The tear load

The mean tear load parallel to the backbone and perpendicular to the backbone in Newtons (N) did not show a significant effect ($p > 0.05$) in our study. The average tear load, considering both parallel and perpendicular directions, was 36.72 N. However, a higher average tear load was observed for DM crossbred lambs (37.58 N) compared to AW crossbred lambs (28.73 N), and this difference was statistically significant ($p < 0.05$). The tear load measured in N/mm did not show any significant difference ($p > 0.05$) among the tested concentrate feeding levels and genotypes. However, the concentrate feeding level did have a significant effect ($p < 0.05$) on the average tear load parallel to the backbone, average tear load perpendicular to the backbone, and average tear load when considering both parallel and perpendicular directions.

These findings align with the results reported by Getachew et al. [6, 7], who also observed no influence of genotype and feeding levels on tear resistance. In summary, the tear load parallel and perpendicular to the backbone did not show significant differences overall, but DM crossbred lambs demonstrated higher tear load compared to

AW crossbred lambs. The tear resistance was not significantly influenced by genotype and feeding levels, consistent with previous findings.

The tear resistance values obtained in our study were 29.23 N/mm for AB, 23.80 N/mm for AW, and 27.63 N/mm for DM sheep breeds. These values were significantly better ($p < 0.05$) compared to the range of 15.01 to 15.99 N/mm reported for Awassi X Menz, Menz, and Washera sheep breeds by Getachew et al. [6, 7]. Additionally, our findings were similar to the tear resistance values reported for Brazilian, South African, and German sheep breeds by Snyman and Jackson-Moss [22] and Oliveira et al. [23]. This suggests that the tear resistance of the AB, AW, and DM sheep breeds in our study was superior to that of the Awassi X Menz, Menz, and Washera breeds studied by Getachew et al. [6, 7], and comparable to the tear resistance values observed in sheep breeds from Brazil, South Africa, and Germany as reported by Snyman and Jackson-Moss [22] and Oliveira et al. [23].

4.4 The chemical properties of leather derived from crossbreed lambs

4.4.1 The moisture content of the raw skin, expressed as a percentage

Table 3 presents the moisture content, expressed as a percentage, for both raw and wet blue skin in this study. The average moisture content of raw skin was determined to be 34%, while for wet blue skin, it was 62%. The breed of the sheep had a significant impact ($p < 0.05$) on the moisture content of the raw skin, with DM lambs exhibiting lower moisture content compared to AB and AW lambs. However, the levels of concentrate supplementation did not show a significant effect ($p > 0.05$) on the moisture content at both the raw and wet blue stages. Additionally, there were no significant differences observed in the moisture content at the wet blue stage among the lamb breeds AB, AW, and DM.

Regarding the moisture content at the wet blue stage, it ranged from 61 to 62% for different levels of concentrate supplementation. These values were slightly lower than the findings reported by Negussie et al. [24], who obtained moisture content ranging from 69 to 74% for Blackhead Ogaden sheep subjected to various feeding regimes. This suggests that the moisture content of the wet blue skin in our study was relatively lower, potentially indicating more efficient processing and reduced water content in the leather.

4.4.2 The fat content of the leather samples, expressed as a percentage

Sheepskin typically contains a natural fat content ranging from 30–40%, which plays a crucial role in the leather's acceptance of fat liquor substances during the tanning process [25]. To remove excess fat, a degreasing operation is performed. If the natural fat is not adequately eliminated, it can hinder the hydrophilic properties of chemicals, specifically liquoring agents. This can result in undesirable quality problems, including decreased physical strength, hardness, imperfect dyeing, and unpleasant odors in the final product [26].

In this study, the fat content of all treatment groups was observed to fall within the recommended standard range of 4 to 10% for the production of upper shoe leather. The average fat content of the skin in this study was determined to be 6%. The lamb genotype and feeding regime did not exhibit a significant impact ($p > 0.05$) on the fat content of the skins. Nonetheless, a minor reduction in fat content was observed across the different feeding regimes, with percentages of 6.29, 6.11, and 5.39% recorded for 300, 600, and 900 g concentrate supplementation, respectively.

DOI: http://dx.doi.org/10.5772/intechopen.1004720

Variable	Average thickness (mm)	Tensile strength (N/mm^2)	Elongation at break (%)	Mean tear load Parallel to the backbone (N)	Mean tear load Perpendicular to the back Bone (N)	Average tear load (N)	Tear-Load (N/mm)
Overall (44)	1.35 ± 0.08	10.26 + 0.81	49.73 + 1.73	32.73 + 0.01	36.72 + 0.45	34.43 + 1.88	27.03 ± 1.32
Breed	*	ns	ns	ns	ns	*	ns
Awassi x Bonga (10)	1.23 ± 0.09^a	12.11 ± 1.05	47.22 ± 2.13	35.14 ± 4.42	35.14 ± 4.42	32.57 ± 3.87^{ab}	29.23 ± 2.96
Awassi x Washera (13)	1.23 ± 0.08^a	10.27 ± 0.86	49.51 ± 1.73	31.91 ± 3.60	31.31 ± 3.60	28.73 ± 3.15^a	23.80 ± 2.42
Dorper x Menz (21)	1.43 ± 0.06^b	9.33 ± 0.68	50.56 ± 1.37	39.84 ± 2.84	39.84 ± 2.84	37.58 ± 2.49^b	27.63 ± 1.90
Treatment	*	ns	ns	*	*	*	ns
Grazing +300 g concentrate (12)	1.17 ± 0.09^a	10.31 ± 0.69	46.44 ± 1.99	23.28 ± 3.72^a	30.31 ± 4.15^a	26.32 ± 3.63^a	25.03 ± 2.78
Grazing +600 g concentrate (16)	1.28 ± 0.07^{ab}	10.22 ± 0.78	50.00 ± 1.57	33.22 ± 2.93^{ab}	32.98 ± 3.26^b	33.16 ± 2.86^b	26.19 ± 1.19
Grazing +900 g concentrate (16)	1.49 ± 0.07^b	11.18 ± 0.78	50.85 ± 1.58	37.66 ± 2.94^b	43.01 ± 3.28^b	39.41 ± 2.87^b	29.43 ± 2.20

*Means with different superscripts for a class within a column differ significantly, *** - P<0.001; ** - P<0.01; * - P<0.05, ns - non-significant. "a" was denoted for lower values and "b" is for the next higher values etc.*

Table 3.
Least squares means (±SE) of skin thickness (mm), tensile strength (N/mm^2), Elongation (%), tear load parallel (N), tear load perpendicular (N), mean tear load (N), tear-load (N/mm) of skins produced from crossbred sheep under different feeding levels.

These results suggest that higher levels of concentrate supplementation contribute to improved leather quality by reducing the fat content.

These findings are consistent with the research by Haroun et al. [27], who reported fat content values of 6 to 7% for Sudan Desert sheep. However, the fat content in our study was lower than that reported by Negussie et al. [24] for Blackhead Ogaden sheep under different concentrate supplementation regimes. In contrast, our study yielded higher values compared to the results reported by Teklebrhan et al. [19] for Hararghe Highland, Black Head Ogaden, Dorper X Hararghe Highland, and Dorper X Blackhead Ogaden sheep.

The fat content in sheepskins can vary widely, ranging from 4 to 50%, whereas in cattle hides, it typically falls between 2 and 12%. These variations depend on factors such as the breed, age, and sex of the animal [28]. During the tanning process, the lower fat content observed in the AB, AW, and DM lamb breeds after degreasing indicates the production of higher-quality leather. This finding aligns with the conclusions mentioned by Sarkar [29], suggesting that lower fat content contributes to the production of superior leather.

In summary, the present study demonstrated that the fat content of the skins fell within the standard range for upper shoe leather production. Lamb genotype and feeding regime did not significantly affect the fat content. However, higher concentrate supplementation levels were associated with lower fat content, indicating improved leather quality. These findings are consistent with prior research, demonstrating that the AB, AW, and DM lamb breeds achieved a low fat content after degreasing, which is indicative of higher-quality leather. These results further support the conclusions mentioned by Sarkar [29].

4.4.3 The hide substance content, expressed as a percentage

The study found that, on average, the hide substance percentage obtained was 33 (**Table 4**). The results indicated that lamb genotype and feeding regime did not have a significant effect on the hide substance of the lambs' skin, as the p-value was greater

Variable	Moisture content for raw skin (%)	Moisture content wet blue (%)	Fat content (%)	Hide substance (%)
Overall (44)	34.06 ± 1.93	61.48 ± 0.68	6.08 ± 0.46	32.46 ± 1.33
Breed	**	ns	ns	ns
Awassi x Bonga (10)	44.16 ± 3.83^{b}	62.12 ± 1.53	5.06 ± 1.06	31.51 ± 3.11
Awassi x Washera (13)	38.64 ± 03.12^{b}	63.09 ± 1.25	6.03 ± 0.87	32.16 ± 2.54
Dorper x Menz (21)	27.42 ± 02.46^{a}	60.20 ± 0.99	6.67 ± 0.68	33.16 ± 2.00
Treatment	ns	ns	ns	ns
Grazing +300 g concentrate (12)	42.03 ± 3.59	61.93 ± 1.44	6.26 ± 0.99	32.64 ± 2.92
Grazing +600 g concentrate (16)	33.33 ± 2.83	61.16 ± 1.13	6.11 ± 0.78	30.53 ± 2.30
Grazing +900 g concentrate (16)	34.85 ± 2.84	62.32 ± 1.14	5.39 ± 0.79	33.67 ± 2.31

*Means with different superscripts for a class within a column differ significantly, *** - P<0.001; ** - P<0.01; * - P<0.05, ns - non-significant.*
"a" was denoted for lower values and "b" is for the next higher values etc.

Table 4.
Least squares means (±SE) of moisture content for raw skin (%), moisture content of skin at wet blue stage (%), fat content of skin (%), and hide substance (%) of skins produced from crossbred sheep under different feeding levels.

than 0.05. As a result, the differences in lamb genotype and feeding regime did not lead to significant variations in the percentage of hide substance.

5. Conclusion

Based on the study presented in this chapter, several significant conclusions can be drawn:

- Concentrate supplementation levels significantly impacted lambs' raw skin weight and size.
- Higher concentrate supplementation (900 g/h/d) resulted in 42% more skin weight and 15% larger size compared to 300 g supplementation.
- Crossbred lambs had better skin thickness (1.35 mm) compared to the standard thickness of 0.60 mm.
- Lambs supplemented with 900 g/h/d had 27% thicker skin (1.49 mm) compared to those supplemented with 300 g/h/d (1.17 mm).
- DM lambs had thicker skin (1.43 mm) compared to AB and AW crossbreeds (1.23 mm).
- Breed and diet did not significantly affect skin tensile strength (ranging from 9.33 to 12.22 N/mm^2).
- Average tear load was higher in DM crossbred lambs (37.58 N) compared to AW crossbred lambs (28.73 N).
- Skins' fat content was within the standard range (6%) for upper shoe leather production and slightly decreased with higher concentrate supplementation.
- Lamb genotype and feeding regime did not significantly affect hide substance percentage.
- In summary, crossbred sheep like DM, AB, and AW demonstrated favorable skin quality that meets industry standards. They have the potential for both meat and skin production, benefiting farmers and sheep raisers in Ethiopia.

5.1 Recommendations and future directions

Based on the results of this study, the following recommendations are suggested:

- Conduct further studies on optimizing concentrate supplementation levels and their effects on skin quality attributes to provide comprehensive guidelines for farmers and sheep raisers.
- Evaluate the economic viability of crossbred sheep production for both meat and skin compared to other livestock production systems.

- Investigate market demand and value chain opportunities for crossbred sheepskin products, both domestically and internationally based on the benefits of feeding systems.
- Assess the potential of crossbred sheep for meat and skin production in different geographical regions based on different levels of feeding systems.
- Conduct economic assessments considering production costs, market demand, value chain opportunities, and profitability for farmers and sheep raisers.
- Facilitate scaling and knowledge transfer through collaboration, capacity building, and adoption of best practices.
- Promote the development of a sustainable and competitive sheepskin industry in Ethiopia through the integration of crossbred sheepskin production into the livestock sector.

Acknowledgements

The authors would like to express their gratitude to the Debre-Birhan Agricultural Research Center and the Ethiopian Agricultural Research Institute (EIAR) for providing financial support for the project, The authors are also grateful to Accelerating the Impact of CGIAR Climate Research in Africa (AICCRA) project and CGIAR initiative on "Sustainable Animal Productivity for Livelihoods, Nutrition and Gender inclusion (SAPLING)" for partially funding this research". They would also like to thank the Leather Industry Development Institute (LIDI) of Ethiopia for their assistance in analyzing the chemical and physical characteristics of the skins. Additionally, the authors appreciate the support received from Mr. Alemayehu H/M and Mr. Deribew Bekele. Their assistance was invaluable to the success of the study. This work is part of a Ph.D. work of Mr. Ayele Abebe derived from the large data set on Dorper crossbreeding evaluation work in Ethiopia.

A. Appendix

See **Figure A1**.

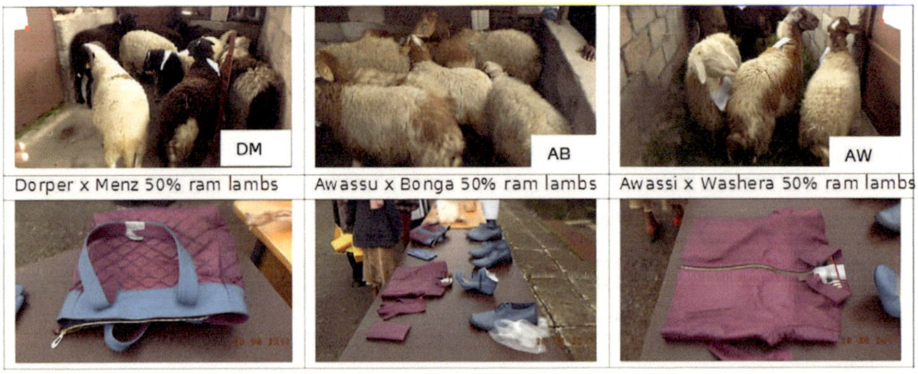

Figure A1.
Pictures of experimental sheep and final products from these breeds at LIDI.

Author details

Ayele Abebe[1,2*], Gebeyehu Goshu[2], Asfaw Bisrat[1], Tesfaye Zewdie[1], Tsegaab Bekele[3] and Tesfaye Getachew[4]

1 Amhara Agricultural Research Institute, Debre-Birhan Agricultural Research Center, Debre-Birhan, Ethiopia

2 Addis Ababa University, College of Veterinary Medicine and Agriculture, Bishoftu, Ethiopia

3 Leather Industry Development Institute of Ethiopia, Ethiopia

4 International Center for Agricultural Research in the Dry Areas (ICARDA), Addis Ababa, Ethiopia

*Address all correspondence to: yemichaeld@gmail.com

References

[1] CSA. Livestock and Livestock Characteristics Agricultural Sample Survey. Addis Ababa, Ethiopia: Statistical Bulletin; 2017. pp. 9-13

[2] Galal ESE. Sheep germplasm in Ethiopia. In: Animal Genetic Resources Information. Rome: FAO; 1983

[3] Gizaw S, Van Arendonk JA, Komen H, Windig JJ, Hanotte O. Population structure, genetic variation and morphological diversity in indigenous sheep of Ethiopia. Animal Genetics. 2007;**38**:621-628

[4] Legese G, Fadiga M. Small Ruminant Value Chain Development in Ethiopia: Situation Analysis and Trends ICARDA/ ILRI Project Report. Nairobi, Kenya: International Center for Agricultural Research in the Dry Areas/International Livestock Research Institute., Trans; 2014

[5] Ayele S, Urge M. Productive and reproductive performances of indigenous sheep in Ethiopia: A review. Open Journal of Animal Sciences. 2019;**09**:97-120

[6] Getachew T, Gizaw S, Lemma S, Abebe A. Quality Parameters of Skin from Menz, Awassi × Menz, and Washera Sheep Breeds for Leather Production 5th Annual Regional Conference on Completed Livestock Research Activities, Bahir Dar. Amhara Regional Agricultural Research Institute (ARARI): Bahir Dar, Ethiopia; 2011a

[7] Getachew T, Gizaw S, Lemma S, Taye M. Breeding practices, growth, and carcass potential of fat-tailed Washera sheep breed in Ethiopia. Tropical Animal Health and Production. 2011b;**43**:1443-1448

[8] FAOSTAT. Food and Agriculture Organization of the United Nations. Rome: Italy; 2012

[9] FAO. World statistical compendium for hides, skins, leather, and leather foot wear. In: Tropical and Horticultural Products Service, Commodities and Trade Division (ESC). Rome: Food and Agriculture Organization of the United Nations; 2010

[10] Association of Official Analytical Chemists (AOAC). Official Method of Analysis. 15th ed. Washington DC: AOAC International; 1990. 1298 p. Available from: https://edgeservices.bing.com/5ec268ae-1f1e-4c29-b273-f3267553e007

[11] Van Soest PJ, Robertson JB, Lewis BA. Methods for dietary fiber, neutral detergent fiber, and nonstarch polysaccharides in relation to animal nutrition. Journal of Dairy Science. 1991;**74**(10):3583-3597. DOI: 10.3168/jds.S0022-0302(91)78551-2 [Accessed: 12 February, 2024]

[12] International Organization for Standardization. ISO 3376-1. Test Methods of Tensile Strength and Percentage Elongation. Geneva, Switzerland: International Organization for Standardization; 2011

[13] International Organization for Standardization. ISO 2419. Leather – Physical and Mechanical Tests – Sample Preparation and Conditioning. Geneva, Switzerland: International Organization for Standardization; 2005a

[14] International Organization for Standardization. ISO 2418. Leather Chemical, Physical, and Mechanical and Fastness Tests – Sample Location. Geneva, Switzerland: International Organization for Standardization; 2005b

[15] International Organization for Standardization. ISO 3377-2. Leather

Physical and Mechanical Tests - Determination of Tear Load Part 2: Double Edge Tear. Geneva, Switzerland: International Organization for Standardization; 2002b

[16] International Organization for Standardization. ISO 2589. Leather Physical and Mechanical Tests - Determination of Thickness. Geneva, Switzerland: International Organization for Standardization; 2002a

[17] Ethiopian Standards. ES 1195. Leather – Determination of Moisture. Ethiopian Standards Agency: Addis Ababa Ethiopia; 2008

[18] Salehi M, Kadim I, Mahgoub O, Negahdari S, Naeeni RSE. Effects of type, sex and age on goat skin and leather characteristics. Animal Production Science. 2014;**54**(5):638-644. DOI: 10.1071/AN13032

[19] Teklebrhan T, Urge M, Mekasha Y. Carcass measurement, conformation, & composition of indigenous and crossbred (Dorper x indigenous) F1 sheep. Pakistan Journal of Nutrition. 2012;**11**(11):1055-1060

[20] BASF. A Factory for Trilon M Opened by BASF in Ludwigshafen, Focusing on Chelating Agents. Philips Parkway, Montvale, NJ: HAPPI; 2010. p. 3

[21] Jacinto MAC, Junior FMDV, Martins CF, Pinto GDS, Reis FA, Oliveira ARD. Influence of genotype on the quality of sheep leather. Revista Brasileira de Zootecnia. 2011;**40**:1830-1836

[22] Snyman MA, Jackson-Moss CA. A comparison of leather properties of skins from ten different south African sheep breeds. South African Journal of Animal Science. 2000;**30**(Supplement 1):129-130

[23] Oliveira RJF, Costa RG, Sousa WH, Medeiros AN, Dal Monte MAB, Aquino D, et al. Influence of genotype on physicomechanical characteristics of goat and sheep leather. Small Ruminant Research. 2007;**73**:181-185

[24] Negussie F, Urge M, Mekasha Y, Animut G. Effects of different feeding regimes on leather quality of finished blackhead Ogaden sheep. Science, Technology, and Arts Research Journal. 2016;**4**:222

[25] Cassano A, Molinari R, Romano M, Drioli E. Membrane processes for the treatment of aqueous effluents from the leather industry. Journal of Membrane Science. 2001;**181**:111-126

[26] Narayan K. Green Approach to Leather Technology, MSC, Masters, University of Applied Science. Finland: Centria; 2013

[27] Haroun HE, Turki IY, Ebrahiem MA. The effect of breed on skin/leather quality of Sudan Desert sheep. Journal of Africa Leather and Leather Products Advances. 2014;**1**:45-53

[28] Bitilisli O, Behzat B, Oscan S, Ahmet A, Gokhan Z. Physical and chemical properties of ostrich skins and leather. Indian Journal of Chemical Technology. 2004;**11**(4):654-658

[29] Sarkar K. Hide and skin processing technique. Madras, India: Indian Leather Producer Association; 1991